Chinese Culture

Globality, Connectivity and Modernity

Volume 15

This book series aims to publish monographs and edited volumes that examine how Chinese culture has been circulated, redeployed and reinterpreted around the world since the 15th century. In this book series, Chinese culture is understood broadly, ranging from canonical texts, philosophical/religious systems and aesthetic tastes of the educated elites to cultural artefacts, festivals and everyday practices of ordinary people. This broad definition of Chinese culture is to serve two purposes. The first is to encourage research that views Chinese culture not just as a home-grown construct serving the Chinese in their native land, but also as a symbol, a site where diverse meanings can be generated for global conversation and transnational exchanges. The second is to provide an opportunity to researchers to publish works that examine how China is used, metaphorically or figuratively, in the recent debates on modernity and post-modernity. The series welcomes proposals from multiple disciplines in connection with the study of Chinese culture, including language and literature, history, philosophy, politics and international relations, media and cultural studies.

Geir Sigurðsson · Tze-ki Hon
Editors

Contemporary Interpretations and Readings of the Yijing

The Changes in Our Times

Springer

Editors
Geir Sigurðsson
School of Humanities
University of Iceland
Reykjavik, Iceland

Tze-ki Hon
Department of History
Beijing Normal University
Guangdong, China

ISSN 2662-9755 ISSN 2662-9763 (electronic)
Chinese Culture
ISBN 978-981-96-0608-5 ISBN 978-981-96-0609-2 (eBook)
https://doi.org/10.1007/978-981-96-0609-2

This Springer imprint is published by the registered company Springer Nature Singapore Pte Ltd.
The registered company address is: 152 Beach Road, #21-01/04 Gateway East, Singapore 189721, Singapore

Contents

Part III Innovative Interpretations

Editors and Contributors

About the Editors

Geir Sigurðsson studied philosophy, sociology, and Chinese studies in Iceland, Germany, Ireland, the United States, and P. R. China. He defended his Ph.D. in philosophy at the University of Hawai'i in 2004 and is currently Professor of Chinese Studies and Transcultural Philosophy at the University of Iceland. Geir is Author of *Confucian Propriety and Ritual Learning: A Philosophical Interpretation* (2015), an annotated translation of the ancient Chinese classic *Sunzi's Art of War* into his native Icelandic (2019), over 50 journal articles and book chapters and Co-editor of three forthcoming volumes on Chinese philosophy and intellectual history. In 2024, he released his first book of fiction.

Tze-ki Hon is Professor at the Research Center for History and Culture of Beijing Normal University, Zhuhai 519087, China. Concurrently, he is Dean of Faculty of Humanities and Social Sciences at BNU-HKBU United International College. Before he relocated to Zhuhai, he taught at City University of Hong Kong, State University of New York at Geneseo, and Hanover College, Indiana. Over the last three decades, he wrote four books and edited six volumes on topics such as the philosophy of the *Book of Changes*, late Qing thought, and the history of Cold War Hong Kong.

Contributors

Jim Behuniak Colby College, Waterville, USA

Bjørn Åge Blix Hunan University, Changsha, China

Jón Egill Eyþórsson Academy of Korean Studies, Seongnam, Republic of Korea

Haipeng Guo Center for Whitehead Studies, BNU-HKBU United International College, Zhuhai, China

Dominique Hertzer Centre for Modern East Asian Studies, University of Göttingen, Göttingen, Germany

Tze-ki Hon BNU-HKBU United International College, Zhuhai, China; Research Center of History and Culture, Beijing Normal University, Zhuhai, China

Rein Raud School of Humanities, Tallinn University, Tallinn, Estonia

Jana S. Rošker University of Ljubljana, Ljubljana, Slovenia

Téa Sernelj University of Ljubljana, Ljubljana, Slovenia

Geir Sigurðsson University of Iceland, Reykjavik, Iceland

Sharon Small Tel Aviv University, Tel Aviv, Israel

Kar Bo Wong BNU-HKBU United International College, Zhuhai, China

Chapter 1
Addressing the Changes in Our Times

Geir Sigurðsson and Tze-ki Hon

1.1 What is in a Title?

The title of the present volume, "The Changes in Our Times," is deliberately ambiguous. On one hand, it points to the focus of our study, namely contemporary interpretations of the ancient manual of divination, the *Yijing* (in English often referred to as *The Classic of Changes* or simply *Changes*). On the other hand, however, the title also highlights the precarious, accelerated, increasingly complex, and seemingly unpredictable nature of our contemporary times. Never have our technical ways of dealing with our surroundings, our norms, and entire societies changed as rapidly as they do today. As the German sociologist Hartmut Rosa has recently pointed out, there is a deep paradox involved in our efforts to make our world evermore controllable or "engineerable" by technological means while it really becomes less controllable:

> We cannot control our late modern world in any way: politically, economically, legally, technologically, or individually. The drive and desire toward controllability ultimately creates monstrous, frightening forms of uncontrollability. (Rosa 2020, ix)

The primary reason for this predicament, Rosa argues, is "social acceleration," our modern societies' structural requirement for increased speed in order only to maintain the status quo. He calls this "dynamic stabilization," which is when a society "systematically requires (material) growth, (technological) acceleration, and (cultural)

G. Sigurðsson (✉)
University of Iceland, Reykjavik, Iceland
e-mail: geirs@hi.is

T. Hon
Beijing Normal University, Beijing, China

BNU-HKBU United International College, Zhuhai, China

T. Hon
e-mail: hon@geneseo.edu

G. Sigurðsson and T. Hon (eds.), *Contemporary Interpretations and Readings of the Yijing*, Chinese Culture 15, https://doi.org/10.1007/978-981-96-0609-2_1

innovation to reproduce its structure and to maintain the institutional status quo." Indeed, this is his very definition of "modernity": "A society can be called modern when its mode of stabilization is dynamic." (Rosa 2017).

In everyday life, we are incapable of grasping adequately the structural dynamism that continuously drives us toward acceleration and unforeseen changes. At the same time, however, most would agree that we cannot avoid experiencing that it has become increasingly difficult to make decisions about what action to take and to make sense of the situations we find ourselves in, even in the most everyday circumstances. Less and less, we feel the support of time-honored norms that can assist us in meeting and responding to the contingent nature of human life. Such circumstances are prone to lead to what the early sociologist Émile Durkheim called "anomie," a breakdown of norms that "no longer carry their normal degree of authority, because they are weakened and no longer as they should be." Durkheim continues:

> The notion of the infinite, then, appears only at those times when moral discipline has lost its ascendancy over wants; it is a sign of the attrition that occurs during periods when the moral system which has prevailed for centuries is shaken, and fails to respond to new conditions of human life, without any new system having yet been formed to replace that which has disappeared. (Durkheim 1972, 174)

Durkheim, writing a century ago about what he perceived as overly swift changes of social norms, refers to "the nature and source of this malady of infiniteness which torments our age." (Ibid. 173) Could he have been able to even conceive of the speed at which we need to continuously adapt and readapt in the present age?

In light of the current situation, we suggest that an exploration of the *Yijing*, originally an ancient Chinese book of divination, could be one way to help us along the way to navigate through the intricacies of the present. Hence, the two meanings of the book title—contemporary interpretations of the *Yijing* and the precarious changes in our times—are united. We propose to use the *Yijing* to help us reflect on our contemporary world, engage with it, and hopefully, initiate changes to make it better. After all, the *Yijing* is precisely about changes, how to understand their patterns, how to anticipate and to respond to them. The essays contained in the volume present different approaches to and suggestions of how to use the *Yijing* to enable us to think through the particularly human challenge of establishing meaning in a constantly changing world and making choices between all the alternatives that continue to unfold before us. The authors of the volume explore and discuss novel and often surprising ways for contemporary readers to interpret and apply this ancient Chinese classic, touching upon diverse fields such as technology, ecology, psychology, aesthetics, ontology, cognition, mythology, and gender issues.

1.2 The *Yijing*

In this introduction, we will refrain from attempting to provide an exhaustive historical or philosophical explanation of the *Yijing*. Such writings abound, of course, but brief and helpful overviews can be found in the contributions to this volume by Hon,

Herzer, and Wong. A sketchy outline will therefore suffice here, including some of our own reflections and ideas about its function and application in our times.

It is well known that the *Yijing* is a seminal source for the early Chinese philosophical conception of cosmology. While it was incorporated into the list of Confucian "classics" during the Han dynasty, it expresses a worldview that predates all the Chinese philosophical schools that operated in the Warring States period and can therefore be regarded as representing something like a pan-Chinese cosmological vision. Most contemporary scholars would agree that both Daoists and Confucians alike shared the philosophy of the *Yijing* as a kind of cosmological foundation.

While the *Yijing* presents an art of divination dating back to the Shang dynasty, the book itself was probably composed and put together during the early Western Zhou period (approximately tenth century BCE), which is why it is also referred to as *Zhouyi* 周易, or *The Changes of Zhou*. A later composition, which became a section of the received version of the *Yijing*, the *Yizhuan* 易傳, perhaps more often referred to as *Shiyi* 十翼 or *Ten Wings*, interprets the prognostications and elaborates on its relation to cosmology, numerology, and moral metaphysics. The *Ten Wings* treatises are traditionally ascribed to Confucius himself, also by the great Han dynasty historian Sima Qian 司馬遷 in his *Records of the Historian* (*Shiji* 史記). This attribution was later questioned and has now been disconfirmed by textual analyses of *Ten Wings* bamboo scrolls excavated among the Mawangdui archeological finds in 1973. These scrolls strongly indicate that at least most of the *Ten Wings* were written not earlier than toward the end of the Warring States period, or around 200 BCE, and certainly by more than one author. However, there is no doubt that the *Ten Wings* are Confucian treatises written in response to Daoist challenges to formulate Confucian views of cosmology.

As a whole, the *Yijing* is an elaborate expression of the Chinese cosmological view that reality is in a constant flux of generative change—that it necessarily exists in ever-flowing time. These changes are symbolized by means of broken and unbroken horizontal lines, which are identified with the cosmic interactive tendencies attributed to *yin* 陰 and *yang* 陽. The 64 hexagrams form the substance of the divinatory symbolism as offering much more detailed possibilities of configurations that can be indicated by single lines or even the eight trigrams. Since the hexagrams embody the processes of reality and are therefore themselves conceived of as being in a constant process of transformation, they should not be taken as fixed representations of the fleeting moments that they signify. Any displayed hexagram is about to yield to a new one as each of its lines, symbolizing *yin* or *yang*, will, eventually, change into its opposite. This means that the constant process of generative (and degenerative) change through time can never be left out of consideration.

The system of the *Yijing* has been regarded as one of the more obscure products of the Chinese tradition. An important reason for this obscurity is beyond doubt the fluidity of the system. Each of the 64 hexagrams is meant to provide an indication as to whether taking certain measures in a particular situation is auspicious or not, depending on the symbolic combination of its broken (*yin*) or unbroken (*yang*) lines. The interpretation proceeds by mutually correlating either the lines or the trigrams that make up the hexagrams. In this way, each interpretive element of the hexagrams represents a complex set of propensities based on the rich symbolic polarity of *yin* and *yang*. Crucial, however, is that there is no one fixed method for such an interpretation. The interpreter can choose from virtually unlimited possibilities of correlation and hence reach practically any desired conclusion. However, as for instance the late philosopher A.C. Graham has suggested, the extreme fluidity of the system does not mean that its application is without significance: Resting upon the Chinese worldview of the unpredictability of events, it has the heuristic and psychological function of unblocking the mind to possibilities that would otherwise not have been envisaged. In this context, it is worth quoting Graham to some length:

> An openness to chance influences loosing thought from preconceptions is indispensable to creative thinking. In responding to new and complex situations it is a practical necessity to shake up habitual schemes and wake up to new correlations of similarities and connexions. … The *Yi* … is designed for responding to unique and complex situations in which correlative thinking must be fluid. … the *Yi* serves to break down preconceptions by forcing the diviner to correlate his situation with a chance sequence of six prognostications. If their meaning were unambiguous, the overwhelming probability would be that the prognostications would be either obviously inapplicable or grossly misleading. Since on the contrary the hexagrams open up an indefinite range of patterns for correlation, in the calm of withdrawal into sacred space and time, the effect is to free the mind to take account of all information whether or not it conflicts with preconceptions, awaken it to unnoticed similarities and connexions, and guide it to a settled decision adequate to the complexity of factors. (Graham 1989, 368; 369–370)

According to Graham's interpretation, the *Yijing* is first and foremost a tool for reflection and insight, not a deterministic predictor. Central to making final decisions are still the intuition and reasoning of the practitioner. The *Yijing* helps by providing a certain structure for exploring the nuances of the situation and stimulating thoughtful consideration before deciding what to do. It is even tempting to designate the *Yijing* as an ancient form of artificial intelligence, for this particular function has an intriguing resemblance to at least one aspect of the continuously developing tool that we refer to as generative artificial intelligence. For instance, when we ask a question to one of its chatbots, such as ChatGPT, we may not necessarily get a truthful or accurate answer, but the answer can inspire and enhance creativity by suggesting associations and ideas that previously did not come to mind. Recent studies suggest that as a dialogue partner, AI can function as a resource that inspires and supports creative flow, as long as it is approached and accessed with such an aim in view (cf. e.g., Lewis 2023).

Philosophically speaking, moreover, Graham's observations underscore the Chinese philosophical emphasis on being conscious and perceptive of all the factors influencing one's immediate environment, resting of course on the cosmological view of reality as being in a continuous process of change and therefore indeterminate and contingent. The German sinologist Gudula Linck (2001, 20) has referred to the Chinese cosmology as a "continuous cosmogony" (ununterbrochene Kosmogonie), which appears to be a most apposite formulation. Tu Weiming 杜維明 has also suggested something similar in his rejection of the commonly found view that the Chinese worldview of temporal sequence should be portrayed as being a cycle or a spiral. Instead, he argues, it is "transformational": "The specific curve around which it transforms at a given period of time is indeterminate, however, for numerous human and nonhuman factors are involved in shaping its form and direction." (Tu Weiming 1985, 39).

The processual and transformational nature of reality necessitates a conscious awareness that excludes the possibility of a fixed or given order. It is therefore open to all possibilities and prepared for anything that might happen. This leads to a high evaluation of the skill to respond to one's environment in the most appropriate or expedient way. It moreover sheds light on the characteristically cautious approach to things in Chinese thought and culture. In responding to a fluid and ongoing process, one always observes carefully before acting. In the midst of creative transformation without an apparently clear direction, hastiness is not to be endorsed.

Having a sound notion of the role of time is obviously central to such an approach. In his discussion of the role of time in Chinese thought, the renowned philosopher Zhang Dainian 張岱年 emphasizes both points mentioned above, i.e., skill and caution. He writes: "Persons of initiative should advance only after having followed the advances of the moment. Moreover, they should be capable of initializing an action that is proper to every aspect of the situation." (Zhang Dainian 2002, 105).

Unsurprisingly, time is also of paramount importance in the ancient *Classic of Changes*. In the *Ten Wings* treatises, which, as already discussed, were composed by Confucian thinkers in the Warring States period, there is much to suggest that the salient but many-sided Confucian idea of *zhong* 中 is closely associated with time and timeliness. The character *zhong* occurs frequently and in various contexts in the ancient Chinese corpus.

Zhong's most common meaning is prepositional, functionally equivalent to the English "in," "inside," or "between," which, in fact, corresponds to the *Shuowen jiezi* lexicon's explanation of it through the character *nei* 內. The *Shuowen* also associates it with the character zheng 正, "upright," "straight," or, as Ge Rongjin (2001, 556), a contemporary commentator, has expressed it, "not biased and not partial, properly placed." Despite the apparent differences between these meanings, we can detect their semantic relationship. To be inside or between, that is to say, to be central, has also the implication of being "properly placed," i.e., being appropriate for the circumstances in question.

There is at least one unambiguous case in which Confucius uses *zhong* in this prescriptive sense, where he claims in the *Analects* 13.3, while explicating his idea of "correcting the application of names" (*zhengming*), that "if government decrees and penal law are not on the mark [*zhong*], the common people will not know where to place their hands and feet." Thus, "not to be on the mark" carries the meaning of being not appropriate in the circumstances or doing something unfitting.

In the *Ten Wings*, the character *zhong* is used to signify the lines occupying the central places of the hexagrams. The central places are the second and the fifth lines, which again are the most important in determining whether the intended action in question will or will not be auspicious. Since a hexagram represents a given situation or "time," the trick consists in making opportunities out of the propensities of the moment as indicated by its central lines. Another way of expressing this in the *Ten Wings* is *shizhong* 時中. It could be translated provisionally as "time centering," where time (*shi* 時) signifies the hexagram as such. But since *shi* refers to the particular point of time under scrutiny, it is perhaps more appropriately translated as "moment." Further, by associating the other discussed meanings of *zhong*, *shizhong* may be construed verbally as "hitting the mark of the moment," which would then make sense of the reference both to the specific prognostications of the hexagrams as well as to one's approach to things in actual reality.

The reference to *shizhong* in the *Ten Wings*, which is found in a commentary on the judgment to hexagram 4, *meng* 蒙, or youthful folly, reads: 蒙亨，以亨行時中也. According to the commentator Tang Mingbang (1997, 12), it can be construed as: "As for youthful folly [*meng*] and good sense [*heng* 亨], it is with good sense that one proceeds to hit the mark of the moment." Tang explains this passage as follows:

> Why the contrasts of youthful folly and good sense? Because things change by following circumstances. Folly is a lack of understanding, but having learned, a lack of understanding is able to turn into understanding, *meng* is able to change into non-*meng*. (Ibid.)

Based on the dynamic interaction of its central lines, the second being unbroken *yang* and the fifth a broken *yin*, the hexagram indicates good conditions for youthful folly to change into good sense. Tang Yinan, a contemporary commentator, argues that the idea of *shizhong* in the *Ten Wings* suggests an approach to reality that is particularly Confucian: that is, to identify things in their temporal moment, observe their transformational development, and then choose the most opportune occasion to realize an appropriate or effective action (Tang Yinan 2000, 286). He quotes the Qing dynasty Confucian scholar, Hui Dong 惠楝 (1697–1758), who identified the notion of *shizhong* as not only the core of the wisdom of the *Yijing* but also as a supreme illustration of the entire Confucian tradition. Marveling at the classic, he wrote: "The way of the *Changes* is indeed profound! To sum up in a word, it hits the mark of the moment." He then continued:

> Pointing out the excellence of Confucius, Zisi wrote in the *Zhongyong*: "A *Junzi* hits the mark of the moment." Mengzi also said: "Confucius was the sage whose actions were timely." The implementation of the *zhong* standard began with the *Zhongyong*, whereby the standard of *shizhong* was illustrated by Confucius, while handed down from Yao and Shun as their model of thinking. (Cited in ibid.)

The vital role of time in Confucian philosophy is also emphasized by Ge Rongjin (2001, 559). He notes that the specific formulation of *shizhong* first appears in the *Ten Wings*, in which, he adds, the notion of time is generally found in the prescriptive context that people's actions ought to try to "hit the mark" (*zhong*) by following the process of time. He further claims that the idea is also prominent in the thought of Confucius himself.

In passage 18.8 of the *Lunyu*, Confucius discusses the steadfastness of some of the more admirable personalities of the ancient era, but then says: "I, however, differ from all these, for I have no 'must not' or 'must'." Ge Rongjin comments on this passage as follows:

> That is to say, not to limit oneself to conventional rules, not to imitate that which is conventionally considered permissible, but to be flexible at all times, and thereby adapt to the variations specific to any situation—this is to "have no 'must not' or 'must'." (Ibid.)

Hence, the concept of *zhong* in its philosophical use, frequent in the Confucian literature in combinations such as *zhongdao* 中道, *zhongxing* 中行, not to forget *zhongyong* 中庸, seems to be closely associated with the notion of *shizhong* and therefore with the idea of conduct involving skill, flexibility, and appropriateness with regard to the particular situation at hand.

Finally, it may be worth touching upon an associated notion, *shi* 勢, which has its most compelling appearance in Sunzi's *Art of War* and is notoriously difficult to translate into European languages. Roger Ames renders it "strategic advantage" but notes that it also comprises meanings such as "aspect," "situation," "disposition," "configuration," "force," "influence," and "momentum." (Ames 1993, 73) The Swiss sinologist Harro von Senger (2011) calls it "siegbegünstigende Kräftekonstellation," which could be explained as "constellations of power conducive to victory." Volker Klöpsch (2013), another germanophone translator of the *Art of War*, calls it "die Schlagkraft" or "the punch power."

While *shi* 時 designates time in general, *shi* 勢 focuses on the moment in question. In a very meaningful sense, *shi* 勢 could be seen as synonymous or at least closely related to *shizhong*, to hit the mark of the moment. Admittedly, it only appears once in the *Yijing*, in the explanations of the hexagram *kun* or earth, which is composed of six *yin* lines. There it says: 地勢坤，君子以厚德載物, or loosely translated: "*Kun* signifies the momentum of earth. Exemplary persons thus use their profound virtue to support all beings."

At least two suggestions can be taken from this sentence: one has to do with the reference to the *junzi*, which demonstrates the Confucian character of the *Yijing* (or at least the *Ten Wings*), and the other concerns the ability and potency to act timely (*shizhong*), which enables the *junzi* to influence the world in a positive manner through flexible or soft (*yin*) means. Softness—the way of *yin*—is therefore perhaps not so much an exclusive Daoist approach, but also a feature of the Confucian way.

Thus, it can be concluded that the *Ten Wings*, containing cosmological treatises added to the original version of the *Yijing*, is an entirely logical appendix to the more practical divination manual contained in the earlier text, intended to provide further insight into the cosmology of change—the continuous cosmogony.

1.3 Chapter Summaries

The eleven authors of the volume propose a number of different approaches to make meaningful use of and, indeed, make sense of the *Yijing*. In the following, an attempt will be made to summarize the main arguments of each chapter.

We have divided the volume into three main sections. The first section is entitled "Divination and Contingency," focusing on the use of the *Yijing* to assist us in making sound decisions in a highly volatile world. In the very first chapter of the volume, "In Search of Possibilities: The Philosophy of Divination in the *Yijing*," Tze-ki Hon provides an interpretation of divination in the *Yijing* through the lens of one of the *Ten Wings* treatises, the "Xici" ("Attached Statements" or "Appended Remarks," also called "Dazhuan" or "Great Commentary"). Through a careful reading of the "Xici," Hon argues convincingly that despite the philosophical and historical readings of the *Yijing*, its core as a divination tool remains crucial for its full appreciation. Pointing out that its divination scheme is not about offering exact predictions of future events, he emphasizes that it should rather be seen as an epistemological medium through which we can come to grasp the continuous unfolding of the universe, or in Hon's own words, the "cosmic dance." In this understanding, divination is first and foremost a helpful tool to navigate through the uncertainties and complexities of life by offering us a system or scheme to facilitate decision-making when faced with adversity. Such divination can reveal previously obscure opportunities in distressing situations and thus lead to psychological alleviation, but it may also bring about a deeper awareness of the inescapable limitations in human life and thereby prevent hubris that otherwise could be potentially catastrophic. Hon underscores this argument by showing how the trigrams and hexagrams are explained in the "Xici" as being deliberately produced to enhance understanding of the changes in the human environment and thus to increase the ability to lead a successful life, thereby promoting self-awareness and confidence to face life's uncertainties with dignity and resolve. In this particular function (as explicated by the authors of the "Xici"), the trigrams and hexagrams are suggestive of Ernst Cassirer's "symbolic forms," although Cassirer envisaged a much broader spectrum of such forms than found in the *Yijing*.

How can we know what we do not know? Dominique Hertzer, in her "Unlocking the Unknown: The Concepts of Intuitive Cognition in the *Yijing*," joins Hon in offering an elaborate discussion and explanation of the epistemological assets of divination, focusing on its ability to stimulate and enhance intuition. While divination has historically been rejected as being irrational or superstitious, Hertzer argues that it occupies an intermediate space between discursive and intuitive knowledge. Even in Western philosophy, which claims to seek understanding of the world through reason only, metaphysical attempts to go beyond rational understanding by asking questions that cannot be answered through human experience abound. Both Plato and Kant pursued such questions, which they considered the highest form of knowledge. Plato even explicitly considered divination as having the ability to bridge the known and the unknown, proposing that it should be integrated into philosophical discourse to attain rational or discursive knowledge of that which we cannot know. In Chinese tradition, as Hertzer points out, the *Yijing* is the tool *par excellence* to guide cognition by intuition. She illustrates this intuitive-cognitive process through the hexagrams *xian* 咸 and *guan* 觀: resonance and contemplation, which exemplify how discursive reasoning and inexplicable insights are bridged in the *Yijing*, whereby divinatory knowledge arises from an intuitive realization of the symbols and at the same time from the internalized knowledge of the text. Both complement and reveal each other. Thus, the *Yijing* illustrates how divination, intertwined with philosophy, functions as a creative impulse for intuitive cognition, offering a unique form of knowledge that transcends ordinary (rational or discursive) understanding by addressing existential questions and guiding human actions.

Sharon Small, in her "Between Divination and Cultivation: Early Daoist Philosophy and the Changes," explores the gradual evolution of abstract thought from the early *Yijing* to the metaphysics found in the *Laozi* and *Zhuangzi*, and further to Huang-Lao philosophy, represented by the recently unearthed text *Fanwuliuxing* ("All Things Flow into Form") and the *Yizhuan* (*Ten Wings*). This process mirrors a shift from divination and ancestral worship to intellectual debates and philosophical systems seeking a unifying principle of heaven and human. By examining the shared cosmological assumptions, cultivation practices, and the ideal sage-ruler concept across these texts, she traces how the dependency on divination gradually gave way to the idea that self-cultivation and the philosophical ability to grasp the *Dao*, or even more commonly, "the One," was considered sufficient for becoming an ideal sage-ruler with the ability to establish just rule and secure a peaceful and prosperous society. Such philosophical views clearly influenced later commentaries on the *Yijing*, for the Huang-Lao manuscripts and the *Ten Wings* share core cosmological beliefs, emphasizing the oneness from which all generation begins. However, the *Ten Wings* text still holds tight to the act of divination and defends it philosophically, while attempting at the same time to synthesize philosophy and divination by absorbing the cosmological ideas found in the *Laozi* and the *Zhuangzi*. By tracing the development of early Daoist thought, the chapter highlights the interplay between divination, self-cultivation, and governance, and the shared cosmological principles that underpin these practices.

The second section, "Transactions with Science and Philosophy," contains four chapters. The first of these, by Jim Behuniak, has the title "Image as Instrument (*qi* 器): *Yijing* Prognostication and 'Knowing' in American Pragmatism," and could also have fitted nicely in the first section as a further elaboration of the epistemology of divination. As Behuniak suggests with his title, he explores the philosophical depth of *Yijing* prognostication through the lens of American Pragmatism. He argues that *Yijing* divination practices in the more human-centered significance that they took on later in the Zhou dynasty, allowing for greater human reflection and interpretation in divination, offer a unique epistemological perspective distinct from both earlier Chinese theories and Greek philosophical traditions. Behuniak draws parallels between *Yijing* divination and American pragmatism, particularly the ideas of Charles Sanders Peirce and John Dewey. Pragmatism views "knowing" as instrumental and purpose-driven, emphasizing the role of human agency in shaping knowledge and its objects. This perspective aligns with the use of "images" (*xiang* 象) and "trends" (*fang* 方) in the *Yijing* to guide action in uncertain situations. In this regard, he associates such knowing with the concept of "not knowing" (*wuzhi* 無知) in the *Zhuangzi*, highlighting an alternative epistemological approach that values spontaneous, non-discursive knowledge in contrast with the tendency toward fixed, unchanging objects of knowledge in Greek philosophy. Behuniak's pragmatic reading suggests that the *Yijing* functions as a sophisticated tool for experimental inquiry, akin to the explicit pragmatic method. It provides a means to navigate doubt and uncertainty, restoring coherence to experience through dynamic, context-sensitive "images" and "types" rather than static forms. This approach underscores the practical, action-oriented nature of both *Yijing* divination and American pragmatism.

How can the *Yijing* offer guidance in our dealings with climate change and the environmental challenges that we presently face? In her chapter, "*Dao* 道 and *qi* 器

in the *Yijing* 易经: Chinese Cosmotechnology and its Implications for a Different Ecology," Jana S. Rošker provides us with plenty of food for thought. She compares Chinese and Western attitudes to ecological thought through the notion of "cosmotechnology," a mode of cultural understanding of—and interaction with—technology, emphasizing its symbolic, economic, and linguistic aspects. In this regard, she focuses on the relationship between the concepts of *dao* 道 and *qi* 器 in the *Yijing*. "Cosmotechnology" is indicative of Yuk Hui's influential theory of "Chinese cosmotechnics," which seeks to recognize diverse cultural approaches to technology to prevent the universalization of Western technological paradigms. Rošker, however, takes issue with Hui's terminology of culturally specific "techniques," which she finds too simplistic, and suggests instead to use "cosmotechnology" as a broader umbrella term to designate large-scale cultural orders and axiological approaches to the world giving rise to specific technologies. She further critiques Hui's interpretation of *dao* and *qi* as being formulated in traditional Western dualistic guise, arguing instead that they represent a dynamic, complementary relationship. She makes a clear distinction between dualisms and binary categories, emphasizing *dao* and *qi* as belonging to a continuous process rather than being static opposites. *Dao*, often misinterpreted as a moral principle, is better understood as a guiding method or principle that ensures harmony and balance rather than morality in the Western sense. She also contrasts Chinese cosmotechnology with the fundamental Greek philosophical concepts *technê* and *aretê*, highlighting that while *technê* (skill or craft) and *qi* (tool or device) may be similar, *dao* differs significantly from *aretê* (virtue) in that the former represents an inherent cosmic order guiding the creation and use of *qi*, aiming for harmony rather than moral control. Thus, Rošker suggests that *dao* and *qi* in the *Yijing*, whose relationship is based on balance and harmony, provide a both vital and viable approach for addressing contemporary ecological crises. They point toward ways to develop and manage technology so that it can promote ecological balance, rather than being driven solely by utilitarian and profit-oriented motives.

Rein Raud's chapter, "The Ideas of Dynamism and Stability in the *Yijing* and Modern/Contemporary Thought," is a comparative exploration of the *Yijing* and contemporary thought, particularly process philosophy and quantum physics. Raud notes that while the methods used in the *Yijing* cannot strictly speaking be considered scientific, they nevertheless have the same objective as our modern natural sciences, that is, to observe the present and predict the future based on certain principles. The *Yijing* uses the interplay of *yin* (flexibility, darkness, and female) and *yang* (rigidity, light, and male) to describe situations through hexagrams, while science traditionally relies on immutable laws governing minimal elements. Unlike the *Yijing*, however, science continuously evolves by questioning its own axioms. Interestingly, such questioning has led modern science, influenced by Heisenberg's uncertainty principle, to abandon the traditional assumption of a "god's eye objectivity" and acknowledge the observer's inevitable impact on measurements, which has in fact aligned it closer to the holistic or inclusive view found in the *Yijing*. Raud proceeds to discuss the expressive style of the *Yijing*, emphasizing its layered textual tradition and the systematic ontological language in the "Dazhuan" or "Xici," one of the *Ten Wings* treatises. He then embarks on a fascinating comparative journey to demonstrate the relevance of the *Yijing* to contemporary scientific thinking, first by applying Algirdas Greimas' "semantic quadrangle" to analyze the discourse of the *Yijing*, illustrating the complexity of its concepts beyond simple binary oppositions; then moving on to Xiong Shili's dynamic ontology, which integrates *Yijing* concepts with Buddhist thought, emphasizing constant transformation without external causes, which parallels Henri Bergson's views on duration and transformation; and finally comparing the dynamic ontology of the *Yijing* with Thomas Nail's process philosophy, which prioritizes change and movement over stability, as well as his concepts of flow, fold, and field, which, despite his focus on Western traditions, highly resonate with the *Yijing*. On the basis of his comparative exploration, Rein convincingly argues that the ontological insights in the *Yijing* are increasingly relevant to contemporary science and philosophy, advocating for a cross-cultural dialogue to enrich both Eastern and Western thought.

In his chapter, "*Yin-Yang* and Whitehead's Process Philosophy," Haipeng Guo also embarks on a comparative philosophical journey, in this case focusing on parallels between Alfred North Whitehead's process philosophy and *Yin-Yang* cosmology. Whitehead's speculative scheme known as "process philosophy" or "philosophy of organism" synthesizes human experience into a dynamic web of relationships, which shows intriguing similarities to Chinese philosophy. Guo points to that affinity as discussed by scholars like Thomé H. Fang, Shih-Chuan Chen, and Chung-ying Cheng. While Fang characterized Chinese thought as "organicism," not unlike in Whitehead's philosophy, Chen and Cheng further explored the parallels between Whitehead's concepts and the *Yijing*, focusing on creativity and the Neo-Confucian concept of *sheng* (creativity). Guo shows how *Yin-Yang*, representing two opposite but interconnected forces in the universe, is mirrored in Whitehead's ideas of dualities such as becomingness and permanence, events and objects, and spatial and temporal relations. He identifies and analyzes such eight pairs of concepts in Whitehead's works that all align with *Yin-Yang*. As he points out, whether the resemblance between Whitehead's philosophy and *Yin-Yang* is coincidental or due to indirect influences from Chinese thought through figures like Leibniz or Whitehead's personal connections, such interdisciplinary exploration greatly enriches the mutual understanding of both philosophical traditions.

The third and final section, also containing four chapters, is entitled "Innovative Interpretations," beginning with Jón Egill Eyþórsson's "Mythic narratives in the *Zhouyi* and the *Guicangyi*." Eyþórsson explores the connections between pre-Qin Chinese mythology, on one hand, and two texts on the other, namely the well-known *Zhouyi* 周易 and the lesser-known *Guicangyi* 歸藏易. Whereas the *Zhouyi* is noted for its lack of mythic elements despite its mantic and shamanic background, this absence is somewhat mitigated by the *Guicangyi*, which shares the hexagram structure of the *Zhouyi* but is exceedingly rich in mythic content. Several renowned scholars, Eyþórsson notes, including Wang Guowei and Gu Jiegang, have reconstructed narrative strands in the *Zhouyi*, linking them to Chinese mythic repositories such as the *Shanhaijing* 山海經 and the "Heavenly Questions" of the *Songs of Chu* (*Chuci Tianwen* 楚辭天問). The chapter investigates mythological and historical elements such as Chinese dragons, semi-historical figures like King Hai 王亥 of pre-dynastic Shang, and other legendary characters. It also delves into the cosmological models represented in Chinese mythology, such as those involving deities like Di Jun 帝俊 and Xi He 羲和, and their connections to the *Yijing*. With its rich mythological references, the *Guicangyi* provides a certain contrast to the more historical and philosophical focus of the *Zhoyi*. Eyþórsson suggests that the latter's lack of mythic narrative might be due to Confucian influences that favored moral stories over myths. The *Guicangyi*, on the other hand, appears to preserve a more mythologically rich tradition. In conclusion, Eyþórsson highlights the potential for further discoveries and reconstructions of mythic elements in the *Zhouyi*, suggesting that these elements were likely included to imbue the text with symbolic meaning for divination. Thus, the mythological content of the *Guicangyi* offers a valuable perspective on the ancient Chinese worldview and its integration into mantic practices.

Moving from mythology to visual art, Téa Sernelj, in her "*Yijing* in Chinese Aesthetics: Shitao's Theory of Individual Creativity and the Holistic Brushstroke," explores the influence of the dynamic ontology of the *Yijing* on the Qing Dynasty painter Shitao 石濤, whose aesthetic treatise on painting, *Huayulu* 畫語錄 (*Remarks on Painting*), is among the most important Chinese works on artistic creativity. In this treatise, he integrates concepts from the *Yijing*, *Daodejing*, and Chan philosophy, emphasizing individual creativity and a holistic approach to art. His theory of the "Holistic Brushstroke" (*yihua* 一畫) is central, advocating for a method that transcends traditional techniques and embraces a natural, spontaneous creative process. Shitao's aesthetic theory critiques the traditionalist school of painting, which focused on imitation and strict adherence to past masters' techniques. Instead, he promotes a return to the aesthetics of literati painters, emphasizing personal or individualist expression and a deep connection with nature. While his approach is predominantly rooted in Daoist philosophy, viewing the artist as a conduit for the universal creative energy, the *Dao*, the chapter focuses primarily on those elements of *Yijing* that were directly addressed by Shitao. By delving into Shitao's biography, highlighting his early life, artistic development, philosophical influences, travels, and personal experiences, Sernelj discusses his embrace of ancient models and nature as primary sources of inspiration. Shitao's "Holistic Brushstroke" embodies the Daoist principle of "method without method" (*wufa* 無法), underscoring the importance of spontaneity and the artist's inner spirit. This concept is explicitly linked to the onto-cosmology of the *Yijing*, where the creative process mirrors the natural world's dynamic and interconnected nature. Shitao's theory also incorporates the idea of transformation and continuity of change (*tongbian* 通變), reflecting the emphasis in the *Yijing* on the interplay of *Yin* and *Yang*. Overall, Sernelj's chapter presents Shitao's aesthetic theory as a profound and innovative approach to Chinese art, deeply influenced by Daoist and *Yijing* philosophies, advocating for a harmonious connection between the artist, nature, and the cosmos.

The final two chapters provide fascinating overviews of how the *Yijing* has been read, interpreted, and applied in North America and Scandinavia in recent times. First, we have Kar Bo Wong's chapter "A Paradigm Shift: *Yijing* Studies in North America, 1980–2020." Wong's study identifies three major approaches that have emerged since the 1970s in American interpretations of the *Yijing*, moving away from the "book of wisdom" perspective popularized by the Wilhelm-Baynes translation. The first approach, which she calls "Foundationalist," focuses on uncovering the original meanings of the *Yijing* through archaeological and philological studies. Scholars such as Edward Shaughnessy, Richard Kunst, and Richard Rutt have emphasized the historical context of the text, arguing that the *Yijing* was initially a divination manual rather than a philosophical treatise. They critique the Wilhelm-Baynes translation for its lack of fidelity to the original text and its heavy reliance on later commentaries. The second approach, the "Commentarial Tradition," examines the diverse interpretations of the *Yijing* that emerged during the Song Dynasty. Scholars such as Richard John Lynn and Joseph Adler have translated and analyzed commentaries by figures like Wang Bi, Cheng Yi, and Zhu Xi. This method highlights the dynamic and evolving nature of *Yijing* interpretations, reflecting the sociopolitical contexts of different periods. The third one, to which Wong refers as "Global Circulation," situates *Yijing* studies within a global historical narrative and is probably best represented in the works by Richard Smith who traces the dissemination and adaptation of the *Yijing* across various cultures, emphasizing its openness and diversity. His research extends beyond China to explore the text's impact in East Asia and the West, challenging the notion of a timeless, universal *Yijing*. Wong concludes that these three approaches collectively provide a comprehensive framework for understanding the multifaceted nature of the *Yijing*. The shift toward a "Global *Yijing*" perspective marks a new trend in the twenty-first century, attracting scholars worldwide to explore the text's cross-cultural significance.

Incidentally, the final chapter may precisely be seen as an instance of such a "global" opening. In his "*Yijing* and Feminism: The Scandinavian Interpretations of the Book of Changes," Bjørn Åge Blix explores how three Scandinavian translators, Jens Windeleff from Denmark, Kristine Tranmark Kossman from Sweden, and Eva Skodvin from Norway, have interpreted the *Yijing* through a feminist lens to align their translations to the dominant social values of their societies and/or ensure that their language has an adequate appeal to Scandinavian readers. In his analysis of the interpretations, Blix takes his cue from Margaret J. Pearson's feminist translation of the *Yijing*, which challenges the traditionally male-centric Western interpretations. Windeleff emphasizes feminine values by altering key philosophical terms to highlight gender-neutrality. Kossman also makes some effort toward gender-neutrality but is less inclined in her focus on feminist themes. Skodvin, however, makes explicit use of the *Yijing* to downright critique Western culture's "*yang*" or male-centric values, advocating for the importance of "*yin*" or feminine values, thus presenting the *Yijing* as a text deserving a place in contemporary feminist literature. Blix's discussion reveals that while the Scandinavian approaches and the extent of their feminist interpretations vary somewhat, Windeleff and Skodvin being more explicit in their feminist agendas, it is evident that gender issues play a significant role to all three translators. Blix's study provides a clear example of the inescapable influence on our own embeddedness and circumstances in our reading and rendering of texts, however, temporally and culturally distant they may be from us.

1.4 Concluding Remarks

The colorful diversity of angles and approaches to the *Yijing* offered in the present volume ought to be evidence of how much this enigmatic and fascinating text still speaks to us and how easily it can adapt to emerging roles in our human lives that at the time of its conception may have been entirely inconceivable. The *Yijing* is therefore far from being an outdated relic, but on the contrary, and in line with its own dynamic ontology, constantly renews its relevance to human living as we have no other choice but continue to go through—and seek to adapt to—the changes in our times.

References

Ames, Roger T. (tr./comm.). 1993. *Sun-tzu. The Art of Warfare*. New York: Ballantine Books.

Zhang Dainian. 2002. *Key Concepts in Chinese Philosophy*. Tr. Edmund Ryden. Beijing: Foreign Languages Press/New Haven, CT: Yale University Press.

Durkheim, Emile. 1972. *Selected Writings*. Tr./ed. Anthony Giddens. Cambridge et al.: Cambridge University Press.

Graham, A.C. 1989. *Disputers of the Tao. Philosophical Argument in Ancient China*. Chicago/La Salle, IL: Open Court.

Klöpsch, Volker (tr./comm.). 2013. *Sunzi. Die Kunst des Krieges*. 5th ed. Frankfurt A.M. and Leipzig: Insel Verlag.

Lewis, Makayla. 2023. AIxArtist: A first-person tale of interacting with artificial intelligence to escape creative block. arXiv.org: https://arxiv.org/abs/2308.11424. Accessed September 10, 2024.

Linck, Gudula. 2001. *Yin Und Yang. Die Suche Nach Ganzheit im Chinesischen Denken*. Munich: C.H. Beck.

Ge Rongjin葛荣晋. 2001. *Zhongguo Zhexue Fanchou Tonglun* 中国哲学范畴通论. Beijing: Shoudu shifan daxue chubanshe.

Rosa, Hartmut. 2017. Living in times of acceleration. Radboud Reflects. Feb 14. Youtube: https://www.youtube.com/watch?v=_BwKasee9Qc. Accessed on August 21, 2024.

Rosa, Hartmut. 2020. *The Uncontrollability of the World*. Tr. James C. Wagner. Cambridge, UK, and Medford, MA: Polity.

Senger, Harro von (tr./comm.). 2011. *Meister Suns Kriegskanon*. Stuttgart: Philipp Reclam jun.

Tang Yinan 唐亦男. 2000. "Cong Rudao Dui Shijian de Kanfa Lun «Yizhuan» "Shi Zhong" yi Gainian Zhi Yiyi 从儒道对时间的看法论«易传»"时中"一概念之意义." In *Ruxue yu 21 Shiji Zhongguo: Goujian, Fazhan "Dangdai Xin Rujia"* 儒学与21世纪中国:构建,发展"当代新儒学," ed. Zhu Ruikai 祝瑞开. Shanghai: Xuelin chubanshe.

Tang Mingbang 唐明邦 Ed. 1997. *Zhouyi Pingzhu* 周易评注. Beijing: Zhonghua Shuju.

Tu Weiming. 1985. *Confucian Thought: Selfhood as Creative Transformation*. Albany, NY: State University of New York Press.

Part I
Divination and Contingency

Chapter 2
In Search of Possibilities: The Philosophy of Divination in the *Yijing*

Tze-ki Hon

Abstract Every day we face serendipity and uncertainty. We plan to do certain things but we end up doing something else. We take actions to solve problems but we do not know whether our actions are effective. We make decisions to end conflicts and controversies but we do not know whether our decisions are helpful. To make matters worse, we know that we have missed a lot of opportunities or overlooked many options because we, knowingly or unknowingly, tend to be fixated on immediate interests, preconceived plans, and well-trodden paths. This quest to be at peace with the complicated world is the main theme in the *Book of Changes* (*Changes* 易經, or *I Ching*). In this essay, I will present a reading of the "Xici" 繫辭 (Attached Statements), a part of the *Ten Wings* of the *Book of Changes*. In this reading, I will explain how the philosophy of divination of the *Book of Changes* can help us overcome our fear of uncertainty. I will argue that the "Xici" offers an understanding of human condition that includes three parts: (1) our finitude due to the limits of our cognitive abilities; (2) our reliance on an artificial system of signs to understand our surroundings and to guide our actions; and (3) our hubris to take full control of our lives, even to the point of planning every step in our daily schedule.

Keywords Change · Fear and anxiety · Philosophy of divination · "Xici" · Yijing

---

T. Hon (✉)
Research Center of History and Culture, Beijing Normal University, Zhuhai 519087, China
e-mail: hon@geneseo.edu

BNU-HKBU United International College, Zhuhai UICR0700007-22, China

G. Sigurðsson and T. Hon (eds.), *Contemporary Interpretations and Readings of the Yijing*, Chinese Culture 15, https://doi.org/10.1007/978-981-96-0609-2_2

2.1 The Philosophy of Divination

As an ancient text in China, the *Yijing* 易經 (or *Zhouyi, Book of Changes*) is unique in two ways.[1] Firstly, it is multi-layered. Traditional accounts claim that the first layer of the core text were graphic symbols—the 8 trigrams and 64 hexagrams. Created by a mythical figure, Fu Xi 伏羲, these symbols mimic the continuous unfolding of the universe and denote the fluidity and complexity of human existence. The second layer of the core text included hexagram and line statements. Allegedly composed by King Wen and the Duke of Zhou during the eleventh century BCE, these written statements invoked concrete historical events—such as the downfall of the Shang dynasty and the rise of the Zhou dynasty—to elucidate the constancy of change in human society. The third layer included seven pieces of writings from fifth century to second century BCE. Divided into ten segments (hence, the name *Ten Wings*, 十翼 *Shiyi*), these writings deduced philosophical insights from the graphic symbols and the hexagram and line statements.[2] By 135 BCE, the core text and the *Ten Wings* were combined to form what we now call the *Yijing*—a composite text consisting of symbols, divination records, historical records, folklores, and philosophical treatises (Nylan 2001, 202–252; Redmond-Hon 2014, 1–157; Smith 2012, 1–47; Shaughnessy 2022, 5–64).

Secondly, because of its multiple layers, the nature of the *Yijing* is hard to pin down. If one focuses on the 64 hexagrams, the *Yijing* resembles a manual of divination. Each hexagram is a record of divination, consisting of a hexagram name describing a specific situation (e.g., marriage, mobilizing an army, or cleaning a well), and six lines detailing the divination results. But if one focuses on the *Ten Wings*, one finds lengthy discussions of process cosmology, the philosophy of symbolic forms, and moral-metaphysics. Since its canonization in 135 BCE, the *Yijing* was often read by the Chinese educated elite as a philosophical text. And it was this philosophical reading that made the *Yijing* a living text in imperial China that constantly posed critical questions to its readers and continuously demanded its readers to reflect carefully on their experiences (Smith 2008, 57–194; Redmond-Hon 2014, 158–180).

Since the end of the imperial system in China in 1911, the *Yijing* became a historical text. Led by scholars such as 顧頡剛 (1893–1980), 高亨 (1900–1986), and 李鏡池 (1902–1975), the *Yijing* became literally the *Zhouyi* (the Book of Changes of

[1] Acknowledgments: 1. the Guangdong Higher Education Upgrading Plan (2021–2025); 2. Project 28810-310432104 supported by "the Start up fund of Research Projects of Beijing Normal University, Zhuhai"; 3. 2024 Rushing to the Top ("冲补强"专项资金项目-粤港澳大湾区文化符号的传播研究), financial code: UICR0400014-24.

[2] The *Ten Wings* are: (1–2) "Tuanzhuan" 彖傳 (Commentary to the Judgments); (3–4) "Xiangzhuan" 象傳 (Commentary to the Images); (5) "Wenyan" 文言 (Words of the Text); (6–7) "Xici" 繫辭 (Appended Statements, also known as "Dazhuan" 大傳, [The Great Treatise]); 8: "Shuogua" 說卦 (Explanation of the Trigrams); (9) "Xugua" 序卦 (Hexagrams in Sequence); (10) "Zagua" 雜卦 (Hexagrams in Irregular Order). Most of these pieces of writings appeared during the Warring States period (481–221 BCE), except that the "Xugua" and the "Zagua" may have appeared in the first century BCE. For the dates of the *Ten Wings*, see Zhu Bokun 1986, volume 1, 39–51. As for the roles of the *Ten Wings* in transforming the *Yijing*, see Redmond and Hon 2014, 140–157.

the Zhou Dynasty) elucidating the historical development of early China. The two archaeological booms in twentieth century China—the discovery of oracle bones in Anyang in the 1930s and the discoveries of *Yijing*-related texts since the 1970s—have further driven this historicization of the *Yijing,* so much so that nowadays the *Yijing* is read in China mainly as a historical text and its roots in divination are ignored (Zhu 1986, vol. 1, 1–105; Jin 1987, 26–65). In the West, the *Yijing* has been known as a "book of wisdom." Helped by the popularity of the Wilhelm/Baynes translation after WWII,[3] the *Yijing* is widely read in the Anglophone world as a philosophical text, elucidating the profound meaning of human existence.

While this historical-philosophical turn to reading the *Yijing* is important in understanding the profundity of the ancient text, it drives readers' attention away from the primordial layer of the text—the use of divination in assisting one to make critical decision. The underlying message of putting Fu Xi (the alleged creator of 8 trigrams and 64 hexagrams) as an author of the *Yijing* is that since time immemorial, human beings must deal with adversity, contingency, and volatility. Whether literate or illiterate, every day they face serendipity and uncertainty. They plan to do certain things, but they end up doing something else. They take actions to solve problems, but they do not know whether their actions were effective. Hence, divination—a ritualistic practice that assists decision-making when someone is at a crossroads—is crucial in allaying the tension and anxiety that ancient people must have. As Chung-ying Cheng puts it: "If there is no other way to know or assess a future event relative to one's purpose at hand, divination becomes important because it provides a certain (albeit randomly chosen) representation and articulation of actuality and implicit reference to a history and a future for one's given concern" (Cheng 2020, 17). For this reason, Cheng argues that although divination is not philosophy, "there is an underlying philosophy or logic to divination" (Cheng 2020, 18). For Cheng, there are at least three aspects of divination that directly link to decision-making: understanding one's limitation, finding one's options, and choosing the best option to resolve the problems at hand (Cheng 2020, 18–23). If we use the language of Paul Ricoeur, these three aspects of divination are equivalent to a *reflection* of the past (to know one's limitation), an *apprehension* of the present (to find one's options), and an *anticipation* of the future (to choose the best option to resolve problems) (Ricoeur 1984, 52–90).

In the *Yijing* text, the "Xici" 繫辭 (Appended Statements) of the *Ten Wings* clearly expresses this philosophy of divination. Although the text of the "Xici" is probably penned by a group of writers, the authors of the "Xici" appear to have shared three

[3] Titled *The I Ching or Book of Changes,* the Wilhelm/Baynes translation was first published in 1950. The translation was a translation of a translation. It was based on the German translation by Richard Wilhelm (1873–1930), published in 1924 with the title the *I Ging.* The German text was rendered into English by Cary J. Baynes during WWII. The Wilhelm/Baynes translation—an English translation of a German translation of a Chinese ancient text—did not receive readers' attention until 1967, when the Princeton University Press reprinted the *I Ching* in a more portable form by combining the original two volumes into one volume. Due to its appeal to the Hippies and the fans of pop song writer Bob Dylan, the Wilhelm/Baynes translation sold a million copies in a decade. It was an unexpected record for a non-fiction in the American book market.

core questions: (1) our finitude due to the limits of our cognitive abilities; (2) our reliance on an artificial system of signs to understand our surroundings and to guide our actions, and (3) our hubris to take full control of our lives, even to the point of planning every step in our daily schedule (Hon 2019). In addressing these three questions, the authors of the "Xici" aim to alleviate our self-inflicted anxiety. It reminds us of our limited ability to know our surroundings. It offers us a system of signs—namely 8 trigrams and 64 hexagrams—to navigate the complicated world. More importantly, they caution us of the danger of unbounded ambitions to have complete control of our lives. By reminding us of our limitations and our hubris, the authors of the "Xici" help us develop an appreciation of ourselves—not only knowing who we are, but also finding out what we can and cannot do. In so doing, we are able to develop self-confidence to face uncertainty with dignity, humidity, and resolve.

In the following, I will trace the steps by which the authors of the "Xici" present their philosophy of divination. As mentioned earlier, the "Xici" is a composite text authored by different hands. Nevertheless, the received text of the "Xici"—divided into two sections and subdivided into passages—offers a systematic view about divination as a tool of decision-making. To their credit, the authors of the "Xici" are aware that their prediction method is an artificial schema of representation. For them, the trigrams and hexagrams are merely a system of signs to navigate the complexity of life. Nevertheless, they believe that the *Yijing* prediction method is effective because it assists readers to endure fear in life and embrace anxiety over the uncertain future. They are confident that their philosophy of divination will not only give hope, but also make people stronger when facing challenges and obstacles.

2.2 The Process Cosmology

If we read the "Xici" from beginning to end, there are three main themes in this collage of writings. The text begins with a declaration that the divinatory techniques in the *Yijing* mimic the natural unfolding in the universe, so much so that they embody all the patterns of the universe including weather, topography, and human culture. And then, the text discusses the application of the divinatory techniques in daily life to avoid calamities and losses. Finally, the text proclaims that the *Yijing* is sacred not only because it was composed by the sages such as Fu Xi, King Wen, and the Duke of Zhou, but also because it connects the known to the unknown, the concrete to the abstract, and the mundane to the spiritual. Together, these themes put forward a coherent argument that includes three components: (1) a process cosmology that describes the world as an organic, dynamic system; (2) a philosophy of symbolic forms that demonstrates the efficacy of trigrams and hexagrams; and (3) a schema of moral practices that is based on the rituals of divination. Collectively, these three components are based on one assumption, namely what one finds in the *Yijing* is an accurate representation of the continuous unfolding in the universe.

In the "Xici," this assumption is spelled out powerfully in the opening paragraph. In a majestic tone, the text opens with a description of a cosmic order that is structurally stable and yet full of motion and movement, creativity, and diversity.

> Heaven is high, the earth is low; thus the Creative and the Receptive are determined. In correspondence with this difference between low and high, inferior and superior places are established. Movement and rest have definite laws; according to these, firm and yielding lines are differentiated ("Xici" I, 1; Wilhelm/Baynes 1967, 280).

Not only is the cosmos meticulously built and elaborately structured, it is also divided into different spheres that are mutually dependent and intricately linked.

> Events follow definite trends, each according to its nature. Things are distinguished from one another in definite classes. In this way good fortune and misfortune come about. In the heavens phenomena take form; on earth shapes take form. In this way change and transformation become manifest ("Xici" I, 1; Wilhelm/Baynes 1967, 280).

In other passages, this cosmic system is described as "heaven and earth" *(tiandi* 天地), "the Way of heaven and earth" (*tiandi zhi dao* 天地之道), or "a great field of action" (*daye* 大業) ("Xici" I, 4:1–2; Wilhelm/Baynes 1967, 293–299). Despite these different descriptions, the cosmos is consistently described as being continuous, holistic, and dynamic. It is continuous because it never stops in renewing itself, driven constantly by the mixing of the *yin* 陰 (receptive) and *yang* 陽 (creative) forces. It is holistic because its self-renewal includes everything in the universe and permeates all aspects of life. It is dynamic because it generates energy and strength all the time, reinvigorating everything in the universe. In this constant process of unfolding, no distinction can be drawn between the natural and human realms, between the observing subject and observed object, and between the inner and outer worlds. Everything is part of a totality, a group dance that never stops.

According to the authors of the "Xici," the deep structure of the cosmos is fully revealed in the divinatory rituals and the graphic symbols of the *Yijing*. In retrospect, this is an ingenious move. What the authors do is transform the original *Yijing,* a manual of divination, into a set of symbols helping readers visualize the cosmic transformation. To achieve this goal, in the same opening passage in the "Xici," we find a juxtaposition of the cosmic patterns with the eight trigrams in the *Changes*.

> Therefore the eight trigrams succeed one another by turns, as the firm and the yielding displace each other. Things are aroused by thunder and lighting, they are fertilized by wind and rain. Sun and moon follow their courses and it is now hot, now cold. The way of the Creative brings about the male. The way of the Receptive brings about the female. The Creative knows the great beginnings. The Receptive completes the finished things. The Creative knows through the easy. The Receptive can do things through the simple ("Xici" I, 1; Wilhelm/Baynes 1967, 283–286).

From here on, we find a continuous expansion in matching the cosmos with the 64 hexagrams and the verbal explanations of the oracles (known as *ci* 辭 "judgments") ("Xici" I, 2; Wilhelm/Baynes 1967, 287–290), until the entire *Yijing* becomes a visualization of the constant unfolding of the universe.

Comparing these "Xici" passages with Whitehead's idea of the co-dependence of God and the World, we see a similar argument for the inseparability of one and many. For Whitehead, God and the World are co-dependent because of the following six conditions:

> It is as true to say that God is permanent and the World fluent, as that the World is permanent and God is fluent.
>
> It is as true to say that God is one and the World many, as that the World is one and God many.
>
> It is as true to say that, in comparison with the World, God is actual eminently, as that, in comparison with God, the World is actual eminently.
>
> It is as true to say that the World is imminent in God, as that God is imminent in the World.
>
> It is as true to say that God transcends the World, as that the World transcends God.
>
> It is as true to say God creates the World as that the World creates God (Whitehead 1929 [1978], 348).

If we use the Whiteheadian language to translate the "Xici," we may come up with six similar conditions simply by replacing "God" with the "Way of Heaven and Earth." However, the question is whether the authors of the "Xici" would approve of replacing the "Way of heaven and earth" with Whitehead's God. Considering their conception of the origin of the cosmic great dance, it is likely that their response would be negative. For them, there is no primal force or the first cause beyond the mixing of the *yin* and *yang*. They are willing to describe "the mixing of the *yin* and *yang* force" as the Way (*dao* 道) because the Way connotes a dynamic process or a co-dependent relationship. But they will not go any further to trace the Way to a single omnipotent, omnipresent Creator, no matter how dynamic and open that Creator may be.[4]

Furthermore, it is beside the point to ask whether the authors of the "Xici" agree with Whitehead. For them, they do not see the process cosmology as an independent subject. Instead, they see it as a precondition for discussing epistemology, namely to what extent human beings can perceive the cosmic great dance and respond accordingly. For this reason, the authors of the "Xici" consistently argue that we must understand the cosmic great dance through the graphic symbols and verbal explanations in the *Yijing*. Take, for instance, "Xici" I, passage 4.

> The *Book of Changes* contains the measure of heaven and earth; therefore it enables us to comprehend the tao of heaven and earth and its order. Looking upward, we contemplate with its help the signs in the heavens; looking down, we examine the lines of the earth. Thus we come to know the circumstances of the dark and the light. Going back to the beginnings of things and pursuing them to the end, we come to know the lessons of birth and death. The union of seed and power produces all things; the escape of the soul brings about change. Through this we come to know the conditions of outgoing and returning spirits ("Xici" I, 4:1-4; Wilhelm/Baynes 1967, 293–294).

For the authors of the "Xici," the process cosmology is important but not their main concern. Their primary concern is affirming the effectiveness of the *Yijing* as a lens to apprehend the ever-changing cosmos.

---

[4] Whitehead certainly expanded the concept of God to refer to a self-generating universe. See Whitehead 1929 [[1978], 18–30. Nevertheless, Whitehead never gave up the concept of God, even though he knew that the concept came with baggage, particularly in theology and religious studies.

2.3 The Philosophy of Symbolic Forms

While scholars generally agree that the authors of the "Xici" see trigrams and hexagrams as symbols of the cosmic group dance, there is no consensus as to how they understand symbolic representation. Do they view symbols as realistic representations of the dynamic unfolding of the universe? Or do they view symbols as selective depictions of the outside world?

The former view is a version of the "copy theory of representation." It assumes that there is an objective world out there, and we develop tools to copy it. And the effectiveness of the tools is determined by how realistically they are in capturing the objective reality. The latter view smacks of the philosophy of symbolic forms of Ernest Cassirer (1874–1945) where symbols are schemas to affirm our images of the world. It assumes that the universe is far more complex and complicated than humans can apprehend, and therefore, the best humans can do is develop the tools to give them a sense of the universe.

From the perspective of the "copy theory of representation," trigrams and hexagrams can be seen as realistic representations of the universe's constant renewal. For instance, the 8 trigrams (☰, ☷, ☵, ☲, ☳, ☱, ☶, ☴) are graphic representations of the mixing of the *yin* and *yang* that drive the constant renewal of the universe. With different combinations of a straight line (—) representing the *yang* cosmic force and a broken line (– –) representing the *yin* cosmic force, a trigram shows empirically a cosmos constantly renewing itself and creating the myriad things. Similarly, a hexagram is also a realistic representation of the unfolding of the universe. For example, a hexagram can be divided into two trigrams: the lower trigram (lines 1 to 3) and the upper trigram (lines 4 to 6). With two trigrams, a hexagram shows the interaction of two sets of *yin-yang* configuration, demonstrating the multiple ways in which the *yin* and the *yang* forces interact with and transform each other in the empirical world. Alternatively, one takes the lower two lines of a hexagram as representing the earth (*di* 地), the middle two lines as representing humankind (*ren* 人), and the top two lines as representing heaven (*tian* 天). Then, we have a trigram within a hexagram. Known as the "three potencies" (*sancai* 三才), the relation of heaven, earth, and humankind highlights the co-dependence between the natural realm (*tian* and *di*) and the human realm (*ren*) that is a given condition and fact in everyday life.

Despite its diverse textual body, underlying the *Yijing* is the notion that the cosmos is an organismic process without beginning or end. As a process, the cosmos resembles a great flow in which "all of the parts of the entire cosmos belong to one organic whole" and all the parts "interact as participants in one spontaneously self-generating process." As such, there are three characteristics of this great flow: continuity, wholeness, and dynamism. It is continuous because it never stops renewing itself. It is holistic because it includes everything in the universe and permeates in all aspects of life. It is dynamic because it is full of motion and movement, generating energy and strength all the time. In this cosmic flow, there is no distinction between the following: the natural realm and the human realm, an observing subject and an observed object, and the inner world and the outer world. Everything is part of a totality, a group dance that never stops.

To the *Yijing* authors, the unfolding of the universe is vividly portrayed in the 8 trigrams and 64 hexagrams. For instance, they see the 8 trigrams (☰, ☱, ☲, ☳, ☴, ☵, ☶, ☷) as graphic representations of the mixing of the *yin* and *yang* cosmic forces (or *qi*, energy). With different combinations of a straight line (—) representing the *yang* cosmic force and a broken line (– –) representing the *yin* cosmic force, a trigram symbolizes the cosmos' constant renewal and its creation of the myriad things.

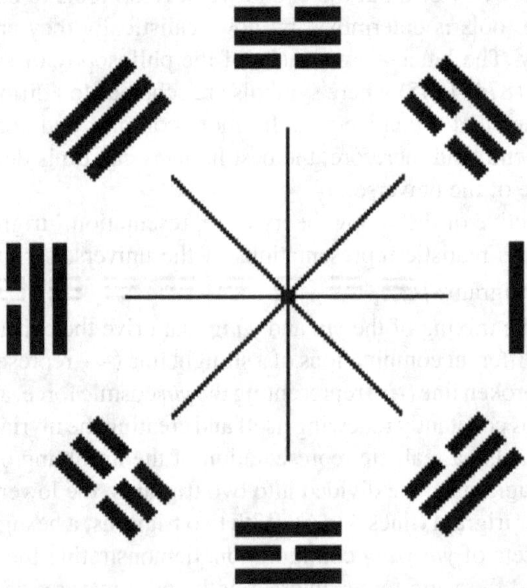

Similarly, a hexagram is also a symbol of the unfolding of the universe. For example, a hexagram can be divided into two trigrams: the lower trigram (lines 1–3) and the upper trigram (lines 4–6). With two trigrams, a hexagram symbolizes the interaction of two sets of *yin-yang* configuration, demonstrating the multiple ways in which the *yin* and *yang* forces interact and transform each other. Or, one takes the lower two lines of a hexagram as representing the earth (*di* 地), the middle two lines as representing humankind (*ren* 人), and the top two lines as representing heaven (*tian* 天). Then, we have a trigram within a hexagram. Known as the "three potencies" (*sancai* 三才), the relation of heaven, earth, and humankind highlights the co-dependence between the natural realm (tian and di) and the human realm (ren).

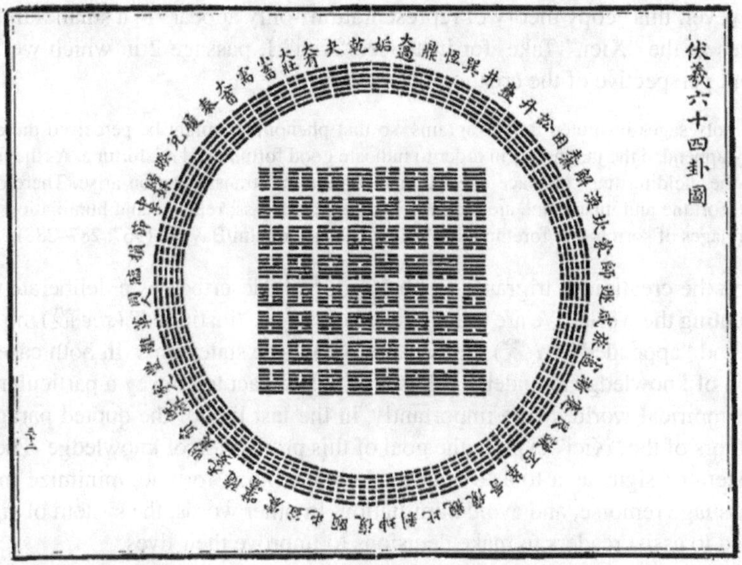

Allegedly developed by Fu Xi, the trigrams and hexagrams can be seen as coded messages from a supernatural power. But they can also be understood as a man-made system of signs that helps users understand the fluidity and complexity of the cosmic flow (more about the symbolism of trigrams and hexagrams later). In the "Xici," we find passages that support the copy theory of representation. The clearest example is the story of Bao Xi 包犧 (another name for Fu Xi 伏羲) in "Xici" II, passage 2. There, Bao Xi reportedly created a system of signs after observing the meteorological patterns in the sky and the geographical patterns on the ground ("Xici" II, 2:1; Wilhelm/Baynes 1967, 328–329). To some scholars, this story not only explains the creation of trigrams and hexagrams but also proves that the graphic symbols are realistic representations of the world. They point out that the two key terms in the Bao Xi story—contemplation (*guan* 觀) and proceeding [from what is close to us to what is far beyond] (*qu* 取)—denote an active quest for empirical knowledge through careful observation and rational deduction that leads to a factual understanding of the workings of the universe (Cheng 2020, 119–148).

Furthermore, the Bao Xi story continues after his death. We are told that another mythical figure, the Divine Husbandman (*shennong* 神農) drew inspiration from the hexagram of *Yi* 益 (Increase, #42) and used his knowledge to teach people farming. He also drew lessons from the hexagram *Shihe* 噬嗑 (Biting Through, #21) to teach people how to exchange goods to improve their lives. After the Divine Husbandman, Yellow Emperor, Shao and Shun continued to draw inspirations from a long list of hexagrams. They used their knowledge to teach people to improve their living conditions, including farming, government, and housing ("Xici" II, 2:1; Wilhelm/Baynes 1967, 330–336). Like a Google Map or a satellite image in our times, trigrams and hexagrams helped the mythical figures navigate the complex reality and achieve what they want in everyday life.

However, this "copy theory of representation" only appears in a small number of passages in the "Xici." Take, for instance, "Xici" I, passage 2 in which we find a different perspective of the creation of symbols.

> The holy sages instituted the hexagrams, so that phenomena might be perceived therein. They appended the judgments in order to indicate good fortune and misfortune. As the firm and the yielding lines displace one another, change and transformation arise. Therefore, good fortune and misfortune are the images of gain and loss; remorse and humiliation are the images of sorrow and forethought ("Xici" I, 2:1; Wilhelm/Baynes 1967, 287–288).

Here, the creation of trigrams and hexagrams is described as a deliberate act of representing the world. We are told that the holy sages "instituted" (*she* 設) the hexagrams and "appended" (*xi* 繫) the hexagram and line statements. In both cases, the creation of knowledge is understood as a calculated act to convey a particular view of the empirical world. More importantly, in the last line of the quoted paragraph, the authors of the "Xici" explain the goal of this production of knowledge. They see the system of signs as a tool to help readers maximize fortune, minimize misfortune, assuage remorse, and avoid humiliation. In other words, the system of signs is intended to assist readers to make decisions to improve their lives.

In another passage, this premediated act of representation is even more explicit. In "Xici" I, passage 12, we find a soliloquy of the Master (presumably Confucius) who questions the efficacy of words and images in conveying reality.

> The Master said: Writing cannot express words completely. Words cannot express thoughts completely. Are we then unable to see the thoughts of the holy sages?
>
> The Master said: The holy sages set up the images in order to express their thoughts completely; they devised the hexagrams in order to express the true and the false completely. Then they appended judgements and so could express their words completely ("Xici" I, 12:2; Wilhelm/Baynes 1967, 322).

Through the Master, the authors of the "Xici" assert that trigrams and hexagrams express the thoughts of their creators rather than the reality of the outside world. Similarly, the hexagram statements (or Judgments) are not the summaries of empirical facts; rather, they are suggestions for taking the appropriate actions to solve problems.

To the followers of Cassirer's philosophy of symbolic forms, the argument in the "Xici" is music to their ears. In his influential article, "Geist and Life," Cassirer describes human existence as a constant battle between the vicissitudes of life (Life) and the symbols that are deployed to make sense of our surroundings (Form). While the former is "objective," involving empirical data and concrete facts in the tangible world, the latter is "subjective," based on artificial schemas that present a picture of external reality to the perceivers (Cassirer 1996, 15–18). For Cassirer, it is this tension between what is external and internal, factual and representational, objective and subjective, and realistic and idealistic that characterize the creativity in human existence. In this continuum between Life and Form, and necessity and freedom, Cassirer urges us to develop our "Will to Formation" to align our understanding of the world with our system of symbols (Cassirer 1996, 29–33). To him, developing the "Will to Formation" is more important than developing the "Will to Power," as

Nietzsche suggests, because it helps us come to terms with the plurality, ambiguity, and conflicts in our lives.

While in principle the authors of the "Xici" would accept Cassirer's active theory of representation, they are totally committed to trigrams and hexagrams as their preferred system of signs. Having invested so much in pairing trigrams and hexagrams with the cosmic great dance, the authors of the "Xici" have no intention to include other systems of symbols to depict the universe, such as visual arts, literature, or poetry, as Cassirer recommends (Cassirer 1996, 34). Herein, perhaps, lies their blind spot. Their unwavering commitment to trigrams and hexagrams leads them to a blind alley where they fail to see the value of other systems of signs.

2.4 Decision-Making

To be sure, the authors of the "Xici" have reasons to commit themselves to trigrams and hexagrams. For them, trigrams and hexagrams are preferable not because they are the perfect symbols, but because they are vivid, flexible, and effective in representing the cosmic great dance. More importantly, trigrams and hexagrams are particularly helpful in sorting out—conceptually and graphically—the complex webs of relations that shape human lives. In "Xici" II, passage 3, we find them rigorously defending the value of trigrams and hexagram.

> Thus the Book of Changes consists of images. The images are intended to resemble [*xiang yezhe xiang ye* 象也者，像也]. The decisions provide the material. The lines are imitations of movements on earth. Thus do good fortune and misfortune arise, and remorse and humiliation appear ("Xici" II, 3:1-4; Wilhelm/Baynes 1967, 336–337).

In this passage, the authors of "Xici" explain their notion of representation. For them, trigrams and hexagrams are not necessarily the perfect tools, but they are the most effective in presenting (*xiang* 像) an image of the intricate cosmic great dance. More importantly, as the last sentence in the quotation indicates, trigrams and hexagrams give readers warnings of the dire consequences of bad decisions and reckless moves. As symbols, trigrams, and hexagrams force readers to reflect on their arrogance, complacency, and self-indulgence. They jolt them to look for ways to come to terms with contingency and serendipity. Above all, they direct their attention to the uncertainty that human beings must live with all the time.

Because trigrams and hexagrams are tools to assist readers to make decisions when they are at a crossroads, in several passages in "Xici" II we find the authors discuss the origin of the popularity of the *Yijing*. In these discussions, they tie the rise of the *Yijing* to the precipitous fall of the Shang dynasty and the unexpected rise of the Zhou dynasty. In crisis, the authors of the "Xici" claim that people look for direction that may lead them out of the chaos. In crisis, the authors of the "Xici" further assert, people reach a moment of truth where human finitude is fully exposed and human cruelty is on full display (*Xic*i I:11).

From the existential danger in a crisis, the authors of the "Xici" extend the argument that trigrams and hexagrams can help readers understand their limitations as well as their opportunities in peace time. At any critical juncture—a career change, a death in a family, or a loss in love—trigrams and hexagrams help readers manage their anxiety and give them hope for the future. Seen in this light, trigrams and hexagrams are no longer oracles. They become the symbols of the constant movements in the universe and the ceaseless changes in one's life.

Consider, for instance, hexagram *Qian* 乾 ䷀ (The Creative #1). The line statements depict the six *yang* lines as a dragon in various positions—a "hidden dragon" in line one at the bottom, an "emerging dragon" in line two, a "worrying gentleman" symbolizing a "worrying dragon" line three, a "wavering dragon" in line four, a "flying dragon" in line five, and an "arrogant dragon" in line six at the top. In addition, the line statements suggest a correspondence between the dragon's position and a proper course of action: the "hidden dragon" should avoid taking aggressive action; the "emerging dragon" and the "flying dragon" should seek help from "a great man;" the "worrying dragon" and the wavering dragon" should take flight over the depths despite the danger and apparent risks; and the "arrogant dragon" will regret being stubborn and excessively confident (for a translation of *Qian,* see Wilhelm/Baynes 1967, 3–10). But, as a hexagram, *Qian* is ambiguous. On the one hand, in five of its six lines, the tone seems to be upbeat, projecting an impression of progress from a hidden dragon to an emerging dragon, a wavering dragon, and finally a flying dragon. On the other, the progression is abruptly cut short by the downfall of an arrogant dragon. Like a Greek tragedy, the rapid fall of the arrogant dragon points to the pitfall of hubris, highlighting the danger of excessive human pride that results in over-exertion and overreach.

If we take seriously the symbolism of the rise and fall of hexagram *Qian*, it makes sense that in the final passage of "Xici" II, a stern warning is issued about failing to discern the signs of good fortune and imminent danger in trigrams and hexagrams.

> The Creative is the strongest of all things in the world. The expression of its nature is invariably the easy, in order thus to master the dangerous. The Receptive [*Kun* 坤, #2] is the most devoted of all things in the world. The expression of its nature is invariably simple, in order thus to master the obstructive. To be able to preserve joyousness of heart and yet to be concerned in thought: in this way we can determine good fortune and misfortune on earth, and bring to perfection everything on earth ("Xici" II, 11, 1–2; Wilhelm/Baynes 1967, 353).

In this passage, the authors of the "Xici" turn trigrams and hexagrams into spatial–temporal grids that reflect our surroundings, offering guidance in our search for alternatives and in developing skills of anticipating perils. As such, trigrams and hexagrams are not only symbols of the ever-changing universe but also reminders of our limitations as well as the opportunities that are potentially present. As shown in hexagram *Qian,* we may be a hidden dragon or an arrogant dragon when we enter the great flow, but as we are swept along by the current, we should find our position, our rhythm, and our trajectory. In the end, the key point is not when and how we enter the great flow of the universe, but what we become and what we achieve after we join the great flow.

2.5 Conclusion

For this reason, Chung-ying Cheng urges us to take seriously the philosophy of divination in the *Yijing*. For him, divination is not superstitious in the sense of a wrongful belief in the existence of a supernatural force. Rather, divination is a ritual, a performance whereby the diviner makes a careful decision on the next step, after a reflection of the past, an apprehension of the present, and an anticipation of the future. Understanding divination as an active act of reflection, apprehension, and anticipation, Cheng argues that divination is inherently philosophy, even though it is not commonly considered as a philosophy. He writes,

> The underlying logic of divination is that one should see divination as understanding both the limitation of the human condition and the freedom of human decision for action. On the one hand, a person is limited by his situation and even by his own purpose, and the future is not dictated by his wishes; on the other hand, a person can seek knowledge by the future or a way of understanding the possibilities of the future and thus make his own decision (Cheng 2020, 18).

For us today, this philosophy of divination reminds us of how far we have progressed from the ancient world, where nothing is certain due to its primitive technological and scientific development. At the same time, this philosophy of divination is refreshing because it encourages us to be spontaneous, creative, and experimental in coping with the complexity of life. Furthermore, it draws our attention to a world that is dynamic, fluid, multi-layered, and multi-causal which we rarely realize because of the humdrum of our daily lives. Most importantly, it reminds us that we are both a subject and an object in decision-making. On the one hand, we are the products of our environment; on the other hand, we are active players in reshaping our environment. Yet, no matter whether we are a subject or an object, what matters is our determination to face uncertainty with courage and dignity. In the end, we must admit that the world is far more complicated than we can imagine. To live, we do our best to move on in life and see how things will turn out.

References

Cassirer, Ernst. 1996. *Philosophy of Symbolic Forms,* vol. 4. New Haven, CT, and London: Yale University Press.

Cheng, Chung-Ying. 2020. *The Primary Way: Philosophy of Yijing*. Albany, NY: State University of New York Press.

Gotshalk, Richard. 1999. *Divination, Order, and the Zhouyi*. Lanham, MD: University Press of America.

Hon, Tze-ki. 2019. The Chinese philosophy of change (*Yijing*). *Stanford Encyclopedia of Philosophy*: https://plato.stanford.edu/entries/chinese-change/

Jin Jingfang 金景芳. 1987. *Xue Yi Sizhong* 学易四种 [Four Pieces of Writings on the *Zhouyi*]. Jilin: Jilinwenshi chubanshe.

Nylan, Michael. 2001. *The Five "Confucian" Classics*. New Haven, CT: Yale University Press.

Redmond, Geoffrey, and Tze-ki Hon. 2014. *Teaching the I Ching (Book of Changes)*. Oxford: Oxford University Press.

Ricoeur, Paul. 1984. *Time and Narrative*. Vol. 1. Tr. Kathleen Mclaughlin and David Pellauer. Chicago: Chicago University Press.

Shaughnessy, Edward L. 2022. *The Origin and Early Development of the Zhou Changes*. Leiden: Brill.

Smith, Richard J. 2008. *Fathoming the Cosmos and Ordering the World: The Yijing (I-Ching, or Classic of Changes) and its Evolution in China*. Charlottesville, VA: University of Virginia Press.

Smith, Richard J. 2012. *The I Ching: A Biography*. Princeton, NJ: Princeton University Press.

Whitehead, Alfred North. 1929 (1978). *Process and Reality: an Essay in Cosmology*. New York: The Free Press.

Wilhelm, Richard, and Cary F. Baynes. 1967. *The I Ching or Book of Changes*. Princeton, NJ: Princeton University Press.

Zhu Bokun 朱伯崑. 1986. *Yixue Zhexueshi* 易学哲学史 [A History of the Philosophy of the *Book of Changes*]. 3 vols. Beijing: Beijing daxue chubanshe.

Chapter 3
Unlocking the Unknown: The Concepts of Intuitive Cognition in the *Yijing*

Dominique Hertzer

> The intuitive mind is a sacred gift and the rational mind is a faithful servant. We have created a society that honors the servant and has forgotten the gift.
> Albert Einstein

Abstract The essay explores the concept of intuitive cognition in the context of divination, focusing on the *Yijing* (*I Ching*). Starting with parallels between the connection of divination and philosophy in Western and Chinese cultural contexts, the text focuses on the question of how we can get to know what we cannot know. The *Yijing* illustrates the cognitive process in the two hexagrams *xian* 咸 and *guan* 觀: resonance and contemplation. They outline the idea of cognition guided by intuition. Intuition cannot be separated from the entire cognitive process, bridging discursive reasoning and inexplicable insights. In the case of the *Yijing*, divinatory knowledge arises from an intuitive realization of the symbols, and at the same time from the internalized knowledge of the text, they complement and reveal each other.

Keywords *Yijing* · Divination · Cognition · Intuition · Resonance.

3.1 Introduction

Any form of divination goes beyond the limits of ordinary knowledge. Fortune-telling always seeks to obtain knowledge about what cannot usually be known, not least because its concern is often—but not necessarily—directed into the future. Whether this is possible at all or is only the result of deception or charlatanry, was and has been the subject of (more or less) scientific investigations for more than 3000 years. Every form of prognostics is just as fallible as it is not always rational or even scientifically verifiable.

D. Hertzer (✉)
Centre for Modern East Asian Studies, University of Göttingen, Göttingen, Germany
e-mail: dominique@zhouyi.de

G. Sigurðsson and T. Hon (eds.), *Contemporary Interpretations and Readings of the Yijing*, Chinese Culture 15, https://doi.org/10.1007/978-981-96-0609-2_3

And yet many people are fascinated by the fact that divination cannot be grasped rationally and must refer to the realm of the unfathomable. From an epistemological perspective, it is not very helpful to speak of a duality of rationality and irrationality. But then how does cognition get into divination? How can we get to know what we cannot know?

Knowledge gained by divination seems to dwell at an intermediate position between a discursively gained and a rationally not comprehensible knowledge, namely a form of intuitive knowledge. Before we discuss the concept of intuition, we will examine to what extent—and this applies equally to the occidental as well as to the Chinese cultural sphere—divination has a close connection to philosophy and thus to thinking accessible to reason.[1]

3.2 Divination and Philosophy in the Occident

In the Occident, philosophy is considered the mother of the individual sciences, because it is not limited to a single specific field of knowledge. Rather, it strives to fathom the world in general, human existence and the meaning of life by means of reason-guided knowledge. Kant (1724–1804) was the first to group the different areas of philosophy into four major questions:

1. What can I know?
2. What should I do?
3. What can I hope for?
4. What is the human being?

Accordingly, philosophy deals with questions of knowledge, with the competence to act as well as its ethical foundations, with the goal and meaning of life and thus also the question of whether and what can be expected after death.

Interestingly, Kant's four questions apply equally to divination, with the difference that the knowledge gained by means of divination goes far beyond purely rational knowledge. For the questions of divination are directed either into the future or into an area about which certain knowledge can usually not be obtained. Especially in the historical beginnings of divination, this kind of knowledge represents a divine knowledge that otherwise remains hidden.

It is precisely here where the connection between philosophy and divination becomes apparent: in the Platonic sense this is not only a transition from, but a connection of *mythos and logos*. Divination was in classical Greece, according to Michael Flower "a primary means of bridging the gap between the known and unknown, the visible and the invisible, the past and the future, and the human and the divine." (Flower 2008, 8).

[1] This connection between divination and philosophy is also intensively discussed by Lisa Raphals (2013) in her comparative work *Divination and Prediction in Early China and Ancient Greece.*

Only when philosophy is to take in the non-discursive irrational elements it may attain true knowledge. Thus, Plato also uses knowledge gained through divination or divine knowledge as a starting hypothesis to be proven or disproven in the course of a logical-discursive argumentation. In the dialogue *Meno,* for example, Socrates speaks of the doctrine of the immortal soul as a "divine matter" (*Meno* 81a-e), the truth of which can be fathomed by means of philosophical investigation:

> Most of the points I have made in support of my argument are not such as I can confidently assert; but that the belief in the duty of inquiring after what we do not know will make us better and braver and less helpless than the notion that there is not even a possibility of discovering what we do not know (*Meno* 86b).[2]

Hence, the goal of philosophy is to discursively verify the knowledge gained by means of divination. In the *Republic,* Plato tells us:

> I will try, I said, to show what seems right to me at least. Now, either concur or dissent, as a co-observer alongside me, to what I distinguish to be or not to be conductive to the sort of things we're talking about, in order that we might see also this more clearly, whether the matter is as I divine it to be. (*Republic* VII 523a; Struck 2018, 56)

Of course, these reflections on the connection between philosophy and divination do not apply to every kind of divination or philosophy. But precisely when it comes to deeply existential questions that bring us to the limits of knowledge accessible to reason and at the same time are not to be answered on the path of (religious) faith, this connection can lead to a special form of knowledge. Thus, for Plato, realization of the Idea of the Good is considered the highest form of knowledge. The latter is difficult to put into words and it resembles divinatory knowledge. He writes:

> That, which every soul pursues and on account of which does everything it does, it divines to be something, although it is at a loss and incapable of grasping sufficiently what in the world it is, nor is it able to feel a steady confidence about it, of the sort which it has concerning other things; and on account of this, even if it got some help from other things, it misses the mark. (*Republic* VI 505e–506a; Struck 2018, 57).

How divinatory knowledge can be attained in detail will be examined in the following. At this point, it should be noted that the integration of divination into philosophical thinking can open doors that usually remain closed to ordinary knowledge.

[2] All Western classical philosophical sources are cited according to the *Perseus Digital Library* and most of the times according to the translation of Peter Struck, 2018. The Chinese classical sources are cited according to the *Chinese Text Project* database. Further commentaries on the *Yijing* are cited according to the Yixue.com database.

3.3 Philosophy and Divination in the *Yijing*

The history of the development of the *Book of Changes* (*Yijing* 易經) reveals another perspective on the multi-layered connection between philosophy and divination that has already been discussed widely in research.[3]

When asked about the primary purpose of divination, Chinese discourse usually refers to a story from the historical work *Zuozhuan* 左傳[4]:

> Divination is used to resolve doubts, if one has no doubts, why consult the oracle? (*Chunqiu zuozhuan*, Henggong, shiyi nian/2, 春秋左傳, 横公十一年)

Seeding doubts, resolving, and dealing with them is one of the most important concerns of philosophy. Here doubt could relate to personal or political issues, often involving questions of health (of an important person), warfare, or any other kind of undertaking. The Xici commentary itself points out that worries, fears, and suffering played an important role for the formation of the *Yijing*:

> The changes came into use in the period of middle antiquity. Those who composed the Changes had great care and sorrow... Without or within they teach caution. They also show care and sorrow and their causes. Though you have no teacher, approach them as you would your parents... (Xici xia, 7–8).

Fears, worries, and doubts are thus an essential motive for consulting the oracle and predicting the future. But even if there are neither doubts nor worries and a decision has already been made by means of one's own will (*zhi* 志), the oracle is still useful. In this case, the oracle serves not only as confirmation of a decision well made, but also an affirmation of realizing one's own will. In this respect, the oracle's statements were also frequently reproduced in the form of prayers in order to enlist the help of the deities and spirits for the realization of one's own wishes and intentions (Shaughnessy 2022, 79–84).

The close connection between divination and divine knowledge that may become philosophical knowledge is reflected in the legendary origin myth of the *Yijing*. The latter attributes the discovery of the original foundations of the *Yijing*—in the sense of the eight trigrams and the 64 hexagrams derived from them—to the mythical emperor Fu Xi (伏羲, ca. 3rd Millennium BC). According to the Xici commentary of the *Yijing*, Fu Xi taught mankind in every form of cultural and social order ("Xici" xia 2). For he derived the eight trigrams (*bagua* 八) and their laws from a precise observation (*guan* 觀) of the heavens—sun, moon, and stars—as well as the earth—geographical features—and applied them to both the macrocosm and the human microcosm. However, this knowledge was not achieved in a discursive-logical way. Rather, it is a *divine knowledge* gained by *observation of nature and the cosmos,* which was embedded in a philosophical system during further historical

---

[3] Shaughnessy (2022, esp. 453–501) has explored the (Confucian) philosophical aspect of the *Yijing* in great detail.

[4] Kidder Smith (1989, 421–463) discusses the *Yijing* from the perspective of different accounts in the *Zuozhuan.*

development. Fu Xi "observed" (*guan* 觀) the eight trigrams, they appeared to him as (primordial) images of nature and he gave them the form of emblems.

The very fact that it is a mythical tale, described in the *Yijing* itself and never doubted in the course of its 2000-year commentary tradition, points to the unquestionable origin of this knowledge. Thus, the 8 trigrams (and perhaps 64 hexagrams) existed for about 2000 years before their symbolic meaning was put into words at the beginning of the Zhou dynasty (eleventh century BC) by King Wen (Zhou Wen Wang 周文王) and his son, Duke of Zhou 周公旦). The added judgments and the instructions for the 64 hexagrams form the oldest and most basic textual layer of the *Yijing*. *Together, they are the first step toward a gradual rationalization of divine knowledge.* The rationalization of divine knowledge is characteristic for the *Yijing* as a method of divination and is responsible for its great popularity up to the present day. By adding text to the 64 hexagrams, the knowledge gained by divination becomes better understandable and accessible for an interested public and is not only reserved for a small elite.

This process has continued to take shape since the second century BC with the addition of the *Ten Wings* commentaries (*Shiyi* 十翼). Together with the classical text, these commentaries form the present version of the traditional text and are as a whole an expression of the multi-layered integration of *the original divine knowledge into philosophical thought*. In this respect, the rich commentary literature is not only evidence of an increasingly differentiated philosophical interpretation of the traditional text, but it also reflects the ongoing attempt to gain new and updated access to an originally divine-spiritual knowledge that transcends rational thought.

What makes the *Book of Changes* so unique is that it is not itself subject to change, since it never loses its validity regardless of any historical changes, but proves itself with every (new) application:

> The *Changes* contain the way of the wise in four ways: In speaking we should be guided by its judgements; in action, we should be guided by its changes; in making objects we should be guided by its images; in seeking an oracle, we should be guided by its pronouncements. When the superior man is about to act and do something, he consults the *Changes* with the help of words. It takes up his communication like an echo; neither far nor near, neither dark nor deep exist for it, and thus he learns of the things of the future. If his book were not the most spiritual thing on earth, how could it do this?
>
> The *Changes* have no thoughts and no actions, they are still and do not move, once stimulated, they permeate all situations under heaven. If they were not the most spiritual thing under heaven, how could they do this? The *Changes* are what has enabled the holy sages to reach all depths and to grasp the seeds of all things. Only through what is deep can one penetrate all wills on earth. Only through the seeds can one complete all affairs on earth. Only with the spirit can one be quick without haste and arrive without moving (*Yijing*, Xici shang/10).

In this respect, the *Yijing* is not only a guide for divination, but its text is a model for speech, its laws of changes are a model for action, and its images are a practical model for the making of tools. As already shown above in the *Zuozhuan,* the *Yijing* is also used as a device for decision-making by providing access to a higher level of knowledge not usually accessible to humans. During the consultation process temporal boundaries are blurring, consciousness and unconsciousness are no longer separated. This is the moment that allows a glimpse into the future.

Since the *Book of Changes* is not subject to change, it is calm and without action. Only when the diviner consults the *Yijing* and puts it into practice, then the resonance between the text and the reader takes place. To describe this "fusion of horizons" between the text and the reader, Richard Wilhelm has compared this mode of action of reading the *Yijing* with an electrical circuit:

> It only has the possibility of illuminating but does not illuminate. Then, by establishing contact with a particular situation through the questioner, electricity is aroused and the situation in question is illuminated (Wilhelm 1981, 292).

To summarize, the connection between philosophy and divination in the *Yijing* appears in different ways. Questioning the oracle is an act of philosophical reflection on the world itself, often initiated by concrete doubts, fears, or worries. The origin myth of the *Book of Changes* reveals that its origins are undoubtedly of a divine-spiritual nature, which is not directly accessible to a rational-discursive understanding. Only through the addition of texts and explanations is the originally divine knowledge integrated into philosophical thought. And finally, the texts and commentaries of the *Yijing* in the last 2000 years are themselves an expression of a philosophical discourse on the world.

Let us recall once again Kant's four basic questions:

1. What can I know?
2. What should I do?
3. What can I hope for?
4. What is the human being?

The questions to the *Yijing*, which are directed toward the future or toward an area that is not accessible to our knowledge, usually move within the scope of Kant's theses. Thus, the oracle either deals with the limits of our knowledge or serves as a support for decision-making ("it serves to resolve doubts"). More importantly, it is directly related to the question of which hopes and expectations will be fulfilled—or whether there is reason to hope at all.

In the context of Chinese philosophy—and this is particularly true for the *Yijing*—the question is about "what should humans do," or "what is their acting and positioning in life." It is about the concrete duties and the specific roles of a human being. In one's relationship to the world, one is not firmly tied to a distinctive individuality. Hence, the art of life is to encounter it with a high degree of flexibility and creativity by taking on different roles in responding to changing circumstances. In this constant response to the changing demands of circumstances, one must decide what action is appropriate to the situation, how best to take advantage of the right moment, and how effectively to seize the right opportunity. Here, the *Yijing*—beyond the concrete divination process—provides the tools for instant and spontaneous responses. It is a philosophical work that deals with life and death, the transformations of macro- and microcosm as well as with the role of human beings in the world.

3.4 The Tension Between Intuitive and Discursive Knowledge in Divination

> Intuitively, or in concreto, every human being is actually aware of all philosophical truths: but to bring them into his abstract knowledge, into reflection, is the business of the philosopher, who neither should nor can do anything more.
> Arthur Schopenhauer

In divinatory use, we are always confronted with knowledge beyond reason. For as soon as we question the *Yijing*, we come into direct contact with divine knowledge for a moment when a certain hexagram is drawn by means of the coins or yarrow stalks. This situation is mainly determined by chance. Chance is the moment when we become permeable to divinatory knowledge, whose origin we cannot rationally name or deduce. But without the use of reason and discursive thinking, neither the elaboration of the question nor the interpretation of the answer will succeed. Ultimately, the *Yijing's* answer can only be revealed thanks to the combination of divinatory and philosophical knowledge.

But what does this mean in practice? And what role does intuition play in this process? Peter T. Struck, in his book *Divination and Human Nature: A Cognitive History of Intuition in Classical Antiquity,* assumes that intuition is essentially involved in the divinatory process of cognition if *cognition is not understood as a dualism of rationality and irrationality* but as the interaction of all factors of the conscious and unconscious involved. Struck writes,

> I have come to the view that trying to measure the rationality of divinatory thinking is actually a stumbling block and not a pathway to understanding it. As I hope to justify in the following pages, the contemporary category of cognition (as used in its broadest sense within the cognitive sciences) allows us to describe such intellectual phenomena better precisely because it allows for a study of thinking that is agnostic on the question of rationality. Cognition, as I will be using it, captures all activities of the mind and allows them an equal share of attention. The modes of thinking that the philosophers speculate about in studying divinatory insight, characterized in multivariant and elegantly subtle ways, is best approached from this broad scope (Struck 2018, 14).

He has convincingly argued that the knowledge gained in divination is a kind of "surplus knowledge" (Ibid., 15). The latter is not the result of discursive thought processes of which we are aware and over which we have self-conscious control. Nor is this "surplus" knowledge an expression of magic or esotericism. Rather, it is a potential inherent in our biological nature, which we define today as *intuition* or *intuitive knowledge*, (Ibid., 23). The characteristic of this intuitive insight is that it appears suddenly and we cannot explain how we came to know it (Ibid.). With Struck's hypothesis in mind, let us outline the psychological and philosophical approach to the notion of intuition before we move on to its role in the divination process itself.

3.4.1 Psychological Approaches to Intuition

Since the Enlightenment philosophy, intuition has been excluded from the vocabulary of epistemology and regarded primarily as a feeling, far inferior to logic and discursive cognition. However, at the end of the twentieth century, intuition conquered space in positions that reject the primacy of cognition as a procedure dedicated primarily to its own content, e.g., in deconstruction as a critique of the logocentrism of the Western tradition and in hermeneutics, in which intuition as a sudden and inexpressible understanding of the "meaning of being" is rehabilitated as an "extra-methodical" experience of truth (Heidegger, Gadamer) (Sandkühler and Borchers 2010, 1167).

Recent research in psychology has further shown that intuition—in the sense of an unconscious process and especially regarding decisions—can be just as important as rational thinking. One of the pioneers in the field of psychology and intuition, Gerd Gigerenzer, describes intuition as a judgment "that quickly emerges in consciousness, whose deeper reasons we are not fully aware of and which is strong enough to act upon" (Gigerenzer 2009, 25.). Thus intuition, which Gigerenzer also calls "gut feeling," functions according to a simple basic principle: "simple rules of thumb that make use of evolved abilities of the brain," (Ibid., 26). These simple rules of thumb help us to make the right decisions quickly, especially in complex and confusing situations, without us being able to name the specific reasons.

Psychologist Daniel Kahnemann describes intuition as one of two phases within the cognitive process. In his work *Thinking Fast—Thinking Slow,* he defines intuition as fast thinking, and distinguishes the area of fast, pre-attentive, preconscious processing from slow, conscious, and logically discursive processing (Kahnemann 2015, 289–302). This research not only shows that intuitive and discursive cognition are two sides of one cognitive coin, but also paints a differentiated picture of intuition. Not every gut feeling is a "real" intuition. For even intuition requires experience in many areas, which shapes implicit and explicit knowledge. Thus, a supposed gut feeling *can be more the result of our hopes and fears than the expression of a genuine intuition.* This aspect is of crucial importance, especially in the various techniques of divination. The interpreter needs a lot of experience with the respective divination technique to arrive at genuine knowledge. Furthermore, this kind of intuition is not given to everyone per se, even if many (esoteric) books and commentaries on divination may suggest this. Rather, intuition is often preceded by a long and arduous process of learning, knowledge, and experience.

3.4.2 Philosophical Approach to Intuition

In this respect, intuition can be a form of cognition in its own right, which is why I take up the distinction between *intuitive and discursive cognition* in the following. In philosophy, the former differs from the latter in that it describes *"the abrupt grasping of the whole object of cognition" in contrast to only "partial cognition"* (Ritter et al. 1976, 524). The word "*intuition*" is derived from the Latin verb "*intueor*," which was transferred from the Greek word *epibole* into Latin and refers to the activity of seeing (Sandkühler and Borchers 2010, 1161). Boethius first uses this term in a technical sense to express "direct apprehension as intellectual vision capable of grasping things in their essence" (Ibid.). The Epicureans used the term *epibole* to refer to the analogy that "already exists between the act of looking and the acquisition of knowledge" (Ibid).

Consequently, *epibole* does not result from cognition assembled from parts, and it is completely different from processual cognition; it is an action that proceeds without the support of language and is not determined by inferences, considerations, and cognitions that one already possesses. It is also an error-free action (Ibid).

Based on what we discuss above, intuition differs fundamentally from discursive knowledge, which can be gained by means of a thinking process or as a result of the combination of individual insights. Based on this meaning of the term in Greek culture, the term "intuition" has been used in two different ways, from which in turn two main traditions have developed. The first goes back to Plato's theory of knowledge and ideas. Here, intuition is understood as *contemplatio,* in which the mind contemplates the ideas—i.e., the ontological structures of reality. The ideas are thereby "grasped through a kind of contact between the mind and the observed" (Ibid.), which means that the entire mind is involved in the process of seeing. This aspect is crucial, especially with regard to Plato's understanding of how knowledge is acquired in divination.

The other tradition, as is often the case in the history of philosophy, is founded by Aristotle. He considers the immediate grasping—in the sense of intuition—to be.

> A form of evident knowledge that concerns only a special faculty or part of the human mind: the logical-rational, which does not grasp the general structures of being in their truth, but first principles and special truths on which the rest of cognition can be built. The characteristic trait is the mutual cooperation between intuition and discursive thinking, (Ibid., 1162).

These two traditions have been elaborated in the course of the history of philosophy, but this outline suffices for the present context. The common ground between these two traditions is that *intuition usually occurs suddenly and does not require any mediation in the form of language or reflection;* its truth reveals itself by virtue of its immediacy and originality (Ibid.).[5]

Plato was the first to speak of knowledge gained by divination as a cooperation of intuition and discursive thinking and in which different parts of the soul are involved.

[5] In his book *Auf den Spuren der Intuition* (On the Tracks of Intuition), Thomas Gonschior (2013) draws a multi-faceted picture of intuition, not only in the above-mentioned psychological and philosophical context, but also with regard to the role of intuition in medicine and the natural sciences, especially physics.

3.4.3 Plato and Divinatory Knowledge

For Plato, the highest knowledge is the knowledge of the ideas. However, this is more like viewing the ideas than an actual knowledge of them. The moment of viewing the ideas appears as a higher kind of knowledge, which Socrates sometimes associates—ironically, playfully, or seriously—with the Oracle of Delphi (Struck 2018, 40). Divination, according to Plato, is the locus of "surplus knowledge" which is non-discursive and often occurs unexpectedly or unintentionally (Ibid., 42). Yet Plato understands divination in most cases not as a profession, but as a way of thinking with the aim of making a correct prediction (Ibid., 47). Thus, in the *Apology,* Socrates is credited with prophetic knowledge shortly before his death, when in a prophetic dream he foresees his own death and the vengeance of his accusers (Ibid.). At the same time, Plato makes use of the phenomenon of divination when it is necessary to express an intuitive insight that far exceeds discursive knowledge. This is revealed, for example, in Socrates' *daimonion* (Ibid., 52).

The *daimonion* is a kind of divinatory guide that—in the guise of a mediator between gods and humans—comes into direct contact with Socrates. It usually speaks to him completely unexpectedly and manifests itself as a voice or a sign, but without him knowing where it comes from. The *daimonion* reliably warns him of danger and restrains him, but never drives him to do anything (Ibid., 68):

> When I was about to cross the stream, my good friend, my daimonion and customary sign that comes to me came—it always holds me back from something I am about to do—and I thought I heard a certain voice from it that forbade me from leaving before I made an expiation, on the grounds that I had committed some sin against the deity. And so I am a seer, not a very good one, but, as the bad writers say, good enough for my own purpose; so I now clearly understand my error (*Phaedrus* 242b–d, Struck 2018, 69).

In the *Timaeus*, one of Plato's most inaccessible dialogues, he concretizes his idea of divination as a special kind of knowledge. Against the background of the creation of microcosm and macrocosm, the *Timaeus* describes the origin and tasks of the three different parts of the soul and their localization in the body. While the immortal part of the soul (*nous*) resides in the head, the lower mortal part of the soul is located in the trunk of the body and in turn consists of two parts. One of these is placed in the chest and is closely connected with the heart, while the other part lies below the diaphragm. The latter is of a fierce nature, it determines appetite and serves to satisfy physical needs as well as the continuation of humanity. But despite—or even because of—its strong impulsiveness, it is at the same time the *center of divination.* Since this part of the soul is deeply unreasonable and tends to completely undermine the *nous*, the liver was created as a kind of protective shield. It protects the other parts of the soul from encroachment and at the same time is itself involved in the production of divinatory knowledge.

This reveals an interesting parallel to the Chinese conception, where the ethereal soul (*hun* 魂) is responsible for dreaming, visions, and fantasies and—as it happens—also finds its home in the liver. For Plato, the lower part of the soul produces images or visions—as we know them from dreams—in the form of material reality:

> And inasmuch as they knew that it would not understand reason, and that, even if it did have some share in the perception of reasons, it would have no natural instinct to pay heed to any of them but would be bewitched for the most part both day and night by images and phantasms,—to guard against this God devised and constructed the form of the liver and placed it in that part's abode; He fashioned it dense and smooth and bright and sweet, yet containing bitterness, that the power of thoughts which proceed from the mind, moving in the liver as in a mirror which receives impressions and provides visible images, should frighten this part of the soul (*Timaeus* 71a–b).

The ability to divine is thus not owed to the intellect but arises directly from the irrational part of the soul. Divination takes place either during sleep—in the form of dreams—or in other extraordinary states, that could even be pathological. The creators of humankind have tried to compensate for the weakness of the soul's irrational part by at least presenting it with the gift of getting in touch with truth by means of divination (*Timaeus* 71e).

But by what means does the lower part of the soul attain divinatory knowledge? Here Plato refers to the moment of the soul's *alignment*. For the most important task of our soul is to *direct* all our movements and strivings for knowledge toward the cosmos. While the uppermost part of the soul (*nous*) does this regularly, the lowermost part of the soul is only able to do so sporadically, for example in predictive dreaming or divination (Struck 2018, 87). In this respect, the unreasonable part of the soul is only able to see the images and visions, but without understanding them or even knowing by what means it has received them. It is rather the task.

> Of a reasonable man to consider what is said and remembered in sleep or in wakefulness by a prophesying being or a being filled with God, and also to think through in a differentiated way all the imaginary images that have been seen, in how far and for whom they indicate something of future, past or present evil or good (*Timaeus* 72a).

The arrival of divine knowledge, in the form of visions or other signs, can therefore *only happen without the participation of reason*, which would rather disturb this process. The work of reason begins only afterward, by translating, understanding, and judging the phenomena or sayings. Reason then shows itself in the person of the diviner, whose task it is to interpret what has been perceived (Ibid., 72b).

According to Plato, the process of divination takes place in two phases: In the first phase, knowledge is gained by a vision, and in the second phase, the images and ideas seen must be interpreted. *Divinatory knowledge*—which is also used metaphorically by Plato for any kind of non-derivative, non-logical or non-discursive knowledge—*arises from the interaction of the highest and lowest parts of the soul.* The person who receives the visions by virtue of his lower part of the soul is, however, not necessarily able to interpret them himself. This is usually the task of the diviner, who can interpret or translate the divination by means of reason (*nous*). Socrates is an exception here in that he knew how to interpret his dreams shortly before his execution or his *daimonion* correctly; he possessed both the gift of receiving the visions and of understanding them.

Therefore, rationality and irrationality or intuition are equally involved in divination. Not to separate the discursive and intuitive cognitive processes with view to divination, but to understand them as complementary opposites, is also a promising approach to the *Yijing*.

3.5 Intuition and Cognition in the Chinese Tradition

In China's classical philosophical tradition, the question of cognition is not primarily a discourse of separation between subject and object. While the process of cognition in the philosophical debate of the Occident strives for a separation and thus also a differentiated definition of subject and object as well as their manifold relationships, the Chinese discourse intends to overcome this division of subject and object. There, cognition is a process of participation in which the subject has a participating interest in in the object to be recognized. This is accompanied by a less strict separation of feeling and understanding, which must be differentiated but not completely separated from each other (Hertzer 2006, 409–411).

In this respect, there is no distinctive concept or explicit discussion on the topic of "intuition" or "intuitive cognition." This does not mean, however, that this discourse is not implicit in many texts, as is the case, for example, with the body-mind discourse (Hertzer, 2006). Correlative thinking, which gradually developed in the first century BC and reached its full flowering in the Han period (202 BC–220 AD), postulates a direct and inseparable connection between humans and the cosmos. The human microcosm is a reflection of the macrocosm of nature, all the laws of the macrocosm work in the cosmos as well as in human beings. In Chinese medicine, the laws of the macrocosm—for example in the form of the alternation of day and night, the cycle of the four seasons, the constellations of the sky or the geography of the earth—serve as window through which the functions of the human organism can be observed and thus provides guidance for diagnosis and therapy (Ibid., 279–284).

In correlative thinking, every kind of phenomena, things and beings in the world are assigned to certain categories. The respective assignment to a certain category is neither purely coincidental nor arbitrary. It is rather an expression of naturally existing resonances (*ganying* 感應) between the human realm and the realm of nature. This is also true for the *Changes* (*yi* 易) and their laws: they too are characterized by resonances.

If we manage to "observe" (*guan* 觀) these resonances that reveal the correlations between heaven, earth, and the human beings and become aware of them, we may also succeed in looking into the future. In the context of divination, it may be no coincidence that the idea of "observing" (*guan* 觀) and that of "resonance" (*ganying* 感應) also appear in the *Yjing* in the context of two hexagrams.

3.5.1 The Phenomenon of Resonance and Hexagram 31 Xian 咸

The Chinese term for "resonance" is composed of the two characters, *gan* 感 and *ying* 應. The character *gan* 感 is first used in the sense of "something that moves the heart" or "stimulate, move" as well as "touch, feel," while *ying* 應 appears in the meaning of "respond, be in agreement with" as well as "should, must."

In principle, two forms of resonance can be distinguished, which complement each other: *resonance by oppositeness* and *resonance by similarity*. Things that belong to the same category correspond with each other because they are in a mutual resonance relationship due to their similarity:

> Beautiful kinds call forth beautiful categories, ugly matters call forth ugly categories, for the things of the same kind emerge in resonance with each other. (*Chunqiu fanlu,* tonglei xiangdong/1 春秋繁露同類相動).

Therefore, they also can stimulate or strengthen each other:

> If water is poured on the earth, it will avoid the dry area and tend to the wet area, whereas if two identical pieces of firewood are exposed to fire, the fire will avoid the wet parts and seek the dry ones. All things avoid that which is different from them and seek that which is similar to them. If the *qi* matches, they meet; if the tones are similar, they resonate with each other (Ibid.).

Essential here is *that resonance is not a matter of cause and effect*. On the contrary, the laws of resonance seem to be completely illogical. In the *Wenyan* commentary to the fifth line of the first hexagram *qian* 乾, the rising of the dragon and the simultaneous appearance of a great man is explained as follows:

> What does the phrase "flying dragon in the sky, advantageous to see a great man" mean? The Master said: The same tones attract each other; the same *qi* seeks each other. The water flows to what is wet, the fire turns to what is dry. Clouds follow the dragon; wind follows the tiger. Thus, the sage rises, and the ten thousand beings follow him with their eyes. What is born of heaven feels related to what is above. What is born of earth feels related to what is below. Each follows its own kind (*Wenyan,* Qian 9/5).

Since things belonging to similar kinds or categories attract each other, *resonance by similarity is mostly* revealed *within the categories of yin and yang*. If *yang* activates *yang* and *yin is* strengthened by *yin*, the increase or decrease of *yin* and *yang* are expression *of resonance by similarity.* This form of resonance is particularly important for Chinese medicine, as it is often responsible for the development of pathologies.

R*esonance by oppositeness,* on the other hand, combines the opposing poles *yin* and *yang* to the very unity from which they originally emerged. The *resonance between opposites is thus caused by the need for mutual perfection and completion—for the completion of the respective missing aspects.*

It is precisely this *resonance by oppositeness* that is spoken of in hexagram 31 (*xian* 咸) of the *Yijing*, where the hexagram text states:

The response is auspicious, advantageous destiny. Taking a wife is auspicious (hexagram 31, hexagram statement).

— —

—— Trigram *Dui* 兑: Lake, joy, youngest daughter

——

——

— — Trigram *Gen* 艮: Mountain, keeping still, youngest son

— —

The symbolism of the trigrams is already a first indication of how to understand this hexagram. For here the trigram *gen* 艮—which stands for the mountain, keeping still and within the family order for the youngest son—is placed below the trigram *dui* 兑, which symbolizes the lake, joy, and accordingly the youngest daughter. This associates the connection between the young man and the young woman, as formulated in the statement of the hexagram text "taking a wife is auspicious." The young man and the young woman are an opposing couple (of *yin* and *yang*) who enter a union thanks to the mutual attraction resulting from resonance. In this respect, resonance by oppositeness is also an expression of the search for mutual perfection. The contrariness is also revealed in the opposition of the three *yin* and *yang* lines in the two trigrams. In the trigram *gen* 艮, there are two *yin* lines at the bottom and one *yang* line at the top. In the trigram *dui* 兑, this is exactly vice-versa.

Almost all hexagram names in the *Yijing* are ambiguous. This is not only because a certain ambiguity is beneficial for a book of divination, but the ambiguity of characters in Classical Chinese is a common phenomenon, not least because many meanings were not yet clearly defined at the beginning of the Chinese writing. The hexagram name *xian* 咸, which originally had the meaning of "complete" or "all-embracing," is interpreted in the commentaries by the addition of the radical for the "heart" (*xin* 心) in the sense of the character *gan* 感 "to stimulate," "to feel" or "resonance." On the oracle bone inscriptions, the two components of "mouth" (*kou* 口) and "axe" (*jian* 戈) can be identified, which is why *xian* 咸 also had the meaning of "kill" or "chop off the head" and, somewhat more generally, "injure."[6]

The character *xian* 咸 is also used as an alternate character for *xian* 緘, which can mean "forbid," "seal" or "stop." In the Mawangdui version of the *Yijing*, the character *qin* 欽 is written instead of *xian* 咸 and usually means "respect" (Hertzer 1996, 237). Originally, however, it is written without the radical *jin* 金 on the left

[6] The different and possible meanings of *xian* are quoted here according to the digital source commentary on the *Yijing*, *Zhouyi quanjie* 週一全解 on hexagram 31. Cf. Yixue.com: https://www.eee-learning.com/book/4834.

side and means "yawn," which in principle indicates a deficiency (in this case of air) that needs to be made up for. Duan Yucai 段玉裁, who in 1815 wrote one of the most important commentaries on the oldest Chinese dictionary, the *Shuowen jiezi* 說文解字, finally defines the character *qin* 欽 in terms of "because one lives simply and serenely, one can receive." Thus, it takes inner emptiness and openness to truly receive other people, as the *xiang* 象 commentary on the hexagram *xian* 咸 states:

> Above the mountain is the lake. The resonance. The superior man receives the people by being empty himself (Hexagram 31, Xiang Statement).

Even if all these meanings are very different or even seem to contradict each other at first sight, the entire field of meaning of *xian* 咸 can be outlined well: The prerequisite for the basic ability to "resonate" or "create resonance" is that one is *empty and open inside,* as the character *qin* 欽 from the Mawangdui version suggests. Out of the need for mutual completion, which is the essence of resonance by oppositeness, the meaning "complete" emerges. At the same time, it is necessary not to exceed a certain level of resonance in the sense of the above-mentioned meaning of *xian* 緘, "to stop," "to seal" or "to forbid." However, should this not succeed, too much resonance may lead to an injury, as indicated by the original use of *xian* 咸 on the oracle bones. In the individual line texts, all these meanings come into play. Contrary to what is often the case in the occidental context and especially in Hartmut Rosa's (2019) reflections on resonance, resonance here is not exclusively a positive phenomenon; too much (or too little) resonance can be just as harmful and hurtful.

In the *Yijing* text presented above, the triggering moment of the marriage is thus the resonance between man and woman, leading to a union of the opposite poles *yin* and *yang* and thus to their *mutual completion.* Another characteristic of *resonance by oppositeness* is that something new emerges from the union of the two opposites, just as children can be born from the marriage of husband and wife. For this reason, the creation of the ten thousand things and beings, their becoming and passing away, can be generally traced back to the relationship of resonance between heaven and earth:

> "Influence" (*xian* 咸) means "stimulation" (*gan* 感). The weak is above and the strong is below. The two *qi* (of hard and soft or heaven and earth) resonate (*ganying*) with each other to unite. Keeping still and joyful, the man is below and the woman is above, for this reason it is successful and of beneficial determination. Taking a wife brings good fortune.
>
> Heaven and earth mutually stimulate each other so that the ten thousand things arise in transformation, the sage stimulates the hearts of the people so that the kingdom is at peace. If we contemplate (*guan*) what makes them resonate, the true qualities of heaven and earth like the ten thousand things are revealed (hexagram 31, Tuan statement).

The commentary on the judgment refers both to the symbolism of the trigrams and to the interpretation of the hexagram text itself. The hard and the soft represent *yang* and *yin as well as* heaven and earth, respectively. As soon as the *qi* 氣 of heaven and earth are in resonance with each other (literally: "stimulate each other and respond to each other"), they unite and complete each other. This relationship of resonance is also evident between the wise man and the people. As soon as it is established, the kingdom is at peace. Finally, the essential quality of every being is at the same time the trigger for the arising of resonances if one is only able to contemplate (*guan* 觀) them.

3.5.2 *Prognostics and Resonance*

Resonances exist between all beings and phenomena of the cosmos; they are always there, and they are primarily unconscious in nature. They cannot necessarily be brought about willingly, and they are partly even unavailable. Therefore, it is even more important to develop inner peace and emptiness in order to perceive and receive them. This also means becoming aware of resonances in which we are involved, especially if we want to withdraw from unfavorable or too strong resonances. Thus, resonance is always the background to be reflected upon for every kind of cognition as well as divination.

The last sentence of the commentary on the judgment ("if you look comprehensively (*guan* 觀) at what makes them resonate, the true qualities of heaven and earth as well as of the ten thousand things are revealed") refers directly to another important aspect of intuition. Comprehensive contemplation (*guan* 觀) not only makes one aware of what resonates with the things in detail or with what they resonate, but also allows one to recognize the essential qualities of the cosmos with all its phenomena and beings. However, this is not a matter of purely discursive knowledge, it is more an immediate perception of the essence of all the beings and things in the cosmos. Precisely, this *ability of direct and comprehensive contemplation* is the subject of the 20th hexagram *guan* 觀, "contemplation."

3.5.3 *Hexagram* **Guan** 觀*—Contemplation*

The character *guan* 觀 initially means "to look at in detail." However, *guan* does not mean the everyday "looking at" of an object or a person. Rather, it is a comprehensive observation that perceives the most diverse aspects and perspectives of a situation.[7] The ability to observe both thoroughly and comprehensively is already evident in the use of *guan* on the oracle bone inscriptions. There it is used for "the owl," referring to its ability to see and observe in the dark.

Moreover, "looking" does not only apply to an external event, but at the same time it denotes the aspect of "introspection" or "contemplation." This meaning is taken up in religious Daoism, for example, where *guan* 觀 is used for the "temple."

---

[7] Cheng Chung-ying (2020, 26) also refers to *guan* 觀 in terms of a comprehensive observation of the entire natural world as the first stage of the development of the *Yijing*. Furthermore, in his *Philosophy of Change* (2023, 233ff.) he explores *guan* as a methodology that even may present a configurational theory of time.

Hexagram *Guan* 觀

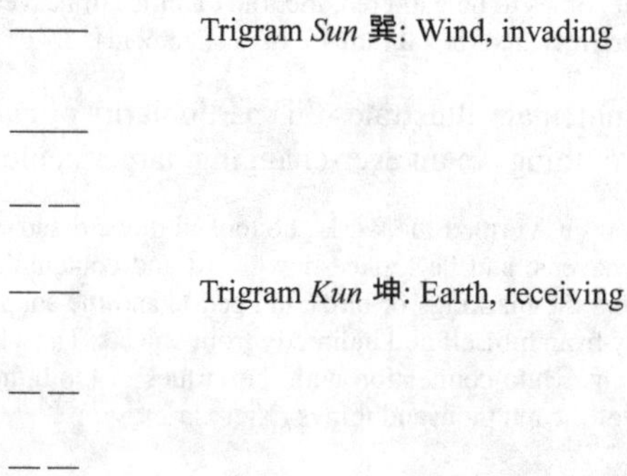

Finally, the character *guan* contains a third level, which is also revealed in the graphic representation of the hexagram. It designates the "spy tower" in front of the imperial court, from which all four directions can be seen and which is visible itself to all others from afar. *Guan* thus combines two opposite directions: The ability to look closely at something (inside or outside) and to make something "visible" to others or to show it to them, with the aim of instructing and cultivating them by example.

In the hexagram text, all these meanings come together. The hexagram *guan* 觀 first illustrates the moment of the sacrificial ritual as it presents itself to the spectators. At the same time, it describes the close observation of the sacrificial ritual, which is to be followed with the utmost attention and which ultimately—due to the seriousness of the situation—leads to introspection by the individual observer:

> The contemplation: The ritual has been made, but not yet the offering of the sacrifice, full of trust they look up to him (hexagram 20, hexagram statement).

The sacrificial ceremony is a great ancestral sacrifice. However, the most important moment is not the offering of the sacrificial animal itself, but the moment before when the water enriched with fragrant herbs is poured out on the ground to invite the spirits and deities to the sacrifice. This moment of utmost concentration and seriousness reveals itself in the vigilant observation of the ritual and implies at the same time introspection by those present. It is precisely this aspect that is examined in more detail in the changing lines, when the "all-embracing contemplation" or "introspection" manifests itself, for example, in the contemplation of one's own life or that of others. As already illustrated above, the commentary on hexagram 31 *xian* 咸 uses the term *guan* 觀 in the sense of an all-encompassing contemplation that leads directly to the essence of things themselves:

> If you contemplate what makes them resonate, the true qualities of heaven and earth like the ten thousand things are revealed (hexagram 31, tuan statement).

We find an almost identical wording in the commentary on the two hexagrams 32, *Heng* 恆 "Duration," and 45, *Cui* 萃 "Gathering together":

> Contemplating what gives them duration, the true qualities of heaven and earth as of the ten thousand things are revealed (hexagram 32, tuan statement).
>
> Contemplating how it comes to be gathered, the true qualities of heaven and earth as of the ten thousand things are revealed (hexagram 45, tuan statement).

The Xici 繫辭 commentary illustrates this particularity of *guan* 觀 as well, where Fu Xi is able to look at things in an ever-changing, larger context:

> In ancient times, when Fu Xi ruled the world, he looked upward and contemplated (*guan*) the symbols in the heavens, and he looked downward and contemplated the patterns on earth. He contemplated the markings of birds and beasts and the adaptions to the regions. He proceeded directly from himself and indirectly from objects. Thus, he invented the eight trigrams in order to enter into connection with the virtues of the light of the gods and to classify the qualities of the ten thousand things (Xici xia 2).

The attentive observation of the outside world and the concentrated introspection that goes with it unites three major perspectives: By observing the symbols in the sky and the laws of the earth, Fu Xi deduces the formation and change of things in time and space as they manifest themselves, for example, as the four seasons and the cardinal directions. Furthermore, all things are subject to permanent change, and they are in turn situated in an ever-changing environment. After all, things are embedded in patterns of order that are on their part integrated into an even more general order of rise and fall. This order reveals the interaction and eternal change of *yin* and *yang* as illustrated in the 64 hexagrams of the *Yijing*.

Considering modern research on intuition, however, *guan* does not distinguish between conscious and unconscious processes. For according to the hexagram *guan*, the conscious and unconscious processes may be differentiated, but not separated from each other, just as the precise observation of external reality can only succeed if it is combined with profound introspection. This is a good example of how cognition results from participation in the object to be cognized rather than from the separation of subject and object. At this point, certain parallels appear with the above-mentioned conception of Plato, who *describes intuition as contemplatio*, when the entire soul participates in the process of seeing and the ideas are "grasped through a kind of contact between the mind and the observed" (Sandkühler and Borchers 2010, 1162).

3.5.4 How Do We Know?

Returning to Peter Struck and his book *Divination and Human Nature*, we can say that intuition also plays an important role in the divination process of the *Yijing*. Beyond this, however, intuition cannot be separated from the entire cognitive process, which includes rational-discursive cognition, not least because any kind of cognition in early Chinese philosophy may only succeed by participation in the object to be cognized and not by a separation of subject and object.

The Yijing illustrates the intuitive aspect of the cognitive process as evident in the two hexagrams *xian* 咸 and *guan* 觀: they are an expression of *cognition guided by intuition*. *Guan* 觀—in the sense of comprehensive observation directed simultaneously toward the outside and the inside—refers to the larger context of individual things or processes and of the way they display themselves to the observer. Every individual thing or being may only be understood against the background of its respective embedding in this larger whole. The phenomenon of resonance (*gan* 感) is the premise for this contemplation, and becoming aware of it enables insight guided by intuition.

Finally, if we look at the two levels of the *Yijing* with its *symbols* and the *text*, we can say that the symbols in the form of the individual *yin* and *yang* lines, the eight trigrams as well as their arrangement into one of the 64 hexagrams act as a creative impulse for intuitive cognition. The corresponding hexagram and line texts as well as the commentaries are both explicit and discursive expressions of the knowledge gained and thus accessible to rational thought. Considering the ambiguity of individual characters of the text, it is perhaps not only due to the possibility of an open or even arbitrary interpretation as is often assumed. Rather, intuitive cognition based on symbolism requires a certain level of freedom when it wants to put the answer of the oracle into words.

In the case of the *Yijing*, divinatory knowledge arises from an intuitive realization of the symbols *and* at the same time from the internalized knowledge of the text; they complement and reveal each other. Of course, this requires a sound knowledge of the text and experience on the part of the interpreter if a serious look into the future is to succeed.

Wang Bi, one of the earliest and most brilliant commentators on the *Yijing*, finally merges the level of symbol and text, intuitive and discursive cognition into a higher level, where the deep understanding of and insight in the *Yijing* is realized by forgetting this very knowledge again in a process of unlearning:

> The words are directed to the symbols. Consequently, one can grasp the symbols by examining the words. The symbols are directed to the ideas. By examining the symbols, one can recognize the ideas. The ideas are fully expressed in the symbols, and the symbols are explained by the words. Consequently, the aim of words is to explain the symbols, but once one has grasped the symbols, the words may be forgotten. The aim of symbols is to preserve the ideas, but once one has grasped the ideas, the symbols may be forgotten. (Wang Bi, *Zhouyi Lueli*/4, 王弼, 周易略例).

References

Cheng, Chung-Ying. 2023. *The Philosophy of Change: Comparative Insights on the Yijing*. Albany, NY: State University of New York Press.

Cheng, Chung-Ying. 2020. *The Primary Way. Philosophy of the Yijing*. Albany, NY: State University of New York Press.

Flower, Michael A. 2008. *The Seer in Ancient Greece*. Oakland, CA: University of California Press.

Gigerenzer, Gerd. 2009. *Bauchentscheidungen: die Intelligenz des Unbewussten und die Macht der Intuition*. 10th ed. Tr. Hainer Kober. Munich: Goldmann.

Gonschior, Thomas. 2013. *Auf den Spuren der Intuition*. Munich: Herbig.

Hertzer, Dominique. 2006. *Das Leuchten des Geistes und die Erkenntnis der Seele: Die medizinische Vorstellung vom Seelischen als Ausdruck philosophischen Denkens—China und das Abendland*. Frankfurt am Main: VAS, Verlag für Akademische Schriften.

Hertzer, Dominique. 1996. *Das Mawangdui-Yijing. Text und Deutung.* Munich: E. Diederichs.

Kahneman, Daniel. 2015. *Schnelles Denken, Langsames Denken.* 21st ed. Tr. Thorsten Schmidt. Munich: Pantheon.

Raphals, Lisa. 2013. *Divination and Prediction in Early China and Ancient Greece.* Cambridge: Cambridge University Press.

Ritter, Joachim, et al. (eds.). 1976. *Historisches Wörterbuch der Philosophie. Völlig Neubearbeitete Ausg. des "Wörterbuchs der Philosophischen Begriffe" von Rudolf Eisler*. Vol. 4. Basel: Schwabe.

Rosa, Hartmut. 2019. *Resonanz: Eine Soziologie der Weltbeziehung*. Berlin: Suhrkamp.

Sandkühler, Hans Jörg, and Dagmar Borchers, eds. 2010. *Enzyklopädie Philosophie.* 3 vols. 2nd ed. Hamburg: Meiner.

Shaughnessy, Edward L. 2022. *The Origin and Early Development of the* Zhou Changes. Leiden and Boston, MA: Brill.

Smith, Jr., Kidder. 1989. *Zhouyi* Interpretation from Accounts in the *Zuozhuan. Harvard Journal of Asiatic Studies* 49 (2): 421–463.

Struck, Peter T. 2018. *Divination and Human Nature: A Cognitive History of Intuition in Classical Antiquity.* Princeton, NJ: Princeton University Press.

Wilhelm, Richard. 1977. *The I Ching or Book of Changes.* 3rd ed. Tr. Cary F. Baynes. Princeton, NJ: Princeton University Press.

Wilhelm, Richard. 1981. *I Ging: Das Buch der Wandlungen.* Munich: E. Diederichs.

Digital Sources

Perseus Digital Library: http://www.perseus.tufts.edu/hopper/
Chinese Text Project: https://ctext.org/
Yixue.com 易學網: https://www.eee-learning.com/

Chapter 4
Between Divination and Cultivation: Early Daoist Philosophy and the *Changes*

Sharon Small

Abstract In this paper, I ask to explore the thread of abstract thought from the early *Yijing*易經 (*Classic of Changes*) to the metaphysics of Laozi and Zhuangzi; from Lao-Zhuang philosophy to the political practice of the Huang-Lao; and to the *Yizhuan* 易傳 (*Ten Wings*) and the art of divination. By observing the key concepts common to the different texts and authors, we find that Huang-Lao manuscripts and the *Ten Wings* share their core cosmological and metaphysical assumptions, their practices of cultivation, and their ideal sage ruler who grasps the principles of heaven and earth. The main difference among them is that for Daoists, self-cultivation was sufficient to grasp the *Dao* and become a sage ruler with penetrating insight to the workings of heaven and earth, while for the *Yi* scholars, self-cultivation was emphasized in the context of the art of divination .

Keywords Pre-Qin Daoist thought · Excavated manuscripts · Self-cultivation · *Yijing* · *Ten Wings* · Divination

4.1 Introduction

To explore the relationship between the Huang-Lao school of thought and the commentaries to the Changes, I carry out an analysis of the excavated manuscript of the *Fanwuliuxing*凡物流形 ("All Things Flow into Form," hereafter FWLX), housed in the Shanghai Museum Collection and dated to the mid-late Warring States Period.[1] The manuscript, as an exemplar of Huang-Lao philosophy that offers an integration between cosmo-metaphysical notions and concrete human affairs, presents a

[1] First published in Chengyuan 2008.

S. Small (✉)
Tel Aviv University, Tel Aviv, Israel
e-mail: ssysmall12@gmail.com

G. Sigurðsson and T. Hon (eds.), *Contemporary Interpretations and Readings of the Yijing*, Chinese Culture 15, https://doi.org/10.1007/978-981-96-0609-2_4

detailed cosmological process using familiar Daoist notions and emphasizes the ultimate origin in oneness from which generation begins and concludes the cosmogonic process with the order of time.[2]

Daoist philosophy after the *Laozi* evolved in two directions: (1) the philosophy of the *Zhuangzi* that expands the cosmological thought and its connection to human life, promotes generation through transformation of *yin* and *yang* energies (*qi*), and brings the notion of transformation into being (*huasheng*化生) onto the frontstage of Daoist thought; (2) Huang-Lao or Jiaxia Daoism that employs the cosmological terminology of the *Laozi* and extracts governmental practices and moral debates from both early Daoist thought and other prominent philosophical systems at the time.

In the golden era of philosophy in ancient China, people began to doubt the practice of divination and renounce ancient feudal religious ancestral worship. This brought thinkers to turn inward, hold intellectual debates, and generate philosophical systems which demand self-reflection, all while eagerly seeking a unifying principle of heaven and human without the need to "resort to divination." In this background, the commentaries to the Changes were compiled. They defend the ultimate position of divination while adopting the theoretical and metaphysical philosophies of early Daoist thinkers and utilizing self-cultivation, as emphasized in Huang-Lao manuscripts.[3]

Zhang Dainian 張岱年 (1996) maintained that early Chinese philosophy can be called the study of heaven and human (*tianrenzhixue* 天人之學), or the "boundaries between heaven and man" (*tianrenzhiji*e 天人之際). The structural connection between heaven and man as embedded in the *Changes* is elaborated in the philosophical argumentation of Daoist philosophers who view this relationship as inherent and necessary.

Prior to the existence of the *Ten Wings* and the era of philosophers, very few sources commented on the *Changes* or the practice of divination. Perhaps one of the best-known comments comes from the Spring and Autumn text of the *Zuozhuan* (*Chunqiu zuozhuan* 春秋左傳), stating that the purpose of divination is to "resolve doubts."[4] Aside from understanding the purpose of divination as a tool for resolving doubts and making decisions, this comment also reflects that divination was a widespread practice that people often used to make decisions when doubts arouse. Following the rise of philosophy in the late Spring and Autumn period and its flourishing during Warring States times, the understanding of the relationship between heaven and

[2] The cosmology of the FWLX resembles that of the *Taiyi* shengshui 太一生水, a manuscript unearthed from Guodian and predates the FWLX by two centuries. For research on comparisons between them, see Huang 2019, 1–26; and Huang 2023, 33–34.

[3] Mainly referring to the *Huangdi sijing* from MWD, the FWLX, and HX in the Shanghai Museum collections, a selection of chapters from the *Zhuangzi*, the *Guanzi*, *Lüshi Chunqiu*, etc., speculated to be affiliated to the Jixia Academy scholars.

[4] In total there are 22 references to the *Changes* in the *Zuozhuan* and the *Guoyu* combined, 16 are in context of practicing divination, the remaining six are explanations. The example above is from *Chunqiu Zuozhuan* 春秋左傳, Huangong shiyinian 桓公十一年: 卜以決疑,不疑何卜 "divination is to resolve doubts, when there are no doubts why use divination?" (Yang 2016, 142).

human radically changed. It no longer demanded the mediation of departed spirits or divination; it could be perceived directly without leaving one's home.

Nevertheless, the cosmology and perception of nature embedded in the hexagrams, hexagram statements or judgments, and the line statements for each of the six lines which compose the *Yijing* 易經deeply influenced Chinese intellectuals in the Spring and Autumn and Warring States Periods. It provided inspiration for Daoist thought in the stage of its formulation, as evident in the philosophical texts of the *Laozi* and the *Zhuangzi*.[5]

4.2 Part One: From External to Internal: The *Changes* and Early Daoist Philosophy

The evolution of the *Changes* throughout the centuries of the Zhou Dynasty from the conquest of Shang-Yin to Spring and Autumn times and to the Warring States Period was also the process of departing from the position of divination in ancient ancestral religion, and distancing from the older framework in which divination was performed at the court of the Zhou and its principalities, praising the authority and sagacity of the ancestral kings of the Zhou. With the decline of the Zhou Dynasty, along with the separation of entire regions into multiple states, divination became widespread practice and formed what was termed a "*Classic*" (*jing* 經) put down in writing. As a subject of both study and practice, there were various editions or "versions" and also distinct divination manuals such as *Rishu* 日書 circulating throughout the different states (Schilling in Legge 2020, 8–9). As archeological evidence suggests, by the Warring States era, there were different copies in circulation, probably a result of each state having their own edition.[6]

In the *Changes,* a distinction is made between three kinds of change: non-change, cyclic change, and sequent change. Non-change (oneness, stillness) is the background against which change (movement) is made possible. Any change must have some fixed point to which the change can be referred; otherwise, there can be no definite order, and everything is dissolved in chaotic movement. This point of reference must be established, and this always requires a choice and a decision. Consequently, at the beginning of the world, as at the beginning of thought, there is the decision, a fixed point of reference. The premise for such a decision is the belief that in the last analysis the world is a system of homogeneous relationships—that is a cosmos, not a chaos. The ultimate frame of reference for all the changes is the non-changing (Lynn 2004, 281).

[5] Chen Guying (2023, 134–144) raises many examples of references to the *Changes* and its influences on Daoist philosophy. Chen further claims that the "Judgments" ("Tuanzhuan" 彖傳) and the "Grand Treatise" ("Dazhuan" 大專 or "Xici" 繫辭) were influenced by Huang-Lao thought.

[6] For an English language study on the recently unearthed *Yijing* manuscripts including their translation, see Shaughnessy 2014.

The Laozi develops this frame of thought into a metaphysical yet concrete philosophy by defining *Dao* as both absence (*wu* 無) and presence (*you* 有), both as the ultimate non-changing, still, unnamed origin (*dao yin wuming* 道隱無名; *dulibugai* 獨立而不改) and the principle of change as a constant ongoing process (*zhouxingerbudai* 周行而不殆).

The order for human beings proposed by the *Laozi* was derived from a metaphysical order of the cosmos, and the way for humans to realize this order and practice it in society begins with cultivating the mind, observing inward, uniting the spirit and the body. The process of inner cultivation may bring one to an understanding of the underlying principle of the cosmos and nature, or in other words—the *Dao*.

Notions from the *Changes* pertaining to ethics such as modesty, the observance of certain restraints; and to cosmic patterns such as return and cyclicality (*fanfu* 反復), the reciprocal relationship between the hidden and the apparent, and the correlativity of gain and loss, are emphasized in the *Laozi*, and appear to have inspired the *Laozi's* own philosophical system. The constant interchange between complementary opposites, the importance of modesty and humility, and the notion of non-reckless and non-rash action are developed into a system that ties heaven, earth, and human through an ultimate origin, the *Dao*. Being a singularity that can be found in all three connected realms, one may divert his attention inward, practice cultivation of the heart and mind, and grasp the way of heaven without ever looking out the window.[7]

In the *Laozi,* we may observe four main strands of thought: one is the method of thinking in complementary opposites; the second, the method of cycles; the third is the deduction of the patterns of nature to human affairs; and the fourth, the unity between heaven, earth, and humans (Chen Guying 2014, 138–166). While the first two modes of thought are apparent in the *Changes*, the latter two tying the universe to one's own self and projecting further onto ruling the state, are developed further by the *Zhuangzi* and Huang-Lao manuscripts and enter the *Changes* only in the *Commentaries*.

The turn inward for comprehending the ultimate principle of the universe marked the divergence of divination and philosophical reflection. In the social-political realm, the ruler no longer needed to resort to divination, rather self-cultivation becomes essential for the ruler to realize the *Dao* of heaven in his own person and practice it in rulership.

Unity and the focus on oneness evolve into a central notion through the developments of the *Zhuangzi* and Huang-Lao works. Huang-Lao, moreover, emphasizes the metaphysical and abstract aspects of *Dao* and strips it of its concreteness. In Huang-Lao thought, the concrete manifestations, i.e., the "presence" and the "named" aspects of *Dao*, are transferred into the concept of oneness (Cui 2023, 19). In this sense, *Dao* becomes more naturalistic and less mystical. It remains a first principle, but it is no longer entirely nameless. It tends to be treated as a natural law of the universe, but at

[7] Chapters 47 and 56 raise clear examples of self-reflection in solitude without the dependence on any external disruptions; in 47 it is expressed in "not looking out the window, the course of heaven is shown" (Ziporyn 2023, 58); in Chap. 56 it appears as instructions: "block the exchanges, close the gates, dull the points, untie the tangles, harmonize with the glares, merge with the dusts—this is called merging into obscure (*xuan* 玄), the obscure merging" (Ibid., 67).

the same time, it loses its position as something beyond heaven and earth.[8] In fact, in Huang-Lao thought, it seems to be a creative force within heaven and earth and emphasis is placed on the relationship between names and forms, timeliness instead of timelessness, law (*fa* 法) that originates from the way, and political methods to establish order.[9] The ideal ruler becomes a Daoist sage, ruling through non-assertive action, practicing techniques of self-cultivation, while the work of administration is performed by his ministers (Rickett 1998, 21).[10] The "Confucian" values of humaneness (*ren* 仁), sense of duty (*yi* 義), and propriety (*li* 禮) are appreciated. In the FWLX, the ultimate origin of oneness becomes so concrete that it can be perceived through the senses:

> You chew it, it has flavors; smell it, it has scents; drum it, it has sounds; close up, you can see it; handle (?) it, you can …(?) it.
>
> 慮(+又=咀)之有味,嗅[之有臭],鼓之有聲(B13b),近之可見,操(?)之可謀(操).[11]

Furthermore, as the manuscript explains, oneness can be found in the self, while the method to realize it in the self is by using *measures*.

> If you want to understand the One, look up then you will see it, look down you will grab it. You don't have to seek it far, just measure yourself and consider it.
>
> 如欲察一,卬(=仰)而視之,俯(?)而揆(?)之,毋遠求,度(B15)於身旨(=稽)之

The notion that *Dao*, or in this case, oneness is found in anything appears as early as the inner chapters of the *Zhuangzi*, yet, the appearance of the method of "measures" marks the difference between Lao-Zhuang and Huang-Lao philosophy.[12]

The *Xinshuxia* 心術下 ("Art of the Heart Part II") and the *Neiye* 内業 ("Inner Workings") of the *Guanzi* 管子 state the preference of self-cultivation and self-reflection over divination:

> Can you concentrate your mind? Can you focus? Without resorting to tortoise shell and milfoil, can you foretell bad fortune from good? Can you tell where to stop? Can you tell when to desist? Rather than asking others, can you find it within yourself? (*Guanzi*, *Xinshuxia*) (Rickett 1998, 60)

---

[8] For further reading on *Dao* as Natural Law, see Peerenboom (1993, 76–84).

[9] The first chapter (*daofa* 道法) in the first book (*jingfa* 經法) of the *Huangdi sijing* 黃帝四經 opens with "*Dao* generates Law" *daoshengfa* 道生法 (Chen Guying 2016).

[10] Four chapters dealing with cultivation in the *Guanzi* are speculated to be authored by Huang-Lao Daoists in the Jixia academy at around 302 BCE. For further discussion on the Huang-Lao authorship of chapters in the *Guanzi*, see Rickett 1998, 15–21. Rickett also mentions that some groupings including two additional chapters: the *zhouhe* 宙合 and the *shuyan* 樞言, ibid., 15. Chen Guying delves further into the Huang-Lao orientation of eight chapters that he affiliates to Daoism in the *Guanzi*. See Chen Guying 2016, 3–27.

[11] The translation and transcription of the Fanwuliuxing cited herein are from Lai 2010.

[12] As Chen Guying (2014, 92) notes, the *Laozi* and the *Zhuangzi* use the term "middle" to describe a state of balance in the heart and mind. Later Huang-Lao Daoists took this and externalized it, shifting from the internal harmony of "middle" to an emphasis on physical balance of "degree" (*du* 度).

In the *Guanzi*, the rhetorical questions mention divination and the prediction of the future, contrasting these arts with the principle of oneness. The sense is that if one is able to grasp the principle of oneness, then the insights about the cosmos that one consequently gains would allow one to navigate their way in the world in a manner that divination cannot. Furthermore, the *Zhuangzi* and Huang-Lao manuscripts not only adopt the notion of the ideal sage from the Laozi, but they also develop methods and practices to achieve this ideal in concrete and daily life.

Among the questions raised in the FWLX, the cultural practice of ancestral worship and serving the dead is questioned with an argument against the remnants of ancient religion:

> Ghosts come from human beings, why do [they] become divinely numinous? After the flesh and bone disintegrate, why does their intelligence become brighter? Where do the departed go? Who knows their borders? Ghosts derive from human beings, why should I serve them? After the flesh and bone disintegrated, no longer can their bodies be seen, why should I voluntarily feed (= offer sacrifices to) them? Their coming cannot be predicted, how can I time [the sacrifices]? Why should [I] perform requital sacrifices? How can I make [them] satisfied? Following the Way of the heaven, what should I treat as the principal? I want to gain the harmony of the hundred clans, what should I do?
>
> 鬼生於人,奚故神明?骨肉之(B4)既靡,其智愈彰,其(B11b)夬(=決、訣[10])奚適,孰知【A5】其疆?鬼生於人,吾奚故事之?骨肉之既靡,身體不見, 吾奚自食之?其來無度,【A6】(B5)吾奚時之?塞[11]祭員(異?=禩=祀)奚 (=登)[12]?吾如之何思(=使)飽[13]?順天之道,吾奚以為頁(首)?吾(B6)欲得【A7】百姓之和,吾奚事之?

This passage questions the authority of spirits and ghosts and questions the very act of serving the departed which was the core of the ancient religion of ancestral worship. This section ends with the conclusion that satisfying ghosts and spirits is not beneficial for the ultimate goal, namely the harmony of the hundred clans. Harmony of the hundred clans is achieved by following the way of heaven (*tiandao* 天道).

As in the passage from the *Guanzi* cited above, introspection is favored over divination. Turning the observation inward to find the principle of heaven is done by focusing the mind on oneness, either as an ultimate origin or a unifying principle of all existence. The *Guanzi* advises its reader to forsake the practice of divination and focus on the self-cultivation of the mind, and the FWLX goes a step further and calls to renounce ancestral worship.

4.3 Part II: From Huang-Lao Daoism to the Commentaries: The FWLX, the *Tuan*, and the "Xici"

The *Daoyuan* 道原 book of the *Huangdi sijing* 黃帝四經 describes *Dao* through four notions: oneness, emptiness, non-action, and harmony: "Oneness is its appellation; emptiness is its dwelling. Non-action is its element; Harmony is its function" (Yates 1997, 175).

Huang-Lao thinkers used oneness or Great Oneness to explain the inherent quality of underlying unity in the myriad beings and worked with the numeral to show the singularity of this quality, thereby establishing a numerical connection between multiplicity as it occurs in the natural and human realms. It becomes a concrete principle one can grasp, hold onto, understand the world, and put into use to govern the state.[13]

The FWLX is relatively late, postdating the *Taiyi shengshui* 太一生水, the *Hengxian* 恆先, and the *Daoyuan* 道原 of the *Huangdi sijing* 黃帝四經 (Wang 2015, 84). It presents a strong philosophical position and unique metaphysical outlook, centering largely on the concept of the one, or oneness. The manuscript explores the cosmogonic process of the one to the many through the correspondence of dual opposites such as heaven and earth, *yin* and *yang*, water, and fire. These relationships are described as crucial for the completion of all things, marked by a full cycle of the four seasons.[14] The FWLX is composed of nine separate passages and thematically distinguished in two parts: the first consists of three passages that raise questions concerning the origins of heaven, earth, and all existence in the world; the second, composed of six passages each beginning with "I have heard it said," offers an analysis of oneness in terms of self-cultivation and rulership.[15] The first three passages are written in a poetic style resembling the poetry of Qu Yuan 屈原 in the "Songs of Chu" (*chuci* 楚辭) and question existence from the source of generation to the essence that gives things life and the lack of something that leads to death.

The emphasis on oneness and self-cultivation with focus on the mind and the ethical relevance of this process in the latter section of the FWLX is traced back to the *Laozi*. However, composed during the mid-to-end Warring States Period, the FWLX reveals textual influences from the *Zhuangzi* and the *Guanzi* as well.[16]

---

[13] For further discussion on the evolution of the notion of Oneness in Daoist thought, see Cui (2023).

[14] This model is found in the Guodian manuscript of the "Great One Generates Water" (*Taiyi shengshui*), with the conclusion of the process marked by *chengsui* 成歲—the completion of a full cycle of the four seasons. In the FWLX we find the phrase "four completes the bond" (*sichengjie* 四成結). Feng (2015, 348–355) interprets "four completes the bond" as the completion of the year and the bond between the four times, which is essentially the same meaning of "completing the year and arresting" (*chengsui erzhi* 成歲而止) in the *Taiyi shengshui.*

[15] For discussion on its structure and style, see Feng (2015, 315–327). In structure, there is an apparent correlation to the "Asking Heaven" (*Tianwen* 天問) poem in the Songs of Chu (*Chuci* 楚辭) in proposing questions on the source of existence for all things and on the mechanism behind all natural phenomena. According to Cao, the first three sections of the FWLX are styled to achieve the literary effect of Qu Yuan's *Tianwen* poem and are not the core of the text, but more of an introduction intended to draw the reader in. The structure of the FWLX is quite loose, seemingly a collection of fragments together to serve a specific purpose. The ideas contained in the text are not original either, rather echo notions from the scholarly tradition connected to the four chapters of the *Guanzi.* The author cites classical works from history to highlight profound philosophical thoughts which make them further accessible and clear and uses poetic devices to facilitate recitation. For the rhymes of the FWLX see Chen Zhixiang (2009). In addition, Scott's (2009) paper on the rhymes of the FWLX is extremely valuable. Despite the existence of rhymes in the text, there has yet to be a unified reading of the rhyme due to inconsistencies in the two manuscript editions.

[16] In overall structure and style, it also resembles the heavenly questions *tianwen* 天問 in Qu Yuan's poetry, and the "Ten Questions" *shiwen* 十問 from the medical corpus discovered in the 1970s in

One is the original number that gives meaning to all objects, and the original cosmic state at the beginning of time. While in the *Laozi*, unity, the one, oneness either stands for *Dao* or as a direct result of *Dao*'s birthing, it also provides a notion of guidance in action, reflection, and comprehension.[17] The *Laozi* does not mention oneness on many occasions, yet one of the most profound instances is in Chap. 10:

> In the midst of the physical vigors bearing you up and those borne up by you, can you hold them together in a single embrace (*baoyi* 抱一) In unifying all your energies of life and breath, can you stay as supple as a new-born? In rinsing clear your obscure purview, can you wipe away every last speck? In caring for the people and ordering the nation, can you remain free of knowledge? In opening and shutting the gates of heaven, can you take the role of the female? In seeing clear through all four directions, can you keep on doing nothing at all? This is the birthing and rearing of things that never possesses what it produces, never expecting anything from its deeds, growing things but never controlling them—the obscure power of remaining obscure (Ziporyn 2023, 12).
>
> 載營魄抱一,能無離乎?專氣致柔,能嬰兒乎?滌除玄覽,能無疵乎?愛民治國,能無知乎?天門開闔,能為雌乎?明白四達,能無知乎?生之、畜之,生而不有,為而不恃,長而不宰,是謂玄德

Although the FWLX mentions the character "*Dao*" three times, including the compound "*Dao* of heaven"; "one" or "oneness" appears on nineteen occasions, including twice the expression "one phrase" (*yiyan* 一言) (Wang 2015). It speaks of "holding on to *Dao*" (*zhidao* 執道) or "oneness" and, very much like other early Daoist works, uses the two terms almost interchangeably. However, here *Dao* is clearly in a secondary position, superseded by oneness.

Three dimensions of oneness emerge in the FWLX: as the creative force of the universe, as the bond connecting the four seasons and five phases, and as the internally structuring potential of the world (and the human).[18] Called "oneness," it forms part of the overall Huang-Lao model of cosmogony, which in many ways echoes that of other Daoist texts. The difference between the model presented by the FWLX and the *Laozi* is the former shifting the focus of the latter—from the metaphysical notion of *Dao* to the ontological notion of oneness. Interestingly, the model in the FWLX resembles the model in the *Taiyishengshui* composed at least two centuries prior to the FWLX. The process begins by oneness, goes through dual opposite and complementary forces, and ends with "the completion of time" (*chengsui* 成歲)—or, in other words: the full cycle of the four times, and not the myriad beings.[19]

Mawangdui 馬王堆. See Feng (2015, 315–325). In addition, due to the existence two separate copies which are essentially the same, some scholars speculate that the FWLX was a widely circulated text before Qin and Han times. See Perkins (2015, 202).

[17] Oneness in the case of Chap. 39 "得一" is used in the meaning of *Dao*; in Chap. 42, oneness is born from *Dao* and hence secondary.

[18] Although a short text of only about 800 characters with two separate editions, the FWLX presents a fundamentally important vision of oneness as pervading the universe, nature, and society. See Chan (2016).

[19] Scholars have compared the cosmology of the TYSS to that of the *Yijing* on several levels. Zheng (2007) argues that the emphasis of TYSS on the cosmic circulation of water between heaven and earth was intended as a kind of corrective to what he sees as the *yang*-centered cosmology of the *Yijing*, one based more primarily on the cyclical movements of the sun. Yao (2002) argues that

The FWLX has:

> I have heard it said: one generates two, two generates three, three generates four, and four completes the bond.[20] Therefore, in having oneness, there is nothing that the world does not have. Not having oneness, there is not a single existence in the world. Know the names without eyes, hear the sounds without ears. This is what the grass and trees get to sprout, the birds and the beasts get to cry. Afar, it extends to heaven; near it is applied on people. Therefore, grasp the *dao*, and through that, cultivate your own person and control the state.[21]
>
> 聞之曰:一生兩,兩生三,三生四,四成結。是故有一,天下無不有;無一,天下亦無一有。無【簡21】〔目〕而知名,無耳而聞聲。草木得之以生,禽獸得之以鳴,遠之步(薄)【簡13A】天,邇之矢(施)人。是故【簡12B】執道,所以修身而治邦家。

This short generative description is followed by: "therefore, having oneness, there is nothing missing in the world; without having oneness, there cannot be a single existence in the world." "Therefore" links the two, making the connection between "bond" and "oneness" significant.

The FWLX emphasizes the importance of five, yet stresses oneness further. By connecting to the five phases through four plus one, it strengthens the Daoist notion of "grasping oneness" 執一, "attaining oneness" 得一, "having oneness" 有一, "able of being one" 能一, and "cherishing oneness" 貴一.

The paragraph illustrates oneness, while grasping oneness means to understand the workings of *yin* and *yang* and the five phases. This cosmogonic model differs from the process described in the *Laozi* Chap. 42 by shifting the focus from an abstract ultimate origin to the phenomenology of the four times and the five elements.[22] Tracing the source of this mode of thought, we may look back at the ancient classics, such as the *Hongfan* 洪範 ("Grand Scheme") chapter in the *Shangshu* 尚書 ("Book of Documents"):

> One is water, two is fire, three is wood, four is metal, five is earth.
>
> 一曰水,二曰火,三曰木,四曰金,五曰土

This is followed by a comment: "all things are born from this" (*jieqi shengshu*皆其生數) (Chen Kang 1986, 296). Likewise, Kong Yida's 孔穎達commentary to the *Changes*, the *Zhouyi zhengyi*周易正義 has:

---

the Xici and the TYSS cosmologies derive from two fundamentally different types of divination methods: the former from an eight trigrams system, and the latter from a nine halls (*jiugong*九宮) system.

[20] The Fudan interpretation reads the character nü as mu 母, Wu (2008). Qin (2009) also renders this character as mother and connects it to Chap. 42 and 1 of the *Laozi*, tying it to the Daoist notion of the mother being the source of generation. The FWLX emphasizes the connection between oneness (or *Dao*) and mother (or *qi*). Shen (2008) reads the character "female" as a loan word for the character "four." Cao (2015) accepts this interpretation and further argues that the four tying the bond is either related to the four times or the five phases.

[21] The translation is my own, based on Cao (2015). Currently there are a number of available translations to English, e.g., Chan (2015) and Wang (2016).

[22] Cao (2015) suggests reading "one generates two, two generates three, three generates four, and four completes the bond" as the sequence of the five elements.

> The Xici says, heaven is one, earth is two, heaven is three, earth is four, heaven is five, earth is six, heaven is seven, earth is eight, heaven is nine, earth is ten. These are the numbers generated from the five elements. Heaven as one generates water, earth as two generates fire, heaven as three generates wood, earth as four generates metal, and heaven as five generates soil. These give rise to multiplicity.
>
> 繫辭傳曰'天一,地二,天三,地四,天五,地六,天七,地八,天九,地十。'此即是五行生成之數。天一生水,地二生火,天三生木,地四生金,天五生土,此其生數也 (Wilhelm and Baynes 2003, 308–310; Yu 2004).

"Heaven as one generates water" in the "Xici" accords with the "great one generates water," which in turn returns to heaven and generates earth, and the observation in the FWLX that water "returns to the sky":

> I heard it said: if you possess extreme tranquility, then you will understand it; examine your understanding, then you will be inspired; examine your inspiration, then you will act on it; examine your action, then you will know the danger; examine the danger, then you will know the difficulty; examine the difficulty, then you can return. This is why the old is new, after people die they become human beings again, and water return to the heaven. The hundred things won't die, just as the moon appears but disappears again, ends but starts again, comes but returns again. Understand these words, all begins with the One.
>
> 聞之舌(=曰)[29]:至情(=靜)而知,[30]【A15】察知而神,察神而同(=動)[31],[察同(=動)]而僉(=險)[32],察僉(=險)而困,察困而復。氏(=是)故陳為新,人死復為人,水復【A24】(B17)於天。凡百物不死,如月出則或(=又)入,終則或始,至則或反。察此言,起於一端【A25】

There are several shared notions between the cosmology of the "Xici," the FWLX, and the TYSS, which are rarely mentioned elsewhere, indicating a scholarly lineage from ancient times to the TYSS, the FWLX, the "Xici," the *Guanzi*, *Zhuangzi*, and the *Lüshi Chunqiu*. Another notion is "flowing into forms" (*liuxing* 流形) that the FWLX shares with the *Tuanzhuan*, the *Guanzi* and the *Zhuangzi*. While the importance of water as a model of morality is stressed in the *Laozi*, the flowing of things into form—a change that generates existence and causes death—can ideologically be traced to the *Zhuangzi* and his theory of *qi* transformation (Huang 2010, 387–398). Oneness as the ultimate origin answers the questions in the first section: things flow into form, what do they get to live, what do they lose to die? The FWLX goes on to explain that it is oneness that is gained and oneness that can be lost as the ground for life and death. This accords both with the idea of "gaining" oneness in the *Laozi* Chap. 39 (*deyi* 得一), and *qi* transformation (*qihua* 氣化) from the *Zhuangzi*.

Another indication of a common lineage between the FWLX, the TYSS, and the "Xici" is found in their cosmologies and practical applications, as the "Xici" states:

> Of changes, there is the great ultimate, and this gives birth to the two models; the two models give birth to the four signs; the four signs give birth to the eight trigrams, the eight trigrams determine good and ill omens; and good and ill omens give birth to great enterprises. Thus there are no greater models and signs than those of Heaven and Earth; no greater adapting through changes than that of the four seasons; no clearer display of signs and illumination than that of the sun and the moon … no greater provider of things and their employment than the sage (Wilhelm and Baynes 2003, 318–19).
>
> 易有太極,是生兩儀,兩儀生四象,四象生八卦,八卦定吉凶,吉凶生大業. 是故,法象莫大乎天地,變通莫大乎四時,縣象著明莫大乎日月…備物致用…莫大乎聖人。

As a singular ultimate origin proceeds to cosmic development, it depends on the interaction of complementary opposites: first of movement and stillness which initiates the process from oneness or nothingness to multiplicity and existence. The logic of grasping the source to realize its outcomes begins with the *Laozi* and is developed into a philosophical, ethical, and practical method emphasized in Huang-Lao texts through *Dao* as the origin of law and principles, oneness as the practice, and names, decrees, and measures for standards. Essentially, the method of self-cultivation and observing from within replaces divination and turns the *Changes* into a metaphysical treatise to be textually analyzed from the Warring States Period to this very day. The ethics are rooted in self-cultivation, which is rooted in cosmic and natural patterns, associating the human being as an integral part of the cosmos and a participant in the generation of things.

4.4 Part III: Metaphysics of *Dao* and *Yi*: Cultivation, Reflection, and Practical Applications

> All under heaven is single in its extent, yet there are a multitude of anxious plans for it. These return to the same home but by diverse routes.
> 天下一致而百慮,同歸而殊涂.

This citation from the "Xici" begins Sima Tan's essay *Yaozhi* 要指 ("Essential Points"), included in the final chapter of his son Sima Qian's *Taishigong* 太史公. In this essay, the school of *Dao* is portrayed through characteristics identified with the Huang-Lao school of thought. It reflects the metaphysical basis of the *Laozi* and self-cultivation further expounded on in the *Zhuangzi*, and the socio-political philosophy and practice of Huang-Lao. Huang-Lao Daoism stresses practical governmental methods, takes Lao-Zhuang philosophy and *Dao* as its core, and in practice, adopts the "best from all schools."

> The Daoist cause the spiritual essence of human beings to be concentrated and unified. Their actions are joined with the formless, their provision sufficient to the myriad things. In the practice of their techniques, they accord with the great sequence of the *yinyang*, select the good of the Ru and the Mo, and adopt the essentials of the Ming and Fa. They move with the seasons and respond to the transformation of things, there is nothing unsuitable. In the practices they establish and projects they carry out. Their points are simple and easily applied, their programs few but results many (Sima Qian 2011, 130: 2479; Watson 1958, 43–44).

Later in the essay Sima Tan expounds on key notions in Daoism, *wuwei* 無為, *xuwu* 虛無, *yinxun* 因循, with focus on methods of self-cultivation and action.

> The Daojia have no doing. It is also said that they have nothing they do not do. Their substance is easy to practice, but their words are hard to know. Their techniques take vacuity (*xu* 虛) and absence (*wu* 無) as their root, accordance (*yin* 因) and conformation (*xun* 循) as their activity …

> Spirit is the root of life, form the instrument of life. To say, before you have first stabilized your spirit and form, "I possess that by which to govern all-under-heaven"—how could one do that? (Sima Qian 2011, 130: 2481).

This description places self-cultivation of spirit and form as the primary requirement for rulers. While we may trace this idea of mind and body cultivation to the *Laozi* Chap. 10, the addition of accordance and conformation is a later development of Daoism as a method of governance. Interestingly, the notions of accordance and conformation, moving in accordance with the times, conforming to change, are key notions shared to early Daoist philosophy, the ancient classic of the *Changes*, Huang-Lao political methods and the commentaries to the *Changes*.

In the FWLX, self-cultivation and its crucial position for gaining knowledge and attaining correct balanced state of heart-mind is the criterion for becoming a legitimate figure of authority—a sage ruler. Continuing the thread of thought which ties cosmos and body as mirrors of one another, the FWLX maintains that one need not leave their own mat to know the world:

> I have heard it said that: They who have grasped the *Dao* need only sit upright, they need not leave the place where they sit. Straightening their cap, they need only stand upright, they need not involve themselves with actual political affairs. (They who have grasped the *Dao*) have a prescience that reaches beyond the Four Seas; their sensitive hearing reaches beyond one thousand li; their developed sight reaches beyond one hundred li. Therefore, the Sage Person need not move from the spot to foresee the stability or downfall of the state, whether there will be disorder.
>
> (聞)之曰:執道,坐不下席。耑(端)文(冕)【14】,箬(舒)不與事,之<先>智(知)四海,至聖(聽)千里,達見百里。是古(故)聖人處於亓(其)所,邦家之【16】危安廌(存)忘(亡),惻(賊)盜)之作,可之<先>智(知)
>
> Therefore, having one, one has all under heaven; losing one, one loses all under heaven. Having grasped one, one knows names without using one's eyes, and can hear sounds without using one's ears.
>
> 是故有一,天下無不有;無一,天下亦無一有。亡【21】目而智知名,無耳而聞聲。

These passages indicate that by grasping *Dao,* and the One can a person transcend everyday sensory perception and manage to be unfettered by everyday affairs, directly laying hands upon the truth of the world, and achieving the state of doing nothing yet leaving nothing undone.[23] Like in the *Laozi* 47, 56, and 10 the emphasis is placed on tranquility, stillness versus motion, and self-cultivation as an art and method of rulership. The FWLX, in resonance to Chap. 64 in the *Laozi*, stresses the action of sitting and reflecting:

> Sit and think about it, one can plan within thousand miles; stand up and use it, one can extend it to the four seas.
>
> 坐而思之,每(=謀)於(B10b)千里;起而用之,申(=伸、陳)於四海.

This self-cultivation which needs no more than self-introspection to grasp the ultimate principle of the cosmos, is also something that is done alone, in solitude

[23] This idea of self-cultivation and gaining knowledge without leaving one's own lodgings is known from chaps. 47 and 56 of the *Laozi*.

or in the darkness, with nothing but one's own mind, as described by Huang (2023, 15–29).[24]

The central passage on self-cultivation in the FWLX places the heart-mind as the locus of the process, the key factor, and the greatest obstacle to overcome:

> This is what I heard: If the mind cannot overcome the mind, great disaster will come; if the mind can overcome the mind, this is called small understanding. What is small understanding? Other people think it is white. But by what means do they know that it is white? For all your life, you possess yourself. Can you say less? Can you concentrate? This is called small accomplishment. One says: what the hundred clans value is only the lord, what the lord values is only the mind, what the mind values is only the One. If you gain it and understand it, you can go up to visit the heaven, and go down to the abyss.
>
> 聞之曰:心不勝心,大亂乃作;心如能勝心,(B19)【A26】是謂小徹。奚謂小徹?人白為察(=識?)。奚以知其白?終身自若。能寡言乎? 能一【A18】乎? 夫(B13a)此之謂小成。曰:百姓之所貴唯君,君之所貴唯心,心之所(B20)貴唯一。得而解之(B21),上【A28】賓於天,下番於淵。

While in the self-cultivation that is conducted in darkness and loneliness, both the FWLX and the "Xici" mention the ability to be clear and pure, being able to reveal oneself and one's character to examination. While in the FWLX the examination mentioned is what the people see in the ruler, while in the "Xici," it is the spirits. The same logic of the process of self-cultivation of the heart-mind is used in the "Xici," yet the goal of this process is to become the ultimate diviner whose predictions are accurate:

> Therefore, the nature of the yarrow stalks is round and spiritual. The nature of the hexagrams is square and wise. The meaning of the six lines is change, in order to furnish information in this way the sages purified their hearts, withdrew, hid themselves in the secret (Wilhelm and Baynes 2003, 316).
>
> 是故,蓍之德,圓而神;卦之德,方以知;六爻之義,易以貢。聖人以此洗心,退藏於密,吉凶與民同患.

Hence, the philosophical turn inward taken in Daoism and the commentaries culminates in the return outward to some sort of political practice, whether as a Daoist sage ruler facing south described in Huang-Lao manuscripts or as divination following the tradition of the *Yi*.

> For comprehending the chaotic diversity of things and exploring what is hidden, for penetrating the depths and extending influence afar, thereby determining good fortune and misfortune on earth and consummating all efforts on earth, there is nothing greater than the oracle (Wilhelm and Baynes 2003, 319).
>
> 探賾索隱,鉤深致遠,以定天下之吉凶,成天下之亹亹者,莫大乎蓍龜。

Recalling the passage from the FWLX which asks us not to resort to divination, the "Xici" shares the desire to comprehend all things and extend influence afar, yet in contrast to Daoist philosophy, the "Xici" maintains that there is no greater method than divination.

---

[24] As Huang shows, the FWLX mentions that the process of lone self-cultivation is also what allows one to expose oneself to examination by others.

The commentaries to the *Changes* philosophically defend the act of divination, yet they do provide an attempt to resonate philosophy and divination by absorbing the natural philosophy and cosmology of Daoist thinkers, equalizing Laozi's notions of *Dao* and *De* and their relationship with the creative forces of *Qian* 乾 and *Kun* 坤 (Chen Guying 2023, 159).

4.5 Concluding Remarks

Daoist philosophy and the *Changes* with their commentaries share the metaphysical assumption that order is found in the cosmos and the epistemological grounds of perception through one's own heart/mind by which one can derive correct actions from the natural course. They share the notion that ethics includes a broader notion of accordance and compliance to heaven and earth and the changes of time, and actions are best done non-coercively or carefully without reckless action, yet the final stages of the process defined by each tradition are remarkably distinct. For *Yi* scholars, the sage is the one who comprehends change, the purpose of cultivation is divination, while divination is a technique used to know fortune and misfortune and thereby benefit the people, whereas for Daoism at the time, especially in its Huang-Lao manifestation, the purpose of cultivation is to become a sage ruler who can establish a *just* government and provide the people with the means of existence so they may thrive and advance on their own without concern over their material needs.

Nevertheless, the early philosophy of the *Laozi* and the *Zhuangzi*, the abstract divination manual with its theoretical explanations, was grouped together under the category of metaphysics once *Dao* and *Yi* were connected. By the time of Wang Bi in the Wei-Jin period, the *Changes*—including the classic and the commentaries—the *Laozi* and the *Zhuangzi* were collectively termed "the three metaphysical treatises" (*sanxuan* 三玄), a term still used by scholars today (ibid., 219). Yet, by the time of Wang Bi, Huang-Lao manuscripts were for the most part buried and unknown, only to be revealed in the twentieth century. In our times, we have a slight advantage over Wang Bi, as Huang-Lao philosophy has been rediscovered, and the ideas found in their manuscripts fill some of the theoretical gaps between the classic, Daoism, and the composition of the commentaries.

References

Cao Feng. 2015. *Jinnian chutu Huang Lao sixiang wenxian yanjiu* 近年出土黃老思想文獻研究. Beijing: Zhongguoshehui kexue.

Chan, Shirley. 2015. Oneness: Reading the "all things are flowing in form" (Fan Wu Liu Xing). *International Communication of Chinese Culture* 2: 285–299.

Chen Guying 陳鼓應. 2014. *Laozhuang xinlun* 老莊新論. Beijing: Shangwu yinshuguan.

Chen Guying 陳鼓應. 2016. *Huangdi sijing* jinzhu jinyi: *Mawangdui Hanmu* chutu boshu 黃帝四經今注今譯: 马王堆汉墓出土帛书. Beijing: Shangwu yinshuguan.

Chen Guying 陳鼓應. 2023. *Daojia zhexue zhuganshuo* 道家哲學主幹說. Beijing: Zhonghua shuju.

Chen Kang 陳抗. 1986. *Shangshu jingu zhushu* 尚書今古文注疏. Beijing: Zhonghua shuju.

Chen Zhixiang 陳志向. 2009. *Fanwyuliuxing yundu* 凡物流形韻讀. Fudan University Research Center of Unearthed Manuscripts, January 10. http://www.fdgwz.org.cn/Web/Show/645. Accessed 15 Sept 2024.

Cook, Scott. 2009. Shangbo qi "fanwuliuxing" jianxu ji yundu xiaobu 上博七《凡物流形》簡序及韻讀小補. Center of Bamboo and Silk Manuscripts of Wuhan University, February 23. http://m.bsm.org.cn/?chujian/5196.html. Accessed 10 Aug 2024.

Cui, Xiaojiao 崔曉嬌. 2023. From Laozi to Lao-Zhuang and Huang-Lao Daoism: The two paths of oneness in the development of early Daoist thought. *Religions* 14 (11): 1390.

Huang Kuan-yun 黃冠雲. 2010. "Liuti," "Liuxing" yu zaoqi rujia sixiang de yige zhuanzhe 流體、流形與早期儒家思想的一個轉折. *Jianbo* 簡帛 6: 387–398.

Huang Kuan-yun 黃冠雲. 2019. Guanyu dao de ming, zi, hao: chongdu taiyishengshui 關於道的名、字、號: 重讀太一生水. *Renwen zhongguo xuebao* 人文中國學報.

Huang, Kuan-yun 黃冠雲. 2023. *A walk in the night with Zhuangzi: Musings on an ancient Chinese manuscript*. Albany, NY: State University of New York Press.

Lai Guolong 來國龍. 2010. *Fanwuliuxing* xinyan 凡物流形新研. Center of Bamboo and Silk Manuscripts of Wuhan University. http://www.bsm.org.cn/?chujian/5461.html#_ftn24. Accessed 2 April 2024.

Legge, James (Trans.). 2020. *I Ching or the book of changes: With a new and extended introduction by dennis schilling.* London: Flame Tree Publishing.

Lynn, Richard John (Trans.). 2004. *The classic of changes: A new translation of the* I Ching *as interpreted by Wang Bi.* New York: Columbia University Press.

Ma Chengyuan 馬承源 (Ed.). 2008. *Shanghai Bowuguan cang zhanguo chuzhushu* 上海博物館藏戰國楚竹書, vol. 7. Shanghai: Shanghai guji.

Peerenboom, R.P. 1993. *Law and morality in ancient China: The silk manuscripts of Huang-Lao.* Albany, NY: State University of New York Press.

Perkins, Franklin. 2015. "Fanwu Liuxing (all things flow into form) and the one in the *Laozi. Early China* 38: 195–232.

Qin Hualin 秦樺林. 2009. *Fanwuliuxing diershiyi jian shijie* 凡物流形第二十一簡試解. Fudan University Research Center of Unearthed Manuscripts, January 9. http://fdgwz.org.cn/Web/Show/642. Accessed 3 Sept 2024.

Rickett, W. Allyn (Trans.). 1998. *Guanzi*: *Political, economic and philosophical essays from early China*, vol. 2. Princeton, NJ: Princeton University Press.

Shaughnessy, Edward. 2014. *Unearthing the changes: Recently discovered manuscripts of the Yi Jing (I Ching) and related texts.* New York: Columbia University Press.

Shen Pei 沈培. 2008. *Lüeshuo shangbo qi xinjian de yi zi* 略說上博七新見的"一"字. Fudan University Research Center of Unearthed Manuscripts, December 31. http://www.fdgwz.org.cn/Web/Show/582. Accessed 2 Sept 2024.

Sima Qian 司馬遷. 2011. *Shiji* 史記. Shanghai: Shanghai guiji chubanshe.

Wang Zhongjiang 王中江. 2015. *Daoism excavated: Cosmos and humanity in early manuscripts.* St. Petersburg, Florida: Three Pines Press.

Wang Zhongjiang 王中江. 2016. *Order in early Chinese excavated texts: Natural, supernatural, and legal approaches.* London: Palgrave Macmillan.

Watson, Burton. 1958. *Ssu-ma Ch'ien grand historian of China.* New York and London: Columbia University Press.

Wilhelm, Richard, and Cary F. Baynes (Trans.). 2003. *I Ching or book of changes.* London: Penguin.

Wu Kejin 鄔可晶. 2008. *Shangbo qi fanwu liuxing chongbian shiwen* 《上博七·凡物流形》重編釋文. Fudan University Research Center of Unearthed Manuscripts, December 31. http://www.fdgwz.org.cn/Web/Show/581. Accessed 31 Aug 2024.

Yang Bojun 楊伯峻. 2016. *Chunqiu zuozhuan zhu* 春秋左傳注. Beijing: Zhonghua shuju.

Yao Zhihua 姚治华. 2002. *Taiyishengshui yu taiyi jiugong zhan* 太一生水与太乙九宫占. In Pang Pu 龐樸. *Gumu xinzhi* 古墓新知, 47–67. Taipei: Taiwan guji chubanshe.

Yates, Robin S. 1997. *Five lost classics: Tao, Huanglao, and Yin-Yang in Han China*. New York: Ballantine Books.

Yu Peide 余培德 (Ed.). 2004. Kong Yida 孔穎達: *Zhouyi zhengyi* 周易正義. Beijing: Jiuzhou chubanshe.

Ziporyn, Brook. 2023. *Laozi Daodejing*. New York: Liveright Publishing Corporation.

Zhang Dainian 張岱年. 1996. *Zhongguo wenhua de sixiang jichu yu ben jingshen* 中國文化的思想基礎與基本精神, vol. 6 in *Zhang Dainian quanji* 張岱年全集. Shijiazhuang: Hebei renmin chubanshe.

Zheng Jixiong 郑吉雄. 2007. Cong Taiyi Shengshui taolun qian tuan suoji liangzhong yuzhoulun 从太一生水试论乾·彖所记两种宇宙论. *Jianbo* 简帛 2 (11): 139–150.

Part II
Transactions with Science and Philosophy

Chapter 5
Image as Instrument (*Qi* 器): *Yijing* Prognostication and "Knowing" in American Pragmatism

Jim Behuniak

Abstract It is difficult to appreciate the philosophical depth of *Yijing* "prognostication" using only original source materials. They do not reveal much about its philosophical underpinnings. In this paper, the American pragmatic tradition will be used in attempting to gain a deeper insight into what this tradition represents philosophically. In locating *Yijing* prognostication in its early Chinese context, reference will also be made to the notion of "Not Knowing" (*wuzhi* 無知) in the *Zhuangzi*, as this may provide insight into how epistemological assumptions in the *Yijing* related to alternative theories of "knowledge" in early China. Suggested here is that *Yijing* "prognostication" makes philosophical assumptions about knowledge and its objects that differ significantly from alternative theories in early China, while also differing sharply from assumptions that are central to the Greek philosophical tradition.

Keywords Prognostication · *Yijing* · Pragmatism · Not knowing (*wuzhi*) · Zhuangzi · John Dewey

5.1 Introduction

The *Yijing* is commonly understood as a tool for "prognostication," an oracle with which to acquire "knowledge" that orients one's actions toward the future. In Chinese antiquity, such divination practices pre-date the *Yijing* by several centuries. Oracle bones and turtle plastrons marked with various "charges" date back to the Neolithic period. Recorded on such objects were propositions such as "We will receive millet harvest," and "In the next ten days there will be no disaster," suggesting that such claims were put forward with the expectation that divination could resolve their veracity and thus see into the future. As David Keightley (2014, 123) suggests, even though early forms of divination remain shrouded in obscurity, "the simple question "What did the Shang diviner think he was doing?" is well worth asking."

J. Behuniak (✉)
Colby College, Waterville, USA
e-mail: jbehunia@colby.edu

G. Sigurðsson and T. Hon (eds.), *Contemporary Interpretations and Readings of the Yijing*, Chinese Culture 15, https://doi.org/10.1007/978-981-96-0609-2_5

As Keightley explains, the nature of such early divination "charges" and their binary "Yes/No" structure suggest that Shang diviners held a worldview in which spirits ultimately determined the future. By displaying virtue and propitiating the spirits, one might persuade them to act in certain ways. Diviners thus operated in a state of what Keightley calls "Neolithic pessimism"—one in which humans were almost completely prone to forces beyond their control.

Such a worldview had evolved by the time the *Yijing* arose, and according to Keightley, the nature of the text and its "prognostication" function reflects this evolution. During the Zhou, humans had begun to understand their place in the world differently. As Keightley explains, "The balance of caution against confidence, of negative doubt against the need for positive action, of religious reflection against secular activity, of Neolithic pessimism against Bronze age optimism, appears, with the passage of time, to have shifted in favor of optimism, confidence, and human control." It is within this context that Keightley understands "the increasing use of *Yijing*-style forms of divination which eventually, if not originally, allowed more scope for human reflection and interpretation." (Ibid. 142–143).

There is little, if any, real philosophical reflection on the act of *Yijing* divination in the early records. Thus, asking what those consulting the text "thought they were doing" requires us to inquire into such practices from a distance, using whatever philosophical resources we have at our disposal. Here, I find the American pragmatic tradition to be particularly insightful. Thinkers like Charles Sanders Peirce and John Dewey helped to formulate theories of "inquiry" and "knowing" that factored human agency and purpose not only into the act of knowing but also into the objects known and the future results of knowing them. "Knowing," for the pragmatist, is thus understood as "instrumental" in that it arises for a purpose and serves to realize that purpose. The notion that "knowledge" makes a difference in how the world unfolds is one of the hallmarks of pragmatic epistemology. Such embedded, "instrumental" forms of knowing are distinct from more standard modes of achieving knowledge through logical deduction or inference. Both the Chinese and Western traditions exhibit alternatives to such approaches, and here the notion of "Not Knowing" (*wuzhi* 無知) in the *Zhuangzi* will be explored as one such alternative providing insight into how the *Yijing* operates. Also, the status of the "objects" of knowledge in this tradition will be considered. It will be argued that the "trends" (*fang* 方) and "types" (*lei* 類) exemplified through the "images" (*xiang* 象) provided in the *Yijing* differ considerably from the "objects" of knowledge most familiar in the classical Greek philosophical tradition.

5.2 Nature and Function of the *Yijing*

The *Yijing* system begins with two primary hexagrams: the "generative" (*qian* 乾) and the "receptive" (*kun* 坤). These two hexagrams represent the most basic, generic traits discernible in the environing world. This is reflected in the following observation:

> Heaven is above and Earth is below; thus, the generative and receptive are determined.
>
> In correspondence with this difference between above and below, inferior and superior places are established. Agitation and equilibrium are constant; and accordingly, firm and yielding lines are differentiated. Trends (*fang* 方) can be sorted into types (*lei* 類). Things and events by their groupings can be distinguished (*fen* 分). This is how the judgments of auspicious and inauspicious come about. (Wilhelm and Baynes 1967, 280)[1]

This passage expounds the original insight that gave rise to *Yijing*'s symbolic cosmology, a cosmology that describes all phenomena and their transformations according to various figurative images and the concrete "trends" to which they correspond. To consult the *Yijing* is to be presented with an "image" along with explanatory commentary on some combination of such primary forms of natural activity.

The most primitive figures are those of the unbroken and broken lines. Together these represent the "constant activity of agitation and equilibrium" (*dongjingyouchang* 動靜有常) exhibited in the behavior of things. According to tradition, the ancient sage Fuxi was the first to observe such patterns of behavior. Among other things, "He observed the patterns of the birds and animals, and how they had adapted (*yi* 宜) to the land." Assumptions tracing back to these primitive observations include that: "directional trends can be sorted by type" (*fangyileiju* 方以類聚), "living beings can be divided by groups" (*wuyiqunfen* 物以群分), and "organic forms mature on earth" (*zaidichengxing* 在地成形). While such forms exhibited regularity, it was also recognized that "change and transformation are manifest" (*bianhuajianyi* 變化見矣) (Ibid., 280ff., 328). Organic forms reflected their "adaptation" (*yi*) to conditions, and the possibility for them to transform (*hua* 化) in the process of maintaining "agitation and equilibrium" within such conditions was understood. Thus, what the text provides is not so much an inventory of fixed "forms," but rather assemblages of characteristic "trends" that dynamic processes tend to exhibit in the natural world. This is what the prognosticator receives.

While the origins of the *Yijing* are unknown, traditional accounts do shed light on how the composition and function of the text came to be understood. According to legend, the Sage-king Fuxi originally composed the hexagram system by "observing" (*guan* 觀) things in the natural world. Each phenomenon exhibited an "image," "symbol," or "representation" (*xiang* 象) that tracked onto larger patterns in Nature. As the text explains:

> The appearance of anything was called an "image" (*xiang* 象). Whenever it took shape it was called a "tool" (*qi* 器). Once these were formulated and employed, they came to be called "patterns" (*fa* 法). Having found their use to be beneficial amidst the comings-and-goings of things, people all used them and regarded them as spirit-like. (Ibid., 318)

Notable here is the "instrumental" language. The *Yijing* provides a set of "tools" that prove useful in coping with problematic situations in ever-changing conditions. Again, traditional accounts can shed light on how this was understood. According to tradition, the bulk of the figurative embellishment on the text's "images" was completed by Ji Chang who, before becoming the illustrious King Wen, was unjustly

---

[1] My citations from the *Yijing* will be referenced according to their location in the Wilhelm/Baynes version of the text. My translations however may differ slightly.

imprisoned by the Shang sovereign, Di Xin. We are told that Ji Chang devoted his years in captivity to formulating the imagery of the text, no doubt ruminating over the myriad social and political complexities that would impinge upon his fate. As the twentieth-century historian, Wu Guozhen, surmises, Ji Chang's own circumstances surely motivated him in this undertaking. As Wu sees it, it was his intention to transform the *Yijing* from an arcane oracle of divination into a manual for navigating real-life situations. Wu (1982, 264) writes of the resultant work:

> The sixty-four hexagrams represent the large contours of 64 possible situations in human life; and the 384 lines represent the varying predicaments in which an individual may find himself within one of these general situations. And through a philosophy of self-improvement and perseverance, humility and patience, Ji Chang sought less to forecast the future than to furnish a guidebook for the 384 possible human conditions, so that, given a particular predicament within a particular situation, an individual might know what dangers or pitfalls he should beware of as well as how to best conduct himself.

Accordingly, the hexagrams of the *Yijing* are not designed to "tell the future" but rather to orient one's actions effectively in the face of immediate problems. Its use was never thought to be therapeutic, recreational, or even necessarily religious. As recorded in the "Great Plan" chapter of the *Book of Documents*, divination was a method for addressing "great doubt" (*dayi* 大疑); and as James Legge notes, it was understood in the commentarial tradition that "the oracle is not to be consulted without the presence of doubt; for to consult the oracle while lacking doubt is considered an insult." (非疑不占非疑而占謂之侮) (Legge 2000, 337–338). Such an offense would be to misuse the imagery presented in the text—to violate its purpose, which is strictly to help resolve the state of doubt.

5.3 Doubt, Inquiry, and Prospective Ideas

The importance of "doubt" in such accounts is what calls to mind the classical pragmatists. In developing "pragmatism" as a method, Peirce began in 1868 by taking issue with how doubt had been treated in the Western tradition. Descartes, famously, and in response to a renascent classical skepticism, suggested in Book One of the *Meditations* that one should begin the quest for certainty by doubting everything. Peirce considered such a method as not only absurd but insulting to the status of doubt in human cognition. "Let us not pretend to doubt in philosophy what we do not doubt in our hearts," says Peirce. (Stuhr 2000, 55) Doubt has its own existential standing and legitimacy. It is not a voluntary state that one can assume on command or direct as one wishes. Doubt arises naturally in the course of human experience, and it has its own nature and purpose. In his landmark 1878 article, "How to Make Our Ideas Clear," Peirce showcases the powerful and central role that doubt plays in the process of thinking. For Peirce, to resolve doubt and attain belief is "the sole function of thought." He immediately points out, however, that such terms need to be understood very broadly. Peirce writes:

> All these words… are too strong for my purpose. Doubt and Belief, as the words are commonly employed, relate to religious or other grave discussions. But here I use them to designate the starting of any question, no matter how small or how great, and the resolution of it. (Ibid., 79)

For Peirce, doubt and belief represent two poles in the everyday thought process—and again, for him, the sole function of thought is to resolve the former and attain the latter. Neither state, for Peirce, is merely cognitive. Belief is not an idle state of affirmation any more than doubt is an inert state of ignorance. Belief and doubt are reciprocal, *active* states, such that, for Peirce, thought itself is "essentially an action." "Most frequently," Peirce writes, "doubts arise from some indecision, however momentary, in our action." (Ibid., 79) Belief is likewise a state that registers in renewed or continued *activity*. "Belief is a rule for action" for Peirce, such that the process of resolving doubts and attaining beliefs has both its impetus and its end in the need to secure an orientation (or re-orientation) from which to act. Peirce describes the cognitive process of resolving doubts as follows:

> However the doubt may originate, it stimulates the mind to an activity which may be slight or energetic, calm or turbulent. Images pass rapidly through consciousness, one incessantly melting into another, until at last, when all is over—it may be in a fraction of a second, in an hour, or after long years—we find ourselves decided as to how we should act under such circumstances as those which occasioned our hesitation. In other words, we have attained belief. (Ibid., 79)

Following Peirce, Dewey develops this into a full-blown "theory of inquiry," whereby doubt, or what he calls the "problematic situation," initiates a cognitive process that ideally terminates in the reconstruction of problematic situations such that action may be restored or renewed within them. The details of Dewey's step-by-step account of such "patterns of inquiry" need not concern us here—in fact, he modifies his account more than once. Important for our purposes is the fact that "inquiry," as Dewey understands it, is always purposeful, action-oriented, and thus, in his words, "experimental." By describing the process as experimental, Dewey means to locate the act of thinking *within* experience, thus obliterating the dualisms that characterize modern philosophy's "Empiricist/Rationalist" dichotomy. Experience is never passive, nor is thought removed. "Knowledge" does not venture beyond experience in pursuit of its objects; instead, knowledge *results* in objects whose meanings register *within* experience in the ongoing activity of thinking. Dewey (1916, 151) explains:

> While all thinking results in knowledge, ultimately the value of knowledge is subordinate to its use in thinking. For we live not in a settled and finished world, but in one which is going on, and where our main task is prospective.

Such thinking is "prospective" or *prospecere*, "looking forward," in that it is a directed activity that concerns itself with the conversion of a doubtful situation into one that is more manageable and secure. As Dewey explains in *The Quest for Certainty*, "the outcome of the directed activity is the construction of a new empirical situation in which objects are differently related to one another, and such that the *consequences* of directed operations form the objects that have the property of being *known*." (Dewey and Boydston 2008, LW 4: 70) Again, such "knowledge" is subordinate to its use in securing situations in which action can take place. Objects, in becoming known, become what they are in our experience, and their meanings *are* what they are experienced *as*. One acts accordingly. When doubt arises, one is unsure about what things *mean*—and accordingly, one is unsure about how to *act*. Here, it is experimental inquiry, which, as Peirce reminds us, might be "slight or energetic, calm or turbulent," that intervenes to restore to experience objects that are *known* sufficiently for action to resume. All activity described as "intelligent" entails having such knowledge in operation. One might say, then, that just as experimental inquiry in the midst of the doubtful situation involves a kind of *prospecere*, "looking forward," intelligent action in the newly restored, empirically reconstructed situation involves a kind of *prognosticare*, "knowing forward." Such "prognostication" is not knowing the future per se but rather knowing a present situation such that the likely consequences of one's actions can be foreseen.

5.4 Prospective Ideas as Instrumental

One must perceive the world in some determinate way if one is to manage situations at all. Otherwise, experience is nothing but a flood of discontinuous stimuli before which one loses all bearing. The *Yijing* works because those who consult it already find themselves in a problematic situation—they have *ipso facto* surrendered certainty as to their interpretation of events. They find themselves in a state of "great doubt" (*dayi* 大疑). The hexagrams and their images invite one to re-orient perception by stimulating the reconstruction of a problematic situation—not randomly, but through ideational patterns that have a certain coherence embedded within them. "Images" (*xiang* 象) thus work like "ideas" in the vernacular sense, as propositions that reconfigure elements in a situation by introducing new relations between them. As such, they operate as "tools" (*qi* 器) in restoring "coherence" (*li* 理) to experience. Dewey describes the instrumental, coherence-restoring nature of ideas as follows:

> Ideas are operational in that they instigate and direct further operations of observation; they are proposals and plans for acting upon existing conditions to bring new facts to light and to organize all the selected facts into a coherent whole. (Ibid., LW 12: 116)

Pragmatically speaking, the accuracy of ideas is measured by how well they organize facts and guide one's action in a satisfactory direction. What prospective ideas reveal, and this is especially true of the "images" in the *Yijing*, is not the static properties of inert objects but the dynamic *relations* that are at play within ongoing situations. Now to be clear, many (and probably most) of our ideas present us with determinate objects in fixed relations. We keep such ideas because they *work*. Such ideas occasion no doubt and present no problems. When such ideas fail us, however, doubt ensues and inquiry begins. Prospective ideas are then utilized in an experimental fashion in order to recover the smooth flow of activity.

There are, accordingly, different types of ideas. Dewey (perhaps over-simplifying things) divides the entire content of human knowledge into two main categories of ideas: the "prospective" and the "retrospective." The former, which requires thinking in the form of inquiry, "occurs when things are uncertain or doubtful or problematic," and the latter gives us "solidity, security, and fertility [in] dealing with the future." (Dewey 1916, 148, 151) The content of the former type of idea differs from that of the latter. The solidity, security, and fertility of well-tested, "retrospective" ideas lend such ideas greater specificity and clarity. "Prospective" ideas, however, must preserve an ample degree of what Peirce calls "vagueness." They must remain open to rich articulation in a variety of situations in order to be experimentally effective. A.C. Graham, in describing the nature of images in the *Yijing*, presents a similar account:

> If [the hexagrams'] meaning were unambiguous, the overwhelming probability would be that the prognostications would be either obviously inapplicable or grossly misleading. Since on the contrary the hexagrams open up an indefinite range of patterns for correlation… the effect is to free the mind to take account of all information whether or not it conflicts with preconceptions, awaken it to unnoticed similarities and connections, and guide it to a settled decision adequate to the complexity of factors. (Graham 1989, 369–370)

Peirce and Dewey would have appreciated this function immediately. Peirce especially, for whom "vagueness" is an essential feature of the prospective idea. "It is vague," Peirce writes, "but yet with such a vagueness as permits of its accurate determination in regard to any particular object proposed for examination." (Peirce, Hartshorne and Weiss 1935, 186) "Images" (*xiang* 象) in the *Yijing* have this quality in great abundance, and such vagueness is crucial to their function.

Read alongside the pragmatists, the *Yijing* amounts to a very sophisticated accessory to experimental inquiry. While it is traditionally regarded as an oracle, and its occult status is long-established, its "spirit-likeness" (*shen* 神) does not stem from its ability to change a problematic situation *objectively* (magic) or deliver insights into reality *subjectively* (revelation). Rather, it operates by reintegrating troublesome situations into novel existential unities wherein meaning is restored to its elements—and almost miraculously, one's purposes and intentions become re-formulated within the newly clarified situation. As Fuxi observed, the natural world is replete with patterns, habits, and regularities. Formulated vaguely in "images," and processed through human imagination, such patterns become "tools" (*qi* 器) in coping with uncertain and doubtful situations. Such tools for "knowing" are what the *Yijing* provides.

5.5 "Not Knowing" (*wuzhi* 無知) in the *Zhuangzi*

The present account raises a number of questions. What does "knowledge" actually mean in this tradition? What kind of cognitive process is it? What are its objects? How does something like an "image" (*xiang* 象) produce different instances of "knowing forward" (*prognosticare*) in different contexts? Assuming that the *Yijing* retains some degree of continuity with other schools of Chinese thought, such questions might be approached by considering how knowledge is understood elsewhere in the tradition. Here, the discussion of "knowledge" in the *Zhuangzi* is particularly insightful.

One of the interesting conceptual features of "prognostication" (*prognosticare*) is that "knowing forward" means to already know. Thus, its infinitive operates as a past participle: to *prognosticate* is to *have prognosticated*, resulting in objects that come to have the property of being known. Such "knowing before" knows the world into stability *in the present* and sets forth from there to see what happens next. Again, this is not about "telling the future." The future cannot be foretold. Rather, it is about exercising prospective knowledge in the immediate present. What is suggested in prognostication is not a discursive process of either logical deduction or empirical inference. As such, it is distinct from other methods of arriving at what is commonly understood as "knowledge."

The *Zhuangzi* describes a primitive mode of *dao* 道-activity that comes before "knowledge" as it had come to be regarded in early China. This is presented as a "knowing without knowing" (*wuzhizhi* 無知知) and it is associated with remote antiquity prior to human artifice and continuous with our animal origins. Empirically speaking, it is highly plausible that knowledge did not (and does not) always "*know* that it knows." As Dewey reminds us, "knowledge has evolved historically out of a state in which there was no mind." (Dewey and Boydston 2008, MW 6: 115) Our pre-human ancestors had brains, but before their brains became organs for "knowing" they served to organize and coordinate their movements, sensations, memories, emotions, and other functions in response to present conditions. Our brains still perform these functions. In the midst of such operations—coextensive, in fact, *with* such operations—knowledge came to be. Between the first twinkling of "knowledge," however, and the advent of the modern epistemological question, "How does one *know* that one knows?" there is a vast spectrum covering 2.8 million years of the genus *Homo*. It strains credulity to think that "knowledge" sprang forth all-at-once aware of its own operations.

According to the *Zhuangzi*, our pre-historic ancestors indeed "knew things without knowing them" (*wuzhizhi* 無知知) and they were perfectly content in doing so. "The ancients who practiced *dao* 道-activity were contented in developing their knowledge," the *Zhuangzi* relates. "Knowledge was for the life process (*sheng* 生), and they did not take it up in order to do or make (*wei* 為) anything with it. So, it might be said that through knowing they were developing their contentedness. Knowing and contentedness, interacting with one another, mutually developed. Thus, their harmony and coherence emerged from their natural dispositions (*xing* 性)." (Zhuangzi 1968, 171) Such an account agrees with Dewey's idea that knowing is not, as he says, "something apart from or added to life." (Dewey and Myer 1984, 115) There is nothing unnatural about knowledge in its primitive form. Its operations retain continuity with the rest of Nature. "The organs, instrumentalities, and operations of knowing are *inside* Nature," Dewey reminds us, "not outside." (Dewey and Boydston 2008, LW 4: 168).

The "primitivist" viewpoint in the *Zhuangzi* is not a simple standpoint. Contemporary scholars understand the *Zhuangzi* to be a multi-authored text comprising different philosophical viewpoints and orientations. In addition to the "Inner Chapters," which are generally believed to be authored by Zhuang Zhou 莊周, subsequent chapters feature the writings of authors commonly referred to as "Yangist," "primitivist," and "agriculturalist"—but the contours of these schools remain unclear. Rather than determine the pedigree of any particular standpoint in the *Zhuangzi*, the focus here is more on the general valuation of "primitivism" in the later chapters and how this relates to "knowing" as a human enterprise. According to the *Zhuangzi*, while knowledge in its primitive form (i.e., *wuzhizhi* 無知知) is continuous with other life activities and with Nature, operations of knowing *can* violate the continuity (*yi* 一) of things and become a force that disrupts such continuity, actually impeding effective human action. The philosophically important distinction in the text is that between a "knowledge" that is disruptive and a "knowledge" that is not.

We are told, for instance, that in pre-historic times, "people had knowledge, but they had no use (*yong* 用) for it. This was called the state of utmost continuity. At that time, no one did/made (*wei* 為) anything with it, and spontaneity (*ziran* 自然) was the norm." According to this narrative, our pre-historic ancestors *did* know things, but "they did not use logical dialectic (*bian* 辯) to ornament their knowledge; they did not try to use it to encompass the whole world; and they did not try to use it to encompass the character of things. They remained aloof and fell back upon their natural dispositions (*xing* 性)." (Zhuangzi 1968, 172–174) According to the "primitivist," once humans departed from this standpoint things began to go wrong. The general concern is that humans have developed an obsession with "knowledge," and this has resulted in impetuous action and overreaching hubris—a species of certainty in which "doubt" never enters the picture. Thus, as Chapter 3 of the *Daodejing* teaches, "the sage is one who compels those who know (*zhizhe* 知者) not to *make* things happen (*wei*)." This circles back to what Zhuangzi identifies as the disruptive enterprise of putting one's knowledge to "use" (*yong* 用).

As an alternative to such disruptive modes of knowing, the Daoist ideal of "primitive" knowledge is to exercise no-knowledge (*wuzhi* 無知), or what David L. Hall and Roger T. Ames call "unprincipled knowing." Hall and Ames do well in turning this negative phrase into a positive ideal. As they explain, *wuzhi* means "the absence of a certain kind of knowledge—the kind of knowledge that is dependent upon ontological presence: that is, the assumption that there is some unchanging reality behind appearance." (Hall and Ames 2003, 40) The kind of knowledge involved in *Yijing* prognostication seems to operate along similar lines. The "objects" of prognostication in this tradition are not fixed ideas or "forms," but rather "images" and relations that become interpreted with respect to the matter at hand. Again, this happens in a uniquely spontaneous manner: to prognosticate is to have prognosticated. The "objects" of such knowledge are not made present in any form other than what becomes known in the newly clarified situation. Strictly speaking, there are no "objects of knowledge" presented in the *Yijing*—rather, there are "tools" (*qi* 器) that convert doubtful situations into ones comprised of known objects.

5.6 "Objects" of Knowledge in Greek and Chinese Thought

Reflection on the status of the "objects" of knowledge typically evokes the Realism/Nominalism debate in philosophy. In making sense of the *Yijing*, similar issues can arise. What *are* the hexagrams? Are they fixed forms instantiated in particular instances? What would that even mean in this context? Here, it is helpful to review how realism develops with respect to "knowledge" in both the Greek and Chinese traditions. In order to understand the notion of "knowing without knowing" (*wuzhizhi* 無知知), it is important to understand the kind of "knowledge" to which it was opposed. Moreover, understanding the Platonic conception of "knowledge" is helpful in making sense of Dewey's own realism, which will become helpful in considering how "images" (*xiang* 象) operate in *Yijing* prognostication.

For Plato, knowledge (*episteme*) is the highest function (*ergon*) of the mind. Like any function, it requires some object upon which to act. Plato's epistemology thus dovetails with his ontology, such that "different functions by nature deal with different things." (Plato 1997, 1104–1105) For each mental operation, there is a corresponding object with a specific grade of reality that serves as subject matter for that particular operation. This theory is most famously outlined in Plato's *Republic.* Socrates asks us to envision a "divided line" that is ultimately composed of five types of mental operation. On the very top is "knowledge," and on the very bottom is "ignorance." Socrates begins by asking the following: "Does someone who knows know something or nothing?" (Ibid., 1103) The answer, obviously, is *something*. Knowledge is thus identified with *something* while ignorance, its complete opposite, is identified with *nothing*.

This distinction makes good enough sense. Were one to ask, "What is the name of Confucius' pet turtle?" Only ignorance can be expected because such a thing does not exist. The object of one's ignorance is literally *no*-thing. One might, however, through imagination, generate an image of Confucius' pet turtle, its size, its color, its domestic accommodations, and so on. Such a mental object is not no-thing—it is *some*-thing—but on the scale of things known, it is not very much. Still, imagination (*eikasia*) is one step above ignorance in terms of the status of its objects.

One step above imagination is belief (*pistis*)—exactly mid-way between knowledge and ignorance on the ontological scale. For the Greeks, this is the middle ground between what "is" (i.e., *something*) and what "is not" (i.e., *nothing*) and thus the region of *change.* Accordingly, the objects of belief are things that undergo transformation over time. Confucius, for instance, believed that the Zhou dynasty was the pinnacle of human civilization. Twenty-five centuries later, things have changed—societies have come and gone, and even Confucius might change his assessment were he alive today. Thus, the truth of every belief is time-stamped, always provisional by virtue of the nature of its ontological conditions and the status of its objects.

The most important division in Plato's "divided line" is that which separates the next function, thought (*dianoia*), from belief—a division that marks a decisive split in Greek ontology. For Plato, the objects of thought are immune from change. He has in mind mathematical objects such as $2 + 2 = 4$ and the Pythagorean theorem.

The signature feature of such objects is that they do not rely upon concrete things in order to be apprehended. Right triangles come and go—they can be carved into the dirt and then scrubbed away. The corresponding object, however, never comes or goes. Thus, the region in which the objects of thought exist is a region above physical things, above time, and above change. With this division, Plato establishes his "two world theory"—one world visible and changing and the other invisible and eternal. The highest mental function, knowledge (*episteme*), connects us to the objects of this invisible world. These are the unchanging forms (*eidos*) that stand waiting to be apprehended through dialectic (*elenchus*), the art of reasoning and logical argumentation.

While Aristotle disagrees with Plato about the degree to which forms are separable from particular things, he never doubts their ontological status as fixed and unchanging. Aristotle's gradation of three types of knowing: the productive (*poiesis*), active (*praxis*), and theoretical (*theoria*), accords both with Plato's epistemic-ontology and with his preferences, such that "the theoretical sciences are more to be desired than the other sciences." (Aristotle 2001, 779) Aristotle subordinates activity and production by noting that their "ends" are not realized apart from the processes that constitute them, locating them squarely in the realm of movement (*dunamis*): this being the bottom half of the "divided line." Alternately, the theoretical sciences deal with "things that have *in themselves* a principle of movement" and thus remain free from temporal passage and its contingencies: this being the top half of the "divided line." (Ibid., 861).

On the face of it, the association of knowledge with fixed, unchanging objects appears arbitrary and strange. Why such an association? Dewey's account of how knowledge attained this connection traces back further than the Greeks, back to a primary distinction in human experience: that between "the ordinary and the extraordinary." (Dewey and Deen 2012, 4) His account goes as follows. Not unlike ourselves, our primitive ancestors went about things in a matter-of-fact way and took daily enjoyment in doing so. There were tasks to be performed, and simple tools were fashioned to perform them. As a species, we have always used tools. The production and employment of stone implements is as old as the genus *Homo*. Recent archeological finds suggest that such tools were produced as long as 3.3 million years ago, pre-dating our human ancestors by at least 700,000 years (Morella 2015, 1). Primitive humans thus had prosaic knowledge about the properties of everyday things, and they could foresee specific ends and plan accordingly. In short, they possessed sufficient intelligence (*ming* 明) to survive: an ability to coordinate means-and-ends creatively and productively.

Pre-historic humans, however, lived under conditions that rendered them extraordinarily exposed to peril. Emotion and imagination transmuted such vulnerability into less prosaic beliefs about gods and other animistic forces beyond their control. "Herein is the source of the fundamental dualism of human attention and regard," writes Dewey. Two operative regions of activity emerged in human consciousness—one was a region of human undertakings that aimed to control the lived environment through simple technologies, and the other was a region of forces beyond such arts that stood apart from human beings and operated independently. "The philosophical tradition regarding knowledge and practice was not original and primitive," Dewey writes. "It had for its background the state of culture that has been sketched." (Dewey and Boydston 2008, LW 4: 11).

Dewey regards this primitive cultural interest, i.e., "the ordinary and the extraordinary," as a human universal, forming "the common matrix out of which emerged all the world's philosophies, Asiatic as well as European." Its two regions, he explains, marked out "by way of anticipation what are later called the natural and the supernatural." It would be a mistake, however, to read into these terms the connotations that they have for us today. For in the primitive mind, these two realms "overlapped and blended," such that there was "no sharp division between heaven and earth [as] separated sources or realms." (Dewey and Deen 2012, 4) Of course, sharper separations between the "Natural/Supernatural" and "Material/Spiritual" would eventually develop. When they did, the region that continued to operate "beyond" the reach of human technology became the less transient realm towards which religious myths, rites, and ceremonies were directed. With the rise of pre-Socratic speculative cosmology in the Greek tradition (and its displacement of *nomos* with *phusis*), philosophy usurped this religious domain. "Philosophy," Dewey explains, "inherited the realm with which religion had been concerned." (Dewey and Boydston 2008, LW 4: 11).

The preceding mental distinction, with human tools on one side and divine forces on another, eventually became incorporated into Plato's "divided line." As Eric A. Havelock establishes, the concept of an "object" of knowledge that is "fiercely isolated from time, place, and circumstance," had crystallized in Greek thinking following a lengthy process. Plato's audience "did not have to have the *Republic* written for them in order to arrive at these elementary and time-honored truths." (Havelock 1963, 223–224) Still, it was with Plato that knowledge evacuated its humbler station explicitly to become a power separated from the simpler arts (*technē*) from which it arose. Its functions and objects are no longer numbered among the "tools" that humans have fashioned for practical purposes since time immemorial. *Episteme* now operated in the realm of intransigent forces (i.e., fixed objects) that were distinct from human activities and purposes. This, in fact, had previously been the region of the gods. As Dewey observes, "the change from religion to philosophy was so great in form that their identity as to content is easily lost from view." (Dewey and Boydston 2008, LW 4: 12).

The story plays out differently in early China, but the concept that knowledge (*zhi* 知) accesses fixed objects nevertheless arose. Like all human groups, the ancient Chinese exhibited a robust religious imagination, worshipping a variety of natural forces and spirits. During the Shang dynasty, worship coalesced around a primary deity, the "High Ancestor" (*shangdi* 上帝). As David Keightley (2014, 63) explains, this deity "may have once been the progenitor of the Shang royal lineage," thus establishing a relationship between humans and deities that was "implicitly genealogical." Accordingly, "there was no sense of radical difference between spirits and humans" in early China. Still, rituals were devised to negotiate two respective, and often antagonistic, fields of operation—tracking on to what Dewey calls "the ordinary and the extraordinary." Some Shang rituals (most notably human sacrifice) would suggest that Chinese divinities were as uncompromising as any other. The Chinese lived in fear of ghosts and spirits and in deference to forces beyond their control, which as Dewey suggests, is consistent with the inherently precarious nature of primitive human experience.

With the advent of the Zhou dynasty, the "High Ancestor" of the Shang was displaced by a more generic force commonly translated as "Heaven" (*tian* 天). The meaning of *tian* would gradually evolve from a roughly anthropomorphic deity to the impersonal forces of "Nature," with texts often oscillating between one conception and the other. The key moment in the development of early Chinese religiousness, however, arrives when Confucius turns away from the spirit realm towards the human-centered world (Analects, 1998, 3.12, 6.22, 7.21, 11.12). The Master would retain his fear and reverence for the inscrutable "mandates of Heaven" (*tianming* 天命), but he directs the use of ritual-custom (*li* 禮) away from divine propitiation to focus on its social and cultural dimensions (Ibid., 16.8, 20.3). As Michael J. Puett (2002, 98) explains, "by decrying the instrumental use of sacrifices by ritual specialists, [Confucius] denied the powers that were used in the Bronze age to mollify divine forces and to make them work for the living. Instead, he urged that we simply cultivate ourselves and accept whatever the divine powers do."

By revolutionizing the function of ritual-custom (*li* 禮) and relegating "extra-ordinary" matters to the inscrutable workings of fate (*ming* 命), Confucius triggered a highly organized, populist reaction led by Mozi. In his critiques of Confucianism, Mozi reasserts the supremacy of an anthropomorphic "Heaven" (*tian* 天) and chastises the Confucians for not believing in the spirit world. Presuming to have divine sanction, Mozi formulates a number of philosophical positions the veracity of which he refuses to doubt—he *knows* that he is right and that the Confucians are wrong. In showing how he "knows that he knows," Mozi becomes the first in China to use the methods of logical argumentation (*bian* 辯)—methods that win him a large number of devoted followers. With Mohism, analytic philosophy becomes refined, expanded, and employed to defend positions on a range of issues with absolute confidence.

As Robert Eno (1996, 131) observes, "Mohist teachings made it possible for China to embark on a philosophical enterprise similar to that of the Greeks." In Mohist technical writings, knowledge (*zhi* 知) thus assumes a new status. "Knowing is a capacity," the *Canons* explain, and "with regard to the capacity of knowing, it is how one knows and knows with certainty." (Mozi 2010, 376–377)[2] This marks a departure from previous notions of knowledge in the Chinese tradition. As Eno says (1996, 131), the Mohists "claimed that what is so could be discovered through argument or through the processes of discursive thinking guided by rules that we call reason."

As in the Greek world, the advent of "reason" in early China involved evacuating knowledge from the more instrumental human realm and stationing it at a level once reserved for the high gods. According to the Mohists, "Heaven's intention" (*tianzhi* 天志) furnishes us with unvarying "standards of rightness" (*yizhifa* 義之法) and such standards guarantee absolute certainty. "I have Heaven's intention just

[2] For citations from the Mozi, Ian Johnston's translations are largely relied upon.

like wheelwrights have compasses and carpenters have squares," declares Mozi. "What conforms to it is right. What does not conform to it is wrong." With such divine and permanent authorization, Mozi likens efforts to refute him to "throwing eggs against a rock." (Mozi 2010, 159–161, 241–243, 673) He thus introduces into Chinese philosophy the notion of a "knowledge that knows" (*youzhizhi* 有知知). Such knowledge is that which the *Zhuangzi* opposes by appealing to a more primitive "knowledge that does not know" (*wuzhizhi* 無知知).

5.7 "Types" (*lei* 類) and Realism

If the *Yijing*, similarly, does not furnish the reader with fixed objects amenable to epistemic certainty, then what does it provide? As the text explains, "trends (*fang* 方) can be sorted into types (*lei* 類). Things and events by their groupings can be distinguished (*fen* 分)." (Wilhelm and Baynes 1967, 280) In the classical Greek tradition, "forms" (*eidos*) are what makes certainty a possibility through deductive reasoning. "All Humans are Mortal; Socrates is a Human; *ergo* Socrates is Mortal." Is there a similar knowledge reached through the apprehension of Chinese "types" (*lei*)? It is crucial to recognize that "types" (*lei*) in classical Chinese philosophy are formulated and come to operate quite differently than "forms" in Greek philosophy.

Recent work in classical Chinese language and logic demonstrates as much. As Chad Hansen argues, the notion of "type" (*lei* 類), even as it is understood in the Mohist *Canons*, is not premised on the notion that universal or abstract properties are ontologically *real* in the Platonic sense. Rather, the tradition rests on the premise that "the world controls projections of linguistic expressions from the outside," i.e., according to "stuff" (*shi* 實) that is actually out there. Formulating "types" commits us to certain behaviors accordingly. The Mohists thus "embed their realistic theory [of "types"] in a pragmatic framework." (Hansen, 1992, 240–241) The formulation of "types" depends on predictable outcomes and behaviors, but it does not track to fixed "forms" in neither the Platonic nor the Aristotelian sense.

A.C. Graham (1989, 418) largely agrees with Hansen in maintaining that, "Chinese philosophy is concerned not with essences but with the fitting of names to objects (*mingshi* 名實)." According to Graham, the Mohist *Canons* teaches that this process demands consistency in identifying similarities and differences, thus obliging us to treat certain things in certain ways—but it does not involve postulating abstract "classes" with individual members (Graham 1978, 36–37, 169). Things actually *do* resemble one another in countless "types" of ways. Generating a "type" (*lei* 類) requires only that we fix some standard (*fa* 法) by which to measure sameness and difference. "The choice of standard is a matter of discretion," Graham (1989, 148) observes. There is no fixed collection that is pre-defined as a "type." As Graham notes, "the Mohist seems to have no other word for definition than 'standard.'" (Ibid.) Thus, establishing "types" is basically a constructivist process of "analogical grouping," as Kurtis Hagen maintains. For Hagen (2007, 41, 154), so ordering the world is an "ongoing process that has no final or perfect articulation." In texts such as the *Huainanzi*, such "types" (*lei*) are assembled according to their practical utility. The text itself is the result of a project undertaken for the purpose of orienting human activity productively in the world. The *Yijing* appears to be formulated in a similar spirit.

Building on the insights of Graham and Hansen, Brook Ziporyn undertakes a comprehensive reconstruction of Chinese thought based on the notion of "coherence" (*li* 理). While "coherence" is a term that enters only gradually into the Chinese philosophical lexicon, Ziporyn demonstrates that its associations are foreshadowed in patterns of thought that precede its emergence as a central philosophical term. One of Ziporyn's main insights is that early Chinese thinkers are not easily divided along "Realist/Nominalist" lines. Rather, there seems to be a common assumption, i.e., "[that] things are neither the same nor different; they can be made as much really one and the same as it is possible to be, or as really different as it is possible to be, by connection with another real thing that connects up with them in a particular situation: that other real thing is human action, designed for human purposes." (Ziporyn 2012, 44–45) According to Ziporyn, rather than being "nominalists" or "realists" with respect to the ontological status of "objects" in the world, Chinese thinkers display "ironic" or "non-ironic" attitudes towards the applicability of "coherences." Ziporyn thus departs from what he sees as the default nominalism that is often ascribed to early Chinese thinkers. For Ziporyn, "the actual approach taken by Chinese thinkers to the question of kinds and categories is neither strictly nominalist nor strictly realist in the Western sense." (Ibid., 56) The notion of coherence (*li*) underwrites this unique approach, which Ziporyn finds significantly different from the nominalism that usually results when Western philosophers deny universal essences as "objects" of knowledge.

In exploring possible avenues towards this Chinese approach, Ziporyn briefly considers the classical American tradition. He notes that Peirce's realism and James' nominalism were both regarded as necessary consequences of the pragmatic method. "This would suggest," he writes, "that pragmatist methodology as such does not supersede the problem of a dichotomy [between realism and nominalism] so much as postpone it; it remains unresolved." Ziporyn mentions Dewey in passing, only to identify him with James—they are "both nominalists." (Ibid., 59) This is incorrect. It is well established that Dewey is not a nominalist. "The defect of nominalism," Dewey says, "lies in its virtual denial of interaction and association… [It] ignores organization, and thus makes nonsense out of meanings." (Dewey and Boydston 2008, LW 1: 145) Ziporyn's aim, to articulate an approach that factors in "human agency and participation in *creating* continuities," such that there are natural qualities that "[emerge] from their coherence with the totality of experience, in a way that evades a dichotomization of nominalism and realism," (Ziporyn 2012, 59, 76) is one that Dewey shares. Dewey's critique of nominalism and partial embrace of Peircean realism positions him squarely in that elusive middle that Ziporyn sees in the Chinese tradition.

For Dewey, "realism is correct in insisting upon universals and upon the fact that they enter in some way into the determination of known and knowable existences." (Dewey and Boydston 2008, LW 11: 111) The problem with realism, says Dewey, is that knowledge (*episteme*) is commonly understood as taking for its "objects" common nouns—fixed in language and presumably fixed in Nature—whereas the content of universals are *ways* of changing and acting, designated by verb forms and variable over time. Dewey's position on "types" grows from his appreciation for Peirce's own approach to universals. "Peirce understands by the reality of a 'general' the reality of a way, habit, disposition of behavior," Dewey explains, "and he dwells upon the fact that the habits of things are acquired and modifiable." (Ibid., LW 6: 276) As Peirce sees it, every generality involves a description of what *may* happen but is not necessarily happening now—as such it involves "potentiality." The capacity of a food plant to nourish, for instance, lies dormant until it is actualized on particular occasions in transactions with herbivores. Thus, giving nourishment is a genuine *way* that the food plant behaves under specific conditions. "So," Dewey notes, "[Peirce] criticizes the nominalists for denying, by implication if not explicitly, that things have *ways* of behaving." Things really *do* have ways of behaving, and such realities provide "the cosmological or physical basis for logical possibilities or universals." Such universals, for Peirce, take the form of "leading principles" that are carried over into the field of inquiry—"modes that with respect to actualization are potential and general, being actualized only under individualized conditions of interaction with other things." (Ibid., LW 11: 89) As Dewey thus sees it, "realism is correct in insisting upon universals and upon the fact that they enter in some way into the determination of known and knowable existences." (Ibid., LW 11: 111).

The "types" (*lei* 類) that come to be cataloged and articulated in the *Yijing* have a similar, non-essential property in being accounts of *processes* and *relations* rather than "objects" or "forms." Also, not unlike Peirce's "universals," such "types" come to be actualized "only under individualized conditions of interactions with other things," namely, in their interactions with the doubtful situations in which prognosticators find themselves. This is not to deny that they stand for something "real." The problem with realism, as Dewey suggests, is linguistic. In coming to know what something is, we classify it under a common noun. Such nouns inevitably become "objects," and are then understood to exist in a constant or uniform manner as the content of knowledge. Such common-noun "objects," however, are not what actually exists in a general way. What exists in a general way are the *verbs* that describe the operations of the common nouns; "for what is designated by a verb is a *way* of changing and/or acting," explains Dewey. Such "ways" are what provide the realist a basis for positing logical possibilities or universals in the form of leading principles—nouns *as such* do not do this. "*A* footrace or *a* fire," Dewey points out, is a singular occurrence expressed in noun form; "but racing and burning are *ways* of acting and changing," and such verbs indicate that which *really* carries the possibility of recurrence (Ibid., LW 12: 249). The *Yijing*, similarly, presents its readers with paradigmatic *ways* of acting and changing. It reveals not the essence of "objects," but rather real "types" of change.

5.8 Conclusion

As Keightley (2014, 142–143) suggests, the shift from "Neolithic pessimism" to "Bronze Age optimism" in early China involved increased confidence in the prospects of "human control" in the face of difficulties, with more scope given to "human reflection and interpretation." While what Dewey identifies as the dynamic between "the ordinary and the extraordinary" resulted in Chinese thinkers positing a realm of "objects" amenable to epistemic certainty, the kind of "prognostication" (*prognosticare*) associated with the *Yijing* is closer to the kind of "knowledge that does not know" (*wuzhizhi* 無知知) with respect to such objects. Those who consult the oracle do so in the midst of activity, upon finding themselves in a state of "great doubt" (*dayi* 大疑). "Images" (*xiang* 象) work like "ideas" in the non-technical sense, as propositions for action that reconfigure elements in a problematic situation by introducing new relations between them. As such, they operate as "tools" (*qi* 器) in restoring smooth-running activity.

In the Daoist tradition, figures like Cook Ding and Carver Qing are tool users as well. Their knives and chisels are employed in such a way that they become a means to "ends" that grow out of the activity that constitutes the process of reaching them. Cook Ding, famously, encounters "trouble spots" or "problematic situations" as he carves his Ox, and so long as his knife navigates the contours of the Ox itself, his knife does not impose anything upon the end result. The "images" (*xiang* 象) of the *Yijing* can perhaps be thought of in a similar, non-imposing instrumental fashion. When "doubt" arises, it allows one to similarly slow down, allowing the "tool" to pass like Cook Ding's knife through the trouble spots—without chopping or hacking or forcing. Smooth-running activity might then be restored, and the natural end reached accordingly. One can then put the *Yijing* away, just as Cook Ding wipes his blade and returns it to its sheath unscathed. The American pragmatic tradition proves insightful in coming to appreciate the depth and nuance that such a tradition exhibits.

References

Analects. 1998. *The Analects of Confucius: A Philosophical Translation*. Tr. Roger T. Ames, and Henry Rosemont, Jr. New York: Ballantine Books.

Aristotle. 2001. *Metaphysics*. In: *The Basic Works of Aristotle*. Ed. Richard McKeon. New York: Modern Library.

Dewey, John. 1916. *Democracy and Education*. New York: The Free Press.

Dewey, John, and Philip Deen. 2012. *Unmodern Philosophy and Modern Philosophy*. Carbondale, IL: Southern Illinois University Press.

Dewey, John, and Samuel Myer. 1984. *Types of Thinking: Including a Survey of Greek Philosophy*. New York: Philosophical Library.

Dewey, John, Jo Ann Boydston, et al. 2008. *The Collected Works of John Dewey*, Early Works, Vols. 1–4. Middle Works, Vols. 1–15. Late Works, Vol. 1–17. Carbondale, IL: Southern Illinois University Press.

Eno, Robert. 1996. Cook Ding's Dao and the limits of philosophy. In *Essays on Skepticism, Relativism, and Ethics in the Zhuangzi*. Eds. Paul Kjellberg and Philip Ivanhoe. Albany, NY: State University of New York Press.

Graham, A.C. 1978. *Later Mohist Logic, Ethics and Science*. Hong Kong: The Chinese University of Hong Kong Press.

Graham, A.C. 1989. *Disputers of the Tao: Philosophical Argument in Ancient China.* La Salle, IL: Open Court.

Hagen, Kurtis. 2007. *The Philosophy of Xunzi: A Reconstruction.* Chicago: Open Court.

Hall, David. L. and Roger T. Ames. 2003. *Dao De Jing: A Philosophical Translation: "Making this Life Significant."* New York: Ballantine Books.

Hansen, Chad. 1992. *A Daoist Theory of Chinese Thought: a Philosophical Interpretation.* Oxford: Oxford University Press.

Havelock, Eric A. 1963. *Preface to Plato.* Cambridge, MA: Harvard University Press.

Keightley, David N. 2014. *These Bones Shall Rise Again: Selected Writings on Early China.* Ed. Henry Rosemont Jr. Albany, NY: State University of New York Press.

Legge, James. 2000. *The Chinese Classics*, vol. 3. Taipei: SMC Publishing Inc.

Morelle, Rebecca. 2015. "Oldest stone tools pre-date earliest humans." BBC News, May 20, 2015: http://www.bbc.com/news/science-environment-32804177. Accessed September 10, 2024.

Mozi. 2010. *The Mozi: A Complete Translation.* Tr. Ian Johnston. New York: Columbia University Press.

Peirce, Charles S., Charles Hartshorne, and Paul Weiss. 1935. *Collected Papers of Charles Sanders Peirce*, vol. 6. Cambridge, MA: Harvard University Press.

Plato. 1997. *Plato: Complete Works.* Ed. John M. Cooper. Indianapolis, IN: Hackett Publishers.

Puett, Michael. 2002. *To Become a God: Cosmology, Sacrifice, and Self-Divinization in Early China.* Cambridge, MA: Harvard University Asia Center.

Stuhr, John, ed. 2000. *Pragmatism and Classical American Philosophy*, 2nd ed. Oxford: Oxford University Press.

Wilhelm, Richard, and Cary F. Baynes. 1967. *The I-Ching or Book of Changes.* Princeton, NJ: Princeton University Press.

Wu, K.C. 1982. *The Chinese Heritage.* New York: Crown Publishers.

Zhuangzi. 1968. *The Complete Works of Chuang Tzu.* Tr. Burton Watson. New York: Columbia University Press.

Ziporyn, Brook. 2012. *Ironies of Oneness and Difference: Coherence in Early Chinese Thought. Prolegomena to the Study of* Li. Albany, NY: State University of New York Press.

Chapter 6
Dao 道 and *Qi* 器 in the *Yijing* 易经: Chinese Cosmotechnology and Its Implications for a Different Ecology

Jana S. Rošker

Abstract In this paper, I will elucidate the basic structure of the correlative and complementary relationship between *dao* and *qi* in the *Yijing*. This relationship not only causes misinterpretations of the term "metaphysics" in the Sinophone world, but also has important—and very topical—implications for contemporary interpretations of the philosophical paradigms of technology in Chinese culture. In environmental studies, technology (including the basic human attitude toward it) is pivotal. In this article, I will focus on questions concerning cosmotechnology in China. In this context, I present a theory by the Hong Kong scholar Yuk Hui whose book on "Chinese cosmotechnics" has been immensely influential in Western academia working on philosophy of technology. In the conclusion, I will show how and why the structure of the relation between *dao* and *qi* is different from the relation between *technê* and *arête* in the ancient Greek philosophy, and why it can be seen as a different kind of an ecological standpoint.

Keywords *Dao* · *Qi* · *Yijing* · *Technê* and *arête* · Cosmotechnics · Yuk Hui · Balance · Ecology

6.1 Introduction: *Yijing* and Cosmotechnology

Given that *Yijing* is one of the most important and paradigmatic classical works of Chinese philosophy and culture, it is by no means coincidental that it has also laid the foundations for the specific kind of Chinese metaphysics. As we shall see, this type of so-called "metaphysics" is very closely connected to the question of what has been coined "Chinese cosmotechnology" or "Chinese cosmotechnics." Therefore, in clarifying the question about the constitution and the function of Chinese metaphysics, we shall start from clarifying its inherent connection to the so-called cosmotechnology.

J. S. Rošker (✉)
University of Ljubljana, Ljubljana, Slovenia
e-mail: jana.rosker@ff.uni-lj.si

G. Sigurðsson and T. Hon (eds.), *Contemporary Interpretations and Readings of the Yijing*, Chinese Culture 15, https://doi.org/10.1007/978-981-96-0609-2_6

The term "cosmotechnology" is used to describe how different cultures understand and interact with technology, emphasizing that this relationship is not merely practical or mechanical but deeply intertwined with the symbolic, economic, and linguistic aspects of society. In other words, it is a part of cosmologies associated with the specific attitudes of individuals and communities toward various specific techniques that are vital to their survival, and toward technology as a coherent, rationally ordered system of those techniques. In this sense, cosmotechnology is a system based on the combination of the cosmic and moral, esthetic or axiological orders in the acts of practicing and passing on techniques. In the history of humankind, many different systems of understanding or explaining the cosmos have evolved, as have many different techniques. Therefore, there cannot be only one cosmotechnology (for instance, only the traditional European one), for there exist as many individual cosmotechnologies as there are symbolic orders of perceiving and comprehending the cosmos. This culturally conditioned practices of techniques and cosmotechnologies are called techno-diversity. It consists of orders that are culturally and linguistically conditioned, while the process of applying techniques and designing their products remains universal.

6.2 The Importance of Techno-Diversity and the Role of Chinese Cosmotechnology

Yuk Hui is a scholar of informatics and philosophy from Hong Kong, who has been living and working in Germany during the last decade. He believes that understanding different culturally conditioned forms of cosmotechnology is important because it can prevent a universalistic equalization of ideas (or ideologies) about the role and manner of interaction between humans and technology. In other words, techno-diversity refers to different patterns of cosmotechnology, i.e., the relationship between humans and technology.

Actually Yuk Hui speaks about cosmotechniques rather than cosmotechnologies[1]: He derives his position from a culturally differentiated consideration of the relationship between humans and technology, and in this context, he emphasizes that "rediscovering multiple cosmotechnics is not to refuse artificial intelligence or machine learning, but to reappropriate modern technology, to give other frames to the enframing (*Gestell*) at the core of modern technology" (Hui 2016, 8).

Here, cosmotechnics emphasizes cultural diversity. It is an understanding based on technological diversity that allows for multi-layered and pluralistic starting points for the study of human-technology relationships. On such foundations, we have produced throughout history a number of different forms of knowledge, linking humans to the world and the earth in different ways and through diverse, specific, multi-faceted

[1] The term cosmotechnics was first used by Gilbert Simondon in his 1965 article "Culture et technique," which was later (2014) included in his book entitled *Sur la technique*. However, Simondon only examined this term in the narrow context of the development of European technology.

relationships not measurable by the criteria of the linear progress of modern science and technology. Only an understanding of the existence of such heterogeneity (as opposed to the isolated contributions of individual "nations" and "cultures") will allow us to resolve the tensions between increasingly isolated social groups.

Thus, Yuk Hui attempts to develop and upgrade it through the prism of the ontological plurality of the relationship between technology, human beings, and nature, starting from the conceptualization of technology within the Chinese tradition of thought. In the following, I will present Hui's theory to clarify the differences between various culturally conditioned perceptions of digital technologies.

Contrary to Hui, I view cosmotechnology as a systemic umbrella field and not only of individual cosmotechnics, since Hui, in my opinion, coins this key term on the basis of a misunderstanding of the difference between these two concepts. In *The Question Concerning Technology in China—An Essay in Cosmotechnics,* he writes:

> I make a distinction between technics, *technê*, and technology. T*echnics* refers to the general category of all forms of making and practice. *Technê* refers to the Greek conception of it, which Heidegger understands as *poiesis* or bringing forth. *Technology* refers to a radical turn which took place during European modernity, and developed in the direction of ever-increasing automation, leading consequently to what Heidegger calls the *Gestell*. (Hui 2016, 4)

However, I disagree with Hui on such a definition of technology. The word is used in most Indo-European languages in the sense of a scientific discipline whose object is techniques (or technics), and not in the sense in which the Hui understand it. Technology derives from the Greek words *technê* and *lógos*. While the former refers to techniques in the sense described by Hui, *logos* means reason or logic. When used as the suffix -logy, it always means the field, discipline, or science of whatever comes before it. Technology, then, is the systematic theory of techniques, not a "radical turn" of techniques that happened in the process of Western modernization.

Yuk Hui attempts to position the concept of cosmotechnics within the theoretical explanation of the relationship between humans, nature (or the external world), and technology. The concept also definitely represents a theory, not simply a category. This applies to his concrete theoretical analyses as well as to technological systems. For instance, the system of traditional Chinese medicine, which Hui (2016, 18) presents as a quintessential example of Chinese cosmotechnics, illustrates this point. One cannot simply speak of Chinese medicine as a specific technique, as it is always also a set of interconnected techniques, methods, and specific approaches to the human body and disease based on a specific cosmology. Therefore, Chinese medicine is a kind of cosmotechnology and not simply a kind of cosmotechnics.

Cosmotechnology, then, is a system based on the combination of the cosmic and moral (or axiological) order in the acts of practicing and passing on techniques. In the history of humankind, many different systems of understanding or explaining the cosmos have evolved, as have many different techniques.

Therefore, as already mentioned, there exist as many individual cosmotechnologies as there are symbolic orders of perceiving and understanding the cosmos. These orders are culturally and linguistically conditioned. And, of course, the process of applying techniques and designing their products is universal. The question of the relationship between universality and the (culturally conditioned) particularity of techniques has long been a subject of debate among philosophers, anthropologists, psychologists, linguists, and scholars of social sciences.

In this context, it is worth mentioning that the French archeologist and anthropologist André Leroi-Gourhan, who introduced the concept of technical tendencies emerging from the interplay between the universal application of technology and the cultural specificity of their practical implementations. In his book *Environment and Techniques* (*Milieu et techniques* 1945), he presents this relationship within the framework of the general theory of dynamic interactions, in which human communities behave as organisms living in the environment defined by external (geography, climate) and internal (culture, tradition) factors. He considers the natural and social environment as external and internal milieu (Leroi-Gourhan 1945, 333). In this framework, the concept of technical tendencies represented a movement or tendency that is formed within the inner milieu and becomes the primary factor influencing the functioning of the community in its natural environment.

Contemporary Chinese theorists have also devoted much attention to determining the relationship between the universal and culturally conditioned factors. One of the most important representatives of philosophical anthropology is Li Zehou, who considers techniques, in the sense of the making and systematic application of tools (as well as the intergenerational transmission of the corresponding techniques), as the basis of becoming human, and thus as the decisive characteristic that distinguishes humans from (other) animals. Li explains this connection with the concept of sedimentation (*jidian* 積澱), which he uses to describe the gradual accumulation of knowledge and experience in the human mind through millennia of evolutionary development (cf. Li Zehou 2016). For him, the process of sedimentation is divided into three levels. The most basic level he calls the "sedimentation of the species (*wuzhong jidian* 物種積澱)," which contains all the universal forms common to all human beings. The second level is "cultural sedimentation (*wenhua jidian* 文化積澱)," which consists of the specific forms of thought, linguistic and behavioral patterns, and techniques peculiar to people living in the same cultural environment. The third and highest level (as well as the narrowest, since this scheme has a pyramidal structure) is "individual sedimentation (*geti jidian* 個體積澱)," which co-creates our intimate value systems or worldviews, feelings, habits, and specific forms of thinking and feeling about people as individuals (Rošker 2018, 33).

Technology as such, however, has evolved in the processes of producing everything necessary for human existence and sustenance. Many theorists consider tools as extensions of human limbs or organs, and thus, Li Zehou speaks of human beings as beings for whom tools or techniques are a "universal necessity," since humans represent "supra-biological beings" who could not survive without all these extensions of their bodies (ibid., 28). Further similarities between the philosophical anthropology of Leroi-Gourhan and Li Zehou can also be found in the fact that they both see technology as a form of externalization of human memory (Leroi-Gourhan 1993, 219 ff.; Li and Cauvel 2006, 3).

For scholars such as Leroi-Gourhan and Li Zehou, the culturally defined dimensions of technology are thus at the forefront of the conceptualization of different cosmotechnologies understood as different externalizations of memory. This is a search for a new frame of reference for technology that will transcend both the ancient Greek concept of *technê* (including its connotation of creation or *poiesis*) and Heidegger's concept of the *Gestell*, which for him marked the essence of modern technology (Heidegger 2000, 21).

On the other hand, as a Sinologist, I will focus on Chinese cosmotechnology. Within this framework, Yuk Hui has set himself the task of systematically examining the ancient concepts of *dao* (the way, method, original principle) and *qi* (vessel, accessory, tool, device). This pair of terms appears together for the first time in the history of written Chinese in the ancient *Book of Changes* (*Yijing*), where it is described as follows: "What is above the forms we call method (*dao*), what is below them we call tool (*qi*)."

6.3 *Dao* and *Qi:* Three Questions Regarding the Nature of Their Relation

For many contemporary Chinese scholars, *Yijing* includes in this aspect the basis of Chinese cosmotechnology. Yuk Hui has elaborated on this question in two of his best-known works. The first one is a book which has been published in English under the title *The Question Concerning Technology in China: An Essay in Cosmotechnics*. The second one is an article, in which Yuk Hui summarizes and explains the core of the relation between *dao* and *qi*, starting from its first mention in the *Yijing*, and tracing its evolution and transformation in the further development of Chinese philosophy. This paper has been published in Chinese under the title "器"与 "道": 超人类主 义未来的一种回应" [*Qi* and *Dao*: A Response to a Transhumanist Future].

Yuk Hui interprets the relationship between *dao* and *qi* as a dualism. But the *dao-qi* dualism is distinct from Cartesian dualism, with *dao* taking precedence. He views *dao* as a moral category, diverging from its original depiction in the *Yijing* and early pre-Qin texts, where it was understood more broadly as a dynamic principle related to nature and the cosmos, without inherent moral implications. This shift toward moral interpretation emerges in Neo-Confucian metaphysics, where *dao* gains significant moral undertones. Yuk Hui's analysis is rooted in this later understanding, transforming the original, neutral concept of *dao* into a heavily moralized framework. Therefore, for him, the relationship between *dao* and *qi* is primarily one between morality and utility. Moreover, he endeavors to compare it with the ancient Greek distinction between *technê* and *aretê*.

Thus, in his search for Chinese cosmotechnology, Hui's starting point is certainly correct and useful, but his interpretation of this pair of terms is problematic. In what follows, I will first critically examine Yuk Hui's interpretation of the relationship between *dao* and *qi* in this *Yijing* quote. I will question his theses through the lens of three central questions.

I start from a distinction between dualisms and binary categories, continue with questions about the moral content allegedly implied in this quotation, and end with a critical elaboration on Yuk Hui's comparison of *dao* and *qi* with the ancient Greek terms *technê* and *aretê*. After this critical confrontation with Yuk Hui, I will answer the question of why and how the specific Chinese cosmotechnology, which manifests itself in this quotation, is closely related to the question of Chinese ecology.

Yuk Hui sees the relation between *dao* and *qi* as a kind of different, i.e., non-Cartesian dualism (Hui 2018, 2). Therefore, my first question for Hui is as follows:

(A) Is this relation indeed simply a different (i.e., a "Non-Cartesian") kind of dualism?

In my view, the reply to this question is a negative one, because when proceeding from the basic paradigms that define ancient and classical Chinese philosophy, we must think about all such relations as parts of its underlying processual paradigm. Dualisms are static models. Even when involved in a dialectical process, it is a dialectic process where movements are composed of distinct static stages of particular static phases. In my view, Yuk Hui fails to see that not every duality is a type of dualism.

On the one hand, he clearly sees that the relationship between *dao* and *qi* cannot be understood as a classical Cartesian dualism. However, for him, it is still a dualism, albeit one of a different kind. For him, the important distinction between the two models can be seen in the fact that Cartesian dualism.

> Generally refers to two opposing and discontinuous entities: mind-body, culture-nature, being-nothingness. This form of dualism is not dominant in China, and Yin-Yang are not conceived of as two discontinuous entities. (Yuk Hui 2016, 54).

I agree with this interpretation, but I also think it is insufficient and fails to capture the essence of the distinction that characterizes the two forms of duality. In my view, *yin* and *yang*, like *dao* and *qi*, cannot be counted as dualisms, even though they represent dualities.

In this regard, we must distinguish between two models of dualities, namely Cartesian dualism on the one hand and the model that I call "binary categories" (*duili fanchou* 对立范畴) on the other.

The most important and crucial differences between the two models are twofold. The first has been correctly identified by Yuk Hui. It concerns the continuous and discontinuous nature, respectively, of the two opposites that constitute these two models of duality. The discontinuous nature of the concepts in the Cartesian model is related to the static paradigm of Hegelian dialectics, while the continuous nature of the binary categories is related to the processual nature of Chinese philosophy and the *Yijing* as its most important starting point. The second distinction is at least as important but has been overlooked by Yuk Hui. It concerns that the Cartesian model is based on the three elementary laws of formal logic that leads to the mutual exclusion of the two opposing concepts and to a synthesis that is a qualitatively new static phase rooted in the unity of contradictions. In contrast, the processual and correlative character of the model of binary categories is based on the mutual complementarity of the two oppositional categories. In this model, the two opposites do not exclude each other. Rather, they complement each other in a continuous process of mutual interaction in which neither of the two opposites can occupy a primary or independent position.

Now, let us turn to the second question regarding Hui's view of the relation between *dao* and *qi* in the *Yijing*. He sees *dao* as a predominantly moral category. Therefore, for him, the relationship between *dao* and *qi* is primarily one of morality and utility. In this context, I will raise the following question:

(B) ***Is this relation really one between morality and utility?***

In my view, this question has—again—to be answered with a decisive no. But for Yuk Hui, Chinese philosophy, which starts with *Yijing*, rests on the paradigmatic nature of morality; hence, *dao*, which is above the forms, is also a symbol of morality. Following this hypothesis, *dao* in the above-mentioned quotation would certainly and necessarily also be a moral principle. Hui tries to prove this hypothesis with an interpretation of another passage from the *Yijing*:

> As the philosopher Mou Zongsan (1909–1995) insisted, the Chinese cosmology was a moral ontology and a moral cosmology, meaning that it did not originate as a philosophy of nature, but as a moral metaphysics, as is stated in the *Qian* (乾) hexagram of the *I Ching*: "The moral of the great man is identical with that of Heaven and Earth; his brilliance is identical with that of the sun and the moon…"[2] (Yuk Hui 2016, 62)

However, the term *de* 德, which has been translated as "moral" in the above quotation,[3] is understood differently by most scholars of etymology and philology. Most scholars believe that the notion cannot be glossed as "virtue" in a limited normative sense. It cannot be limited to such a connotation, while it can certainly also imply the best and most positive potential in a more general sense. According to the authoritative expert of classical Chinese etymology, Peter A. Boodberg, the usage of the term in earliest sources is essentially free of any moral connotations, which have only been added in later Confucian texts. Boodberg explains:

> We can now move on to the consideration of the term *de* 德, perhaps the most significant word, next to *dao* 道, in ancient Chinese macro- and microcosmology. The standard translation for it is "virtue," both in the sense of inherent quality and in that of moral excellence, but with the validity of the traditional rendering somewhat shaken by Arthur Waley's insistence on interpreting it as "power." Indeed, it is believed by many scholars that the term originated in the mytho-magical period of Chinese speculation when it was conceived as a kind of mana-like potency inherent in substances, things, and human beings, a potency which, on the one hand made them true to their essence, and, on the other, made possible their influencing of other entities. (Boodberg 1953, 324)

---

[2] 大人者、與天地合其德，與日月合其明.

[3] The term has clear moral connotations in modern Chinese, for it is the second part of the compound *daode* 道德, meaning morality in contemporary language. However, this meaning has no direct link to its ancient connotations in the classical Chinese language.

Thus, in the *Yijing*, the term was mostly understood as the potential of realization of *dao* in the individual. There are also differences between later Confucian and Daoist interpretations of the character.[4]

Moreover, Mou Zongsan, on whose theory Yuk Hui's argument is based, cannot be considered the sole or most authoritative interpreter of traditional Chinese philosophy. As the most influential representative of the second generation of Modern New Confucianism,[5] his idealistic interpretation has its roots in the Neo-Confucian philosophies of the Song and Ming dynasties. At the same time, Mou has neglected all other major currents of Confucianism,[6] and has been severely criticized by numerous renowned Chinese scholars as a result (see e.g., Li Zehou 1999, 9).

But in the context of Yuk Hui's thesis, the focus should be on *dao* rather than *de*. And with respect to the former, it is even clearer that the term (as used in the *Yijing*) does not carry any normative or moral connotations. Most often, it is used in a much broader sense, as a principle, a way, or a method that cannot be directly linked to moral content in any way.

Let us look at some examples from the *Yijing*. *Dao* appears in this work over one hundred times, so I will limit these examples to the respective passages from the commentaries to the first diagram *Qian*, which is represented by the hexagram of pure *yang*, and to the last one, the hexagram *Kun*, which represents pure *yin*.[7]

> The principle (or method) of *Qian* is to change and transform, so that everything obtains its appropriate nature in accordance with the mandate of life.[8]
>
> Active and vigilant all day, guided by this original principle (or method) over and over again.[9]
>
> Something is leaping up, while still being in the deep; a profound transformation is taking place in the method indicated by (this) *Qian* diagram.[10]

In the last hexagram *Kun*, *dao* becomes the principle or method which guides the elements connected to *yin*. The hexagram is described in the following way:

> The principle or method of *Kun* is to follow. It receives the influences of heaven and acts according to different situations.[11]

In the Confucian commentaries, this principle is then applied to social norms:

---

[4] While the later Confucian scholars indeed mostly translated it as "moral character; virtue; morality," the Daoist philosophers applied it in the sense of "inherent character; inner power; integrity.".

[5] For a comprehensive explanation of the main philosophical agenda of this generation of Modern New Confucian scholars, see for instance Sernelj 2014, 84–85.

[6] For example, Mou completely neglects the important school of thought based on Xunzi's interpretation of original Confucianism, which has been the basis of dominant, political, or institutionalized Confucianism throughout Chinese history (see e.g., Rogacz 2017 and Du 2017).

[7] For a standard translation, please see Wilhelm and Baynes 2011.

[8] 乾道變化，各正性命.

[9] 終日乾乾，反復道也.

[10] 或躍在淵，乾道乃革.

[11] 坤道其順乎，承天而時行.

> Although *yin* has excellent qualities, their implementation in rulership cannot complete it. This is the principle (or method) of the earth, the wife, and the minister. The method or principle of earth is without completion but can only be accomplished through transformation via successive replacements.[12]

In my view, this means that any activity can only be completed through mutual complementarity between both principles, that of *Qian* with that of *Kun*, that of *yang* with that of *yin*, and so on.

But what we have seen from all these fragments is that *dao* can hardly be compared to morality as it is commonly understood.[13] Although the cosmic principles can be projected to society in the sense that one has to act in accordance with principles guiding the paradigm that defines one's own social role, they can only function in reciprocal relations with their respective other. This is not about morality in the sense of a free will of an autonomous subject, nor a morality implemented by a moral subject of virtue ethics.

However, because Yuk Hui sees *dao* primarily as a moral category, he tries to compare it with the ancient Greek distinction between *technê* and *aretê*. Hence, my third question is the following:

(C) Is the comparison with the ancient Greek relation between *technê* and *aretê* suitable?

Again, my answer is negative. As we have seen in the previous discussion, *dao* is quite different from *aretê*, for it is neither a virtue nor a moral category. The term *qi*, on the other hand, is quite comparable to the ancient Greek notion of *technê*. It includes both the connotation of a skill as well as the narrow utilitarian perspective that can lead to pure instrumental rationality if not controlled by moral or rational principles. This insight has profound implications for grasping the distinct Chinese relationship between technology and nature. It informs our understanding of the Chinese system of cosmotechnology and science, highlighting its significance. Furthermore, it sheds light on the traditional Chinese perspective on the relationship between human beings and nature, thereby enriching the discourse on Chinese ecology.

However, Yuk Hui's comparison between the terms *dao* and *qi* on the one side, and the ancient Greek terms *technê* and *aretê* on the other, is particularly problematic for two reasons. As we have just seen, *dao* cannot be reduced to moral connotation, but rather represents an all-pervasive cosmic order, and simultaneously a method through which every phenomenon can be brought into coherence with this natural cosmic order.

---

[12] 陰雖有美「含」之以從王事，弗敢成也。地道也，妻道也，臣道也。地道「无成」而代「有終」也。

[13] Such a meaning was ascribed to the word *dao* only much later, through Confucian commentaries on this work, and thus also exclusively in the context of the Confucian view of the cosmos. Of course, we must take into account here that such an understanding, within which the universe is saturated with moral principles, had, due to the dominant position of Confucianism, already acquired a paradigmatic status in the early Middle Ages. This moral component is particularly noticeable in the compound word *rendao* 人道, which refers to the "Way of humankind" and describes human ethical maxims. In the *Book of Changes* itself, which is much older, *dao* is seen only in its most basic meaning of the Way, that is, the methods, principles, and modes of action.

Secondly, Yuk Hui portrays *dao* as superior and primary relative to *qi*, contrasting with the ancient Greek perspective, which, from Aristotle onward, he perceives as more instrumental, emphasizing the means to achieve ends. According to Yuk Hui (2016, 89), this distinction highlights the essence of what would, in the last two centuries of the previous millennium, become foundational to Western modernization: instrumental reason.

But while both *technê* and *qi* 器 are similar in that they both can evolve toward pure utility when not guided by controlling forces, *aretê* is very different from *dao* 道. Being the guiding principle of ancient Greek *technê*, *aretê* is relying on morality. It is the external moral subject, the bearer of virtue, that controls the faceless and heartless *technê*. In the Chinese case, on the other hand, the utilitarian element contained in *qi* must be guided by the creative principle, *dao*, inherent in the method of its creation, which always aims to establish the harmonious flow and balance between nature and culture, human beings, and technology.

6.4 Conclusion

Thus, the proper relationship between *dao* and *qi* in the *Yijing* is based on a continuous, dynamic process of unceasing adjustment. The criteria or the main standard for such tendencies are not based on any kind of normative morality, but on the principle of balance, which is typical of the classical Chinese worldview and manifests itself in many different terms, such as harmony (*he*), equilibrium (*zhong*), or the proper measure (*du*). Since all these concepts are the foundations of the elemental paradigms that make up the Chinese worldview, balance between people and their environment[14]is actually built into the basic structure of the frames of reference that defines most dominant Chinese philosophies and systems of ideas. This idea of balance seems to be at the core of what might be called the specific Chinese teleology.

Nowadays, it has become quite clear that technological development, which—if left to its own devices and guided only by the narrowly utilitarian, profit-oriented tendencies of our current political and economic systems—can lead to serious ecological disasters, must be managed and controlled in the most life-enhancing way possible. Here, we might ask ourselves whether it is better to let technology develop at its own pace and to intervene in this development from the outside through subsequent application of *aretê*, or whether it would be better to follow an inherent teleological principle in this development, adhering to an organism-friendly paradigm of equilibrium (*dao*), instead of following the instrumentally rational, capitalist laws of profit-maximization.

---

[14] Roger Ames, Cheng Chung-ying, Chen Guying, along with other scholars, refer to the pursuit of harmony between the natural world and human society as "the study of heaven and humankind" (天人之學). This pivotal idea was initially introduced by Wang Fuzhi, as documented by Liu (2003). Cheng Chung-ying further developed this concept in his 1987 work. For significant contemporary explorations of this notion, refer to the works of Ames (2023) and Chen (2018).

And what does this mean for today's global world, so burdened by acute, all-encompassing ecological crises of planetary proportions? At least for the near future, it could open our eyes to the fact that prevention is better than cure. In this context, however, we must also realize that it is not only the application but also the very nature of the production or creation of technology that affects our environment in the most severe and problematic ways. This includes rethinking and possibly changing the utilitarian and profit-oriented nature of our current political and economic systems.

Acknowledgements The research for this chapter was financed by ARIS, grant numbers P6-0243 and J6-50202.

References

Ames, Roger T. 2023. Zoetology: A new name for an old way of thinking. *Royal Institute of Philosophy Supplements* 23: 81–98.

Boodberg, Peter A. 1953. The semasiology of some primary Confucian concepts. *Philosophy East and West* 2 (4): 317–332.

Chen, Guyin. 2018. Tracing the Origins of Humanist Philosophy in Early China. In Chen Guyin. *The Humanist Spirit of Daoism.* Tr. Hans-Georg Moeller. Leiden: Brill, 138–168.

Du, Lun. 2017. The early Zhou period: origin of the idea of political legitimacy and the political philosophy of Confucianism. *Asian Studies* 5 (1): 67–80.

Heidegger, Martin. 2000. Die Frage nach der Technik. In *7*, ed. Gesamtausgabe I. Vol, 5–36. Frankfurt am Main: Vittorio Klostermann.

Hui Yuk 许煜. 2018. "Qi" yu "dao": chao renleizhuyi weilaide yizhong huiyi '器' 与 '道': 超人类主义未来的一种回应 [*Qi* and *Dao*: A Response to a Transhumanist Future]. *Shehui kexue bao*: https://www.sohu.com/a/228200401_550962. Accessed December 12, 2022.

Hui, Yuk. 2016. *The Question Concerning Technology in China: An Essay in Cosmotechnics.* Falmouth: Urbanomic.

Leroi-Gourhan, André. 1945. *Milieu et Techniques.* Paris: Albin Michel.

Li, Zehou, and Jane Cauvel. 2006. *Four Essays on Aesthetics: Toward a Global View.* Lanham, MD: Lexington Books.

Li Zehou. 1999. A few questions concerning the history of Chinese aesthetics (Excerpts). *Contemporary Chinese Thought* 31 (2): 66–76.

Li Zehou 李澤厚. 2016. *Renleixue Lishi Bentilun* 人類學歷史本體論 [Anthropo-historical ontology]. Qingdao: Qingdao chuban she.

Liu Xingbang 刘兴邦. 2003. Lun Wang Fuzhide "Tian Renzhi Xue" 论王夫之的 "天人之学". *Chuanshan Xuekan* 船山学刊 4: 9–13.

Rogacz, D. 2017. In the shadow of the decay. The philosophy of history of Mencius and Xunzi. *Asian Studies* 5 (1): 147–715.

Rošker, Jana S. 2018. *Following His Own Path.* Albany, NY: State University of New York Press.

Sernelj, Tea. 2014. The unity of body and mind in Xu Fuguan's theory. *Asian Studies* 2 (1): 83–95.

Wilhelm, Richard and Cary F. Baynes (tr.). 2011. The I Ching or Book of Changes. Princeton, NJ: Princeton University Press.

Chapter 7
The Ideas of Dynamism and Stability in the *Yijing* and Modern/Contemporary Thought

Rein Raud

Abstract It has often been pointed out that the Chinese philosophical tradition as a whole resounds more with process ontologies than object-oriented ones, and a vocabulary for the description of reality as a dynamic plenum is indeed to be found in the *Yijing*, particularly in the *Ten Wings* treatises. In this chapter, I am going to have a look at some passages in the "Xici" (or "Dazhuan") treatise and compare them to certain ideas expressed by Xiong Shili, the founder of New Confucianism, as well as Thomas Nail, one of the proponents of dynamism-based philosophy active at present. In order to do this, I will also introduce a way of analyzing multi-layered Chinese philosophical concepts that relies on the theories of Algirdas Greimas and his "semiotic quadrangle" in particular. As a result, I hope to show that the ontological language of the *Yijing* prefigures several crucial insights on which varieties of modern and contemporary process philosophy rely.

Keywords *Yijing* · Algirdas Greimas · Xiong Shili · Thomas Nail · Process philosophy

7.1 Introduction

While it would most certainly be incorrect to characterize the methods used by the *Yijing* as "science" in the proper sense of the word, there are nonetheless certain similarities between the basic dispositions of these two knowledge systems. Both natural science and the divination system elaborated in the *Yijing* propose technologies of observation of any present situation and set themselves the goal of extrapolating the most probable possible futures from it. Both presuppose an ontology, or axiomatically accepted claims about how the world is, as well as a set of methodological principles for extracting and interpreting the necessary data that allows them to make their predictions. The *Yijing* assumes that the world is available to us in situations,

R. Raud (✉)
School of Humanities, Tallinn University, Tallinn, Estonia
e-mail: rein.raud@tlu.ee

G. Sigurðsson and T. Hon (eds.), *Contemporary Interpretations and Readings of the Yijing*, Chinese Culture 15, https://doi.org/10.1007/978-981-96-0609-2_7

which share certain sets of defining features that can be exemplified in patterns of interpenetration of two primary ontological poles, the *yang* (rigidity, light, male) and the *yin* (flexibility, darkness, female). These situation patterns can be represented by symbols consisting of six lines (hexagrams), each of which refers to either of these two poles. Science, for most of its history, has relied on the assumption that reality is decomposable into indivisible, self-identical solid minimal elements, which relate to each other in measurable ways governed by immutable laws. Both systems assert that we can find these laws and patterns out and make predictions about the behavior of the world on their basis.

All of this is not to say that the methods of the *Yijing* system are well-grounded and can produce the promised results, unlike the better part of science. The ways in which the correlation between the system of situation patterns and the actual affairs of daily life is determined according to it are without any doubt illegitimate. Assuming that the random occurrences (coin tosses, separations of yarrow stalk bunches) that guide the divination process have any relation to how things really stand at the moment is an axiomatic presupposition that lacks any foundation except belief. However, similarly illegitimate beliefs have also been firmly held by earlier representatives of the Western scientific tradition, such as the alchemists or the phrenologists, and are still held by the currently active creationists and racists. What natural science does, and the tradition of the *Yijing* does not, however, is the systematic questioning of its axiomatic claims. For example, when the results that experimentation has yielded are consistently incompatible with the currently endorsed theoretical paradigm, then it is the paradigm that has to be at fault. This has allowed science to evolve by discarding previous firmly held beliefs in favor of new, often more complex, but also more adequate and more readily applicable narratives about the nature of the world.

As a result of that process, science has now, somewhat surprisingly, also abandoned quite a few of those tenets that have strictly opposed it to other regimes of knowledge production in the past. In particular, this applies to the view that the act of measuring the processes of nature is somehow itself beyond nature and, given the increasing precision of measurement apparatuses, can attain absolute accuracy at some point. The classical paradigm of science appealed to god's-eye objectivity, but contemporary philosophy of science, since Heisenberg, admits the embeddedness of the scientist and the impact of the measuring systems on what is measured (Heisenberg 1958, 52). This brings the pattern of thought in contemporary scientific practice closer to some of the axiomatic formal assumptions that the *Yijing* tradition has held, and which have been incompatible with science in the past. The *Yijing* divination technique posits a clear link between the act of predicting the future from extrapolations of the present situation, which is seen holistically, while the Pre-Heisenbergian scientific practice of the West has always denied the link between the act of measuring any aspects of the present situation and that situation itself, which is seen as objectively carved up according to a number of parameters and categories. We now know that this latter assumption has been false. If we accept the consequences of that realization—namely the view that the scientists involved in the experiments and measurements are themselves also elements of it, "kinetic operators," as Thomas Nail (2021, 214) has called them—then we should have no trouble in simultaneously accepting the view that the ancient Chinese divination expert is also not engaged in finding out the details of a pre-determined future, but rather in the act of *producing* it. Indeed, the description of the sage in "Xici" I 4 suggests precisely that: 範圍天地之化而不過, 曲成萬物而不遺 "he contains the transformations of heaven and earth and does not go beyond them; he brings to completion the myriad things and does not leave any of them out."

When we think of how predictions can influence an actual state of affairs—for example, how a rumor that a certain (completely solvent) bank is about to go bankrupt may prompt its customers to withdraw their money and thereby actually cause its bankruptcy—we are in a better position to see how both scientific and divination-based observations about reality, regardless of their accuracy, can influence the course of the very transformations they study. Again, this is obviously not to put them on an equal footing or even on the same side of a watershed between the rational and the irrational, but to show that a gradient exists on which they can both be situated, even if at considerable distance from each other. It is this gradient that makes the comparison between scientific and *Yijing* discourses possible and lets us think of their philosophical underpinnings in the same vein.

In what follows, it will be my aim to have a look at the notions of dynamism and stability and how they are conceptualized in the *Yijing* as well as in recent and contemporary process philosophy which, in turn, has been co-developing with quantum physics. I will not be making claims that the *Yijing* somehow anticipates quantum physics or that recent developments in science somehow vindicate alternative (i.e., non-scientific) forms of knowledge. What interests me here is a certain modality of thought, which privileges change and dynamism over stability and stasis. The *Yijing* is certainly one of the earliest texts in the collective human heritage that explicitly manifests this modality, and this is why it has remained relevant as a source of serious philosophical study to this day.

7.2 The Yijing and its Expressive Style

The *Yijing*, just like the Bible or the Avesta, is not a single text, but a cluster of multiple textual strata, in which later ones clarify and modify earlier ones, and cryptic remarks (initially written down perhaps as memory aides for preserving a primarily orally transmitted knowledge) gradually gave way to more systematic elaborations of philosophically relevant thoughts. In particular, a treatise included in the latest layer of the book called the *Ten Wings*, a rather short and self-contained text entitled "Xici" ("Appended Remarks," often referred to as the "Dazhuan" or "Great Commentary"), presents us with a systematic construction of ontological language, even if it remains largely undeployed in other layers of the text, perhaps due to its practical rather than speculative orientation. It has been noted that after the Han dynasty nearly all references to the *Yijing* in philosophical texts refer to this treatise (Nylan 2001, 209).

The earliest extant manuscript of the "Xici" is dated 168 BCE (Ames 2015, 2), and the decades preceding that date are also the most likely time of its appearance, although traditionally it has been claimed that the ideas therein were already in circulation at the time of Kongzi and may have been distilled into their current shape over time (Peterson 1982, 73–77). In form, it is written on the topic of the two extremities of the spectrum of patterns that make up the world—the hexagram *Qian*, which consists of pure *yang*, and the hexagram *Kun*, which is pure *yin*.

However, neither pure *yang* nor pure *yin* can be met in reality. It has been suggested that the limitation of situation patterns to the canonical number of 64 hexagrams is itself an arbitrary move to keep the conceptual apparatus manageable, but yet sufficiently precise (Cheng 2020: 40): the system of eight trigrams from which the tradition of divination is supposed to have evolved is too crude to make accurate characterization of situations possible, but further precision, such as a possible system of 512 "nonagrams," which would render the characterizations slightly more accurate, would be too complicated to master. The latter consideration here outweighs the former. Just as we use a rough approximation of π in our calculations of the relation between the diameter and the circumference of a circle, the results of divination are considered to be both detailed enough and accurate enough within the paradigm of 64 situation patterns. Therefore, situations considered to fall under *Qian* or *Kun* are indeed possible, but not because they would fully correspond to the appropriate extremities of the range, but because the presence of the opposite element in them is negligible.

Another factor that dislodges any approach to this ontology that wants to rely on rigid binary oppositions is the relevance of the composition of every situation pattern. We know from chemistry that different substances can have the same chemical composition. Both ethanol and dimethyl ether, two substances that exhibit quite different behavior, fall under the formula C_2H_6O, but ethanol is more correctly represented as CH_3CH_2OH and dimethyl ether as CH_3OCH_3. Similarly, there are 18 hexagrams in which there are three *yin* lines and three *yang* lines, with very different explanations attached.

One final thing to mention about the modality of thought in which the "Xici" has been written is characteristic of Classical Chinese works in general: it is the paratactic rhythm of parallels and oppositions that facilitates the transmission of meaning, helping to determine the role each particular character assumes in otherwise often ambiguous phrase structures. If all the phrase structures were strictly parallel, however, then long passages of text would become exceedingly monotonous (and that would limit the expressible meaning considerably), thus parallels are balanced with oppositions on various levels. The evolution of this technique culminated in the so-called "parallel prose" (駢文 *pianwen*) that appeared during the Han dynasty, but the tendencies that led there can be observed from early writings onward. The effects of these stylistic features on the expressive-interpretive field of a Chinese text have been well documented and analyzed by Vladimir Spirin (2006); on the whole we can say that, in contrast with the primarily unilinear Western textual paradigm, Chinese texts present us with a multidimensionality that requires a different analytic approach.

7.3 The Greimassian Semantic Quadrangle and the Ontological Discourse of the "Xici"

What I would now like to propose as a methodological tool for the analysis of the ontological discourse that has been tentatively formulated in the "Xici" is the so-called "semantic quadrangle" proposed by Algirdas Julius Greimas (1983, 1987). Unlike any analytical tools relying on simple binary oppositions, Greimassian semantics makes the simultaneous consideration of parallelisms and oppositions feasible. Generalizing from the works of various structuralist thinkers (Barthes 1990; Lévi-Strauss 1983a, 1983b), who were all in pursuit of minimal meaning-carrying units, Greimas has proposed the concept of a *seme*, or atomic carrier of meaning, which, in the structuralist tradition, is always definable as one pole in a binary opposition. Instead of the usual singularly defined binary opposition, however, Greimas distinguishes between contradiction and contrariety, which both allow for the construction of an oppositional axis (1987: 49). As a result, a minimal unit of signification always has both a contrary and an implied opposite—the former being its negative counterpart and the latter its absence. Thus, the contrary of "life" is "death," while the opposite of "life" is "non-life" (or the realm of the anorganic). Logically, the fourth corner of the quadrangle has to be simultaneously the opposite of the first contrary (or "death" in the example) and the contrary of the first opposite (or "non-life")—which, in the present case, would amount to ghosts and zombies, the "undead." These, according to Greimas, are the contradictories, or categories to which a term cannot simultaneously belong. Figure 7.1 presents the result:

Greimas also applies this framework to normative rules, discussing these in detail, using the example of sexual relations in traditional French society (1987: 52–58), showing how the poles of "prescribed" (= heterosexual matrimony) and "prohibited" (= incest and homosexuality) correlate with "not prohibited" (= infidelity by men) and "not prescribed" (= infidelity by women).

As we can see, this view presumes a certain ambiguity at the heart of any carrier of meaning, an inherent tension between two axes of signifying, both of which become

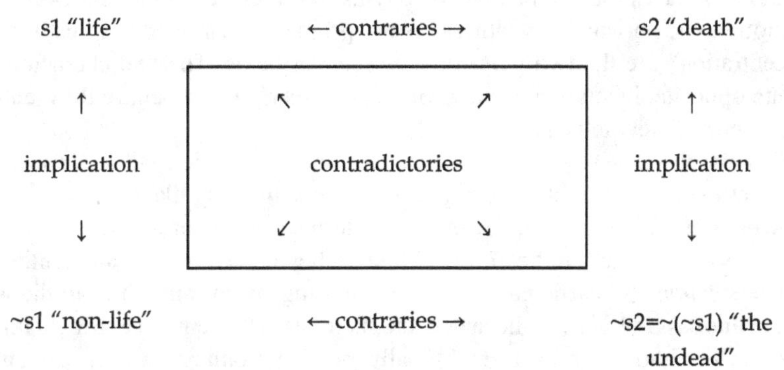

Fig. 7.1 The semantic quadrangle according to A. J. Greimas

manifest through the act of negation. If we envisage each instance of contextualized signification as the intersection of two equally defining binary axes, then either of those can be taken as primary (substantial) and the other as secondary (accidental) for the construction of parallels and oppositions. For example, if we think of snow as cold and soft, then it can be parallel to ice on the cold-hot axis and oppose it on the hard-soft axis, and at the same time be parallel to sand on the soft-hot axes and oppose it on the cold-hot axis. In the actual semantic system, of course, it is never just two binary axes that define a unit of meaning, but the imagining of a duplicity is already an important step ahead of simple, singular binaries.

This duplicity is very similar to the double character of the context-embedded Chinese character, which has both parallel—and opposition-building capacities in relation to other characters that occur in similar positions in structurally corresponding phrases elsewhere in the text. This is why it seems that the semantic quadrangle of Greimas is indeed well suited for a close reading of passages that expound discourses about the nature of the world, such as the following extract from the “Xici” (I 6):

> 夫易, 廣矣大矣, 以言乎遠, 則不禦。以言乎邇, 則靜而正。以言乎天地之間, 則備矣。夫乾, 其靜也專, 其動也直, 是以大生焉。夫坤, 其靜也翕, 其動也闢, 是以廣生焉。廣大配天地, 變通配四時, 陰陽之義配日月, 易簡之善配至德。
>
> Speaking of the change-process [as a whole], it has great extension and great intensity. When we say it reaches distances, this indicates that it cannot be controlled. When we say it takes place near us, this indicates its stability and authenticity. When we say it fills the space between Heaven and Earth, this indicates its completeness. Speaking of *Qian*, its stability is particular, its dynamism is linear. This is how intensity acquires its generative power. Speaking of *Kun*, its stability consists in folding, its dynamism consists in unfolding. This is how extension acquires its generative power. The polarity of extension and intensity corresponds to the polarity between heaven and earth. The complementarity of transformations and resilience corresponds to [the principle governing the alteration of] the four seasons. The logic of *yin* and *yang* corresponds to [the principle governing the alternation of] the sun and the moon. The goodness of the simplicity of the change-process corresponds to the highest degree of virtuous energy.

This passage needs to be read carefully. For example, it might seem that *guang* 廣 and *da* 大 are simply repetitive synonyms, but they act in the text as poles on a semiotic axis, on which "greatness” is the primary given, while “spreading” and “concentration” are the two poles of the secondary axis. The two characters thus indicate opposite, incompatible ways of being “great,” which behave differently, as the text immediately tells us.

When we place the key terms of the passage into a semantic quadrangle according to the method elaborated above (Fig. 7.2), we get something like this:

It would be incorrect to assert that these terms are part of a discourse that has been widely elaborated in the *Yijing*, although they do create such a potential. The characters *zhuan* 專 “particular” and *xi* 翕 “folding” occur only once in the whole work, in this passage; *zhi* 直 “linear” occurs six times in the sense of a straight line and twice for “straightforward, sincere.” Finally, *pi* 闢 “unfolding,” is only encountered in the “Xici” and not in other parts of the *Yijing*, but in the other context of this text, too, it simply refers to the opening of a door. It may therefore be legitimately claimed

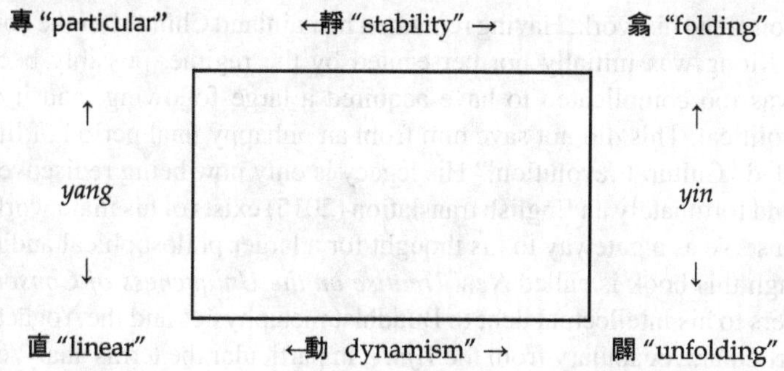

Fig. 7.2 The semantic quadrangle of the *Yijing*

that this single passage is insufficient for the description of an ontological discourse, but, as we shall see, the terms have been picked up for precisely that purpose in the twentieth century by Xiong Shili, and that alone should be considered sufficient ground for their analysis in their original context.

What we observe here are two axes of parallel-opposition forming, one of them between the polarity of stability and dynamism, the other between *yang* and *yin*. We are accustomed to thinking of *yang* as stable and *yin* as dynamic, but in this passage both of them (in the form of the hexagram consisting of only *yang* or *yin* lines) have a stable as well as a dynamic aspect. *Yang* here stands for singular, self-identical things as opposed to the general flux, movement along distinct lines with a specific direction, while *yin* refers to a movement occurring even in stability, which can consist both in a retreat into itself and a movement coming from the inside and spreading out, perhaps even occurring in multiple directions simultaneously. We need to leave the actual square empty here, because this is where each individual occurrence of being would be located: any single thing consists of both *yang* and *yin*, and is therefore heuristically somewhere within the square, its identity or being-itself-ness consisting in the balance of its particularity/folding on one hand and its embeddedness in the flux, which takes place, in turn, as a balance of linear and unfolding movement on the other. This rather complicated scheme of things nonetheless reflects a consistent ontology of a dynamic plenum, which can serve as a basis for a practical discourse of sociocosmic order.

7.4 The Dynamic Ontology of Xiong Shili 熊十力 (1885–1968)

In an ideal world, Xiong Shili would certainly stand in line with the great thinkers of the twentieth century such as Henri Bergson, Edmund Husserl, Alfred North Whitehead, Ludwig Wittgenstein, Martin Heidegger, and Nishida Kitarō. As things stand, very few people even among the specialists in Chinese studies have heard of him, let alone read his work. Having remained in mainland China after the communist takeover, Xiong was initially not persecuted by the regime, possibly because his thought was too complicated to have acquired a large following, and it was also fairly unpolitical. This did not save him from an unhappy final period of life during the so-called "Cultural revolution." His legacy is only now being rediscovered little by little, and fortunately an English translation (2015) exists of his main work (2008), which can serve as a gateway to his thought for a larger philosophical audience.

Although this book is called *New Treatise on the Uniqueness of Consciousness*, which refers to his intellectual debt to Buddhist metaphysics and the Yogācāra tradition in particular, vocabulary from the *Yijing*, in particular the terms analyzed above, play a central role in his thought, and the discourse expounded in the passage quoted above is taken up at the very beginning of his discussion of "transformation": "It is transformation alone that moves but cannot be controlled; that changes but cannot be fathomed." (2015, 94).

In Xiong's ontology, there is no external cause to change, which is all there is, a "great thing" (大物 *dawu*) that is undergoing constant transformation and is the only reality (2015, 95). The nature of that transformation is described as a simultaneous unitary 翕 *xi* "folding" and 闢 *pi* "unfolding." John Makeham has translated these terms as "contraction" and "expansion," respectively: "One contraction and one expansion is called transformation" (2015: 96). Xiong's (2008, 32) own formulation is rather cryptic: 一翕一闢之謂變. It is unclear how the "one" should be read—does it refer to one total cosmic movement, or one minimal movement in the constitution of a prospective entity? Xiong's autocommentary is also not very helpful here, simply saying "These two 'one' words simply highlight different tendencies (勢 *Shi*) in dynamism" (2015, 96).

Unlike the Buddhist impermanence, Xiong's constantly transforming reality is a plenum, "because nothingness cannot transform" (2015, 95). It seems appropriate to interpret the "folding" taking place within this plenum as referring to a tendency to become wholly material, a movement toward an unreachable state of solidity, while "unfolding" is a force that acts within that folding as a sort of self-assertion over the environment, tendency to establish itself, to rule (Xiong actually equates this to the ruler, 2015, 98). While Xiong emphasizes that the words "material" and "mental" lack stable referents and therefore only such transformation takes place (2008, 33; 2015, 98), he nonetheless derives what we perceive as material and mental from "folding" and "unfolding," respectively. It should also be noted here that notwithstanding his affirmation of the Chinese-style plenum of being, Xiong is also a presentist in the Buddhist tradition and sees reality as the constant arising and ceasing of dimensionless, momentary being-instances that occur without intervals; thus, any talk about "matter" and "mind" is secondary to these two tendencies that make up the constant transformation.

When we look at the two *Yijing* concepts in Xiong's interpretation, a further parallel suggests itself with the intuitions of Henri Bergson, in particular as expressed in a passage of *Introduction to Metaphysics*, where he discusses the extremities of duration (which in Bergson's parlance occupies the role that transformation plays for Xiong):

> …The intuition of our duration, far from leaving us suspended in the void as pure analysis would do, brings us into contact with a whole continuity of durations which we must try to follow, whether downwards or upwards; in both cases we can extend ourselves indefinitely by an increasingly violent effort, in both cases we transcend ourselves. In the first we advance towards a more and more attenuated duration, the pulsations of which, being rapider than ours, and dividing our simple sensation, dilute its quality into quantity; at the limit would be pure homogeneity, that pure repetition by which we define materiality. Advancing in the other direction, we approach a duration which strains, contracts, and intensifies itself more and more; at the limit would be eternity. No longer conceptual eternity, which is an eternity of death, but an eternity of life. A living, and therefore still moving eternity in which our own particular duration would be included as the vibrations are in light; an eternity which would he the concentration of all duration, as materiality is its dispersion. Between these two extreme limits intuition moves, and this movement is the very essence of metaphysics (1912, 63–64).

It seems that the two described ways of advancement, in spite of the obvious differences, bear distinct conceptual similarity to the two movements of Xiong's change, "expansion" being parallel to the attenuated duration reaching for the pure homogeneity of absolute matter, and "contraction" to the movement toward eternity as the concentration of all duration.

For considerations of space, I will not be able to engage in a further comparative analysis of Bergson's and Xiong's views here, but I hope that these cursory parallels show how the metaphysical vocabulary of the *Yijing* and its elaborations by Xiong have an important place in the evolution of process philosophy also outside the context of Chinese thought.

7.5 Movement and Folding in the Philosophy of Thomas Nail

One further thinker to be addressed here is one of the currently most influential process theorists, namely Thomas Nail, whose works (2019, 2021, 2024) have proposed an original ontology that privileges change and movement over identity and stability. As this is also my own position, I consider myself to be on his side as far as the principal divide between object- and process-oriented philosophy is concerned, but nonetheless there are certain major differences between his ontology and mine as it has been expressed in *Being in Flux* (2021). It seems, in fact, that the ontological discourse of the *Yijing* and its derivates in Xiong's philosophy constitute a very good background for clarifying them.

Nail has repeatedly stressed that his philosophical inquiries, speculative and historical, do not venture beyond the Western tradition (2019, 445; 2021, 285; 2024, 11, n.13) although he readily acknowledges the existence of non-Western dynamism-based philosophical systems. In his writings, he has also provided a pedigree of the Western minority tradition that reaches down to the Minoan civilization of pre-classical Greek antiquity, although his analyses of the latter (2024, 21–31, 73–78, 111–125), based as they are on pictorial material rather than texts (which are not available), remain somewhat speculative. With the Chinese case, on the other hand, we stand on a much firmer ground. It remains to be hoped that Nail will turn his attention toward the non-Western traditions at some point, which could serve to strengthen his theory in a considerable way.

The structure of Nail's ontology is more complicated than can be presented in a brief summary, but, at least for the present purposes, we can form an idea of it through its central concepts of *flow*, *loop/fold,* and *field*. The three are co-primary and inseparable (2019, 67). When Nail speaks about matter, he insists that it is not substantial (2021, 25), but consists in the flow, understood as the twinning of movement and continuity, the latter being a prerequisite of the former (2019, 68). However, in order to rescue the concept of the self-identical individual object, a "metastable formation of matter in motion" (2021, 4), Nail introduces the idea of the fold, which "is produced by the junction or intersection of a flow *with itself*… A fold is like an eddy or whirlpool in the flows of being. It is a relative stasis that is always secondary to the primacy of the flows and events that compose it… Flow and fold are thus co-constituted in the same immanent kinetic process… A fold is the repetition of a kinetic differential: a cycle" (2019, 99–100, italics in original). This is how metastable individuals come into being: objects "fold" into relatively stable patterns or cycles (2021, 31) which never repeat precisely (2021, 37)—there is no discrete unity, but only "a series of material processes of folding and unfolding" (2021, 38). Together, these processes create an environment in which they can relate to each other. "Flows join into metastable folds, and folds are conjoined into things, but things are also arranged and ordered together through a field of circulation… If flows intersect and folds periodically cycle, fields organize them all in a continuous feedback loop" (2019, 129).

Each individual, constituted in this manner, is constantly undergoing two types of motion simultaneously: extensive, which takes an object from one spatial location to another, and intensive, which occurs within a localized situation (2021, 25). These movements are not random, but also not determinate—they are *pedetic*, that is, they occur within a range of possibilities, but remain unpredictable, as they are caused by the interaction of infinitely many heterogeneous trajectories of movement (2021, 26–27); pedetic movements are generative of order, and the patterns of order "are what we call objects" (2021, 28).

It seems to me that the similarities of Nail's ontology to the language of being deployed in the *Yijing* and in particular the interpretation of its concepts in the work of Xiong are striking precisely because Nail has never interacted with the Chinese tradition. Yet the parallels are obvious. The idea of folding, or contraction, of a holistic movement-continuity form the basis of all three systems discussed here. Contraction produces cyclically repetitive, locally stable processual knots that, if their movement patterns follow the same rhythm, interrelate with each other as if in stasis. Fundamentally, however, no stasis is possible, because continuous transformation undermines it on a more basic level. Nail's extensive and intensive movement parallel the *yang*- and *yin*-type movements, respectively. The resulting ontological systems allow for a treatment of the relatively stable in fundamentally dynamic terms and establish a middle position between the received object-centered metaphysics of the

Western tradition and the more radically dynamic ontology proposed by Buddhist philosophy, especially in the Chinese forms of it that came into being through its creative encounter with Lao-Zhuang thought.

What the three systems of the *Yijing*, Xiong, and Nail also share is the axiomatically postulated dynamic substance, or the primacy of the mover over the process of movement. In the vocabulary of the traditional Chinese worldview, this primal stuff is called *qi* and is neither material nor energetic, but forms both through its contractions and expansions. For Xiong, as said, the monistic "great thing" also constitutes a plenum, because he, too, rejects the idea that nothingness can be in transformation. Finally, Nail, in defining the fold, postulates the continuity of what moves to the extent that intersect "with itself," which cannot be read otherwise than as a claim that past phases of a process share their being with the present as well as the future phases of the process in a substantial way. It is therefore entirely correct to call Nail's ontology *kinetic* (as he does) and not *dynamic*: just as most of the Western tradition, it does not think of movement without a mover.

This is also where I have to part company with Nail because I do not think that the axiomatic requirement of a primal, substantially understood being is justifiable as self-evident, especially if physical matter is only considered to be its derivative. As I have argued elsewhere, any entity, any "it" that can intersect with itself is the result of an act of entification, or extraction of certain segments of the flux of being from it; there is no selfsame continuity in that flux, but only significant overlap, and the significance of the overlap is determined by the perspective of the observer (Raud 2021, 18–23, 36–39, 45–48). I do therefore completely agree with Nail that scientists can be considered "kinetic operators" (Nail 2021, 216–19) who co-create their objects through their acts of observation, but, unlike Nail, I do not think it is justified to credit objects with a self-sameness that is independent of any observers at all. My reason for rejecting such a claim is simple: I believe that one of the imminent tasks of contemporary philosophy is to evolve beyond the anthropocentric worldview that characterizes most of the Western tradition (as well as a rather significant part of the Chinese one), and this simply cannot be done by assuming that reality has observer-independently the same structure as the human mind discerns in it.

7.6 Conclusions

What I hope to have shown here is that the ontological language of the *Yijing* prefigures several crucial insights on which some versions of modern and contemporary process philosophy rely. Importantly, as we now know, these ideas are in a better accord with the views advanced by contemporary natural science than are the classical ontological discourses of the West, even if the conceptual language is not deployed and developed in the *Yijing* in a systematic manner. Nonetheless, we can say that the paradigmatic changes of Western science have given the pre- or protoscientific intuitions and ideas of the *Yijing* a higher degree of relevance than they would have had in the context of classical Western science. Up to now, however, these ideas have been discussed mainly within the framework of the Chinese tradition, and, in the case of Xiong Shili, in dialogue with the Buddhist branches of it, but it seems evident—as demonstrated by the parallels with the philosophy of Thomas Nail—that they have a significant potential also for a dialogue with Western thought and need to be taken seriously also by those philosophers who are not engaged with specifically cross-cultural projects. It remains to be hoped that this dialogue is now finally beginning.

References

Ames, Roger T. 2015. The great commentary (Dazhuan 大傳) and Chinese natural cosmology. *International Communication of Chinese Culture* 2 (1): 1–18.

Barthes, Roland. 1990. *The Fashion System*. Tr. Matthew Ward and Richard Howard. Berkeley, CA: University of California Press.

Bergson, Henri. 1912. *An Introduction to Metaphysics*. Tr. T. E. Hulme. New York and London: G. P. Putnam's sons.

Cheng, Chung-Ying. 2020. *The Primary Way: Philosophy of Yijing*. Albany, NY: State University of New York Press.

Greimas, Algirdas Julien. 1983. *Structural Semantics: An Attempt at a Method*. Tr. Daniele McDowell, Ronald Schleifer, and Alan Velie. Lincoln, NE: Nebraska University Press.

Greimas, Algirdas Julien. 1987. *On Meaning: Selected Writings in Semiotic Theory*. Tr. Paul Perron and Frank H. Collins. Minneapolis, MN: University of Minnesota Press.

Heisenberg, Werner. 1958. *Physics and Philosophy; the Revolution in Modern Science*. New York: Harper.

Lévi-Strauss, Claude. 1983a. *Structural Anthropology*. Tr. Claire Jacobson and Brooke G. Schoepf. Chicago: University of Chicago Press.

Lévi-Strauss, Claude. 1983b. *The Raw and the Cooked*. Tr. John and Doreen Weightman. Chicago: University of Chicago Press.

Nail, Thomas. 2019. *Being and Motion*. Oxford: Oxford University Press.

Nail, Thomas. 2021. *Theory of the Object*. Edinburgh: Edinburgh University Press.

Nail, Thomas. 2024. *Matter and Motion. A Brief History of Kinetic Materialism*. Edinburgh: Edinburgh University Press.

Nylan, Michael. 2001. *The Five "Confucian" Classics*. New Haven, CT: Yale University Press.

Peterson, Willard J. 1982. Making connections: Commentary on the attached verbalizations of the *Book of Change*. *Harvard Journal of Asiatic Studies* 42 (1): 67–116.

Raud, Rein. 2021. *Being in Flux: A Post-Anthropocentric Ontology of the Self*. Cambridge: Polity.

Spirin, Vladimir. 2006. *Postroenie Drevnekitaiskikh Tekstov*. St. Petersburg: Peterburgskoie Vostokovedenie.

Xiong, Shili. 2008. *Xinweishilun*. Beijing: Shijichuban.

Xiong, Shili. 2015. *New Treatise on the Uniqueness of Consciousness*. Tr. John Makeham. New Haven, CT: Yale University Press.

Chapter 8
Yin-Yang and Whitehead's Process Philosophy

Haipeng Guo

Abstract This paper explores the connections between Alfred North Whitehead's process philosophy and traditional Chinese philosophy, focusing on the *Yin-Yang* concept from the *Book of Changes*. By analyzing Whitehead's earlier works on the philosophy of nature and his later writings on metaphysics and cosmology, we identify eight conceptual pairs that align with the *Yin-Yang* binary: becomingness and permanence in the duality of nature; events and objects in human experience; spatial and temporal relations of extension; many and one in the ultimate category; actual entities and eternal objects in the categories of existence; mentality and physicality of actual entities; the primordial and consequent nature of God; God and the world in the final interpretation. These findings highlight significant parallels between Whitehead's process philosophy and Chinese philosophy, providing a comparative perspective that deepens our understanding of both traditions.

Keywords Process philosophy · *Yin-Yang* · Creativity · Actual entities · Eternal objects

8.1 Introduction

Alfred North Whitehead (1861–1947) was a British mathematician and philosopher, one of the deepest and creative thinkers of the twentieth century. Whitehead's academic life can be divided into three successive periods, spent, respectively, in Cambridge, London, and Harvard. He began his career at Cambridge University as a mathematician with strong philosophical interests; then he made very important contributions to the philosophy of science and theoretical physics in his middle period in London; finally, he ended at Harvard as a constructive metaphysician with strong mathematical and scientific background. Whitehead's *magnum opus*, *Process and Reality: An Essay in Cosmology* (1929), was one of the major philosophical texts of

H. Guo (✉)
Center for Whitehead Studies, BNU-HKBU United International College, Zhuhai, China
e-mail: hpguo@uic.edu.cn

G. Sigurðsson and T. Hon (eds.), *Contemporary Interpretations and Readings of the Yijing*, Chinese Culture 15, https://doi.org/10.1007/978-981-96-0609-2_8

the twentieth century. In it, he presented a speculative scheme, known as the "Process Philosophy" or "Philosophy of Organism," to synthesize the various elements of human experience into a dynamic, complex web of relationships. In *Process and Reality,* Whitehead made a well-known statement highlighting the commonality between his process philosophy and Eastern thoughts. He wrote: "In this general position the philosophy of organism seems to approximate more to some strains of Indian, or Chinese, thought, than to western Asiatic, or European, thought. One side makes process ultimate; the other side makes fact ultimate." (Whitehead 1978 [1929], 7) However, he never explicitly elaborated this point in any of his works.

The affinity between Chinese thought and Whitehead's process philosophy has been widely acknowledged and discussed by many scholars, including Thomé Fang (1899–1977), Shih-Chuan Chen (1909–2005), Lik Kuen Tong (1935–2012), Chung-Ying Cheng (1935–2024), Joseph Needham (1900–1995), John Cobb Jr. (1925–), and others. Thomé H. Fang used the term "organicism" to characterize the general mode of Chinese thought as found in Confucianism, Taoism, and Mahayana Buddhism (especially Hua Yan Buddhism), in which the universe is understood as an organic whole and all things are related to each other just as in Whitehead's process philosophy (Fang 1980). Following Fang's direction, his student Shih-Chuan Chen investigated more deeply the similarities and differences between Whitehead's process philosophy and the *Yijing*, or *Book of Changes*. He understood *yi* 易 as creativity and translated the title of the *Book of Changes* into "*The Classic on Creativity*," wherein the concept of "creativity" is the most ultimate notion in process philosophy (Chen 2002 [1973]). Chung-Ying Cheng compared Whitehead's category of creativity with the Neo-Confucian concept of *sheng*生 (creativity) in the *Taiji tushuo* 《太极图说》(*Discourse on the Diagram of the Great Ultimate*) as developed by Zhou Dunyi 周敦颐 (1017–1073), the founder of neo-Confucianism in the Song dynasty (960–1279) (Cheng 1979). In the same vein, Joseph Needham, in *Science and Civilization in China*, considered the traditional Chinese worldview to be "organic naturalism," which is for him also an appropriate description of Whitehead's process philosophy (Needham 1962). In the 1970s, John Cobb summarized three commonalities between Whitehead's philosophy and Chinese thought: their common realization of the primacy of process; their common style of thinking in terms of polar opposites that nonetheless require each other, like *Yin* and *Yang*; and there are harmonies of *Yin* and *Yang* in both (Cobb 1979).

Among the similarities between the *Book of Changes* and Whitehead's process philosophy, the *Yin-Yang* bipolarity is crucial to understanding the affinity between the two philosophical systems. As John Cobb said, "Chinese philosophers and Whiteheadians are drawn together by their common realization of the primacy of process; … they share a style of thinking in terms of polarities as over against the dualistic model of thought so common in the West." "There is a bipolarity in all occasions; and this is described as physicality and mentality." (Ibid.) This polarity is called *Yin* and *Yang*, or *Yin-Yang*, which is the most important concept that originated in Chinese philosophy, and it is articulated clearly in the *Book of Changes*. As we know, *Yin* and *Yang* represent two opposite but interconnected, mutually perpetuating forces in the universe. *Yin* is retractive, passive, and receptive, while *Yang* is active, repelling, and

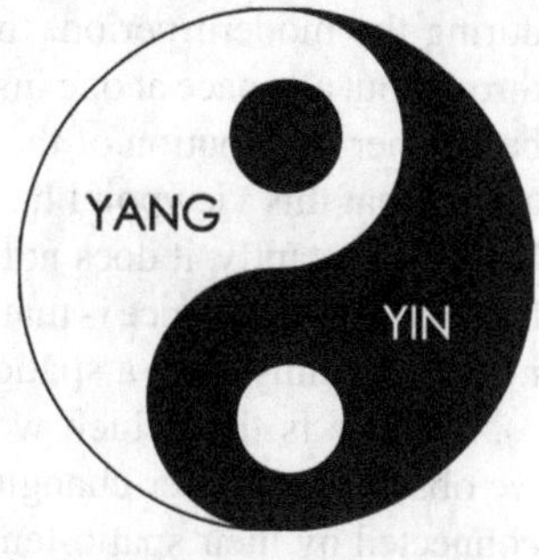

Fig. 8.1 *Yin-Yang Taiji* diagram

expansive. In principle, this dichotomy is seen in all things in various forms. And the *Yin* and *Yang* together is called the *Taiji* 太极, or the Supreme Ultimate, which is the ultimate principle that governs the cosmos in Chinese thought. The principles of *Yin-Yang* and *Taiji* are commonly represented in the "*Yin-Yang Taiji* diagram" as shown in Fig. 8.1. The diagram is a circle consisting of one white and one black half, both swirling around and merging into each other. The "*Yin-Yang Taiji* diagram" depicts an organic, holistic, dynamic, and dialectical world view. It has become one of the fundamental concepts in Chinese thought.

For us, the question is: beside the above-mentioned polar opposites of physicality and mentality, are there any other pairs of *Yin-Yang* in Whitehead's process philosophy? John Cobb has noted that, "Whitehead's less fluid use of concepts precludes the understanding of all polarities in terms of a single pair of terms. Hence there can be no exact equivalent to *Yin* and *Yang*." (Ibid.) This paper aims to illustrate that Whitehead's writings indeed contain more polarities reflecting the nuanced perspective of the *Yin-Yang* philosophy. By scrutinizing Whitehead's early works on the philosophy of nature, as well as his later writings focusing on metaphysics and cosmology, this paper explains the subtle interplay between various polarities, shedding light on the intricate fabric of his thought. Through this interdisciplinary exploration, this paper explores the explicit and implicit connections between Chinese philosophy and Whitehead's process philosophy. It offers evidence that shows the resonance and mutual enrichment between these two philosophical traditions.

8.2 The Discussion of *Yin-Yang* in Whitehead's Early Writings

Whitehead's philosophy of nature is largely presented in his early works, such as *An Enquiry Concerning the Principles of Natural Knowledge* (1919), *The Concept of Nature* (1920), and *The Principle of Relativity* (a response and criticism of Einstein's own theory, 1922). In these early writings the notion of "event" was central. There, the roles of events are analogous to those played by actual entities or actual occasions in his later works on metaphysics and cosmology. In the traditional point of view during the modern period, the ultimate fact of nature is a distribution of material throughout all space at one instance of time, and at another instance of time there will be another distribution of the same material throughout the same space. Whitehead argues that this viewpoint has difficulty explaining the notion of change in physics. More importantly, it does not allow room for expressing the concept of organism in biology, whose essence is that it is a thing which functions and spreads through space, i.e., it is a unity with a spatio-temporal extension. According to Whitehead (1920, 3), "Nature is that which we observe in perception through the senses"and what we observe is an ever-changing process. And the ultimate facts of nature are events connected by their spatio-temporal relations. Hence, for Whitehead, the traditional scientific concepts of time, space, and material are merely abstracts and adjuncts of actual events. From his early writings on the philosophy of nature, we can identify the following three pairs of *Yin-Yang* bipolarity: the becomingness and the permanence as the duality of nature; events and objects in the passage of nature; and the spatial and temporal relations (extensions) connecting events and objects.

8.2.1 Becomingness and Permanence

In his *An Enquiry Concerning the Principles of Natural Knowledge* (1919), Whitehead discusses the duality of nature as follows:

> There are two sides to nature, as it were, antagonistic the one to the other, and yet essential. The one is development in creative advance, the essential becomingness of nature. The other side is the permanence of things, the fact that nature can be recognized. Thus nature is always a newness relating objects which are neither new nor old." (Whitehead 1919, 98)

In reality, no one could ignore the passage of nature. What has gone, has gone forever. Whitehead has called this as the "creative advance of nature." On the other hand, there are also certain permanent recognizable features in this creative advance of nature, such as sunrise, sunset, and the cycle of the seasons. These two sides of nature, becomingness and permanence, can be considered as a pair of *Yin-Yang* as shown in Fig. 8.2, in which becomingness is *Yang* and permanence is *Yin*. This can easily remind us of a famous similar statement in the *Book of Changes*: "Three are three meanings of *Yi* 易: mutability; immutability; ease and simplicity." Here, mutability and immutability correspond exactly to the becoming and permanence of the duality of nature as described by Whitehead. In *Process and Reality*, Whitehead also uses "flux and permanence" to refer to this pair of notions:

> In the inescapable flux, there is something that abides; in the overwhelming permanence, there is an element that escapes into flux. Permanence can be snatched only out of flux; and the passing moment can find its adequate intensity only by its submission to permanence. Those who would disjoin the two elements can find no interpretation of patent facts. (Whitehead 1978 [1929], 338)

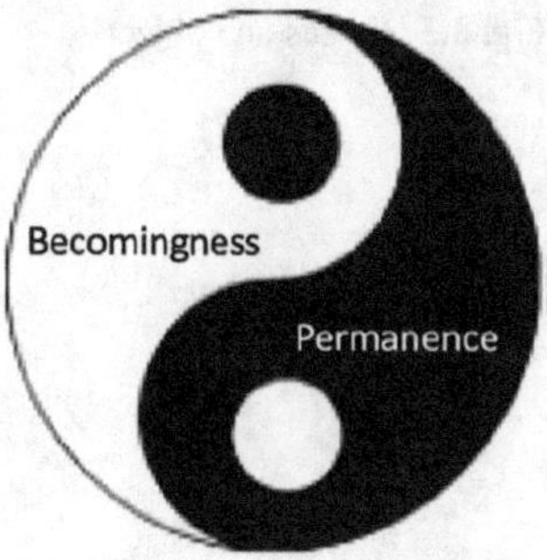

Fig. 8.2 Duality of nature: becomingness/flux and permanence

8.2.2 Events and Objects

In Whitehead's philosophy of nature, nature is not a static system; rather, it is an evolving, ever-changing process. It is always a becoming or a spatio-temporal happening. Whitehead gives the name "event" to such a becoming. For the permanence recognized in events, Whitehead uses the name "object" to represent them. Objects have the possibility of recurrence in experience. The same object is recognized as related to diverse events. For example, the color green is an object, and the awareness of the color green is a recognition. Therefore, the self-identical object maintains itself in the flux of events. Strictly speaking, objects are without time and space because they can occur there and then, also here and now. In other words, events pass but objects do not pass. The continuity of nature is to be found in events; while the atomic properties of nature can be found in objects. As for the relationships between events and objects, objects can be seen as qualities of events and events as relations between objects. On one hand, events signify objects in mutual relations. There can be no events without related objects. On the other hand, related objects signify events as well. There are no objects without such events. In this sense events and objects can be considered as a pair of *Yin-Yang* where events are *Yang* and objects are *Yin* (Fig. 8.3). The theory of events and objects was first developed in *An Enquiry Concerning the Principles of Natural Knowledge* (1919, 61–67). In his later writings, events and objects were replaced by actual entities or actual occasions and eternal objects.

8.2.3 Spatial and Temporal Relations

In Whitehead's theory of events, each event encompasses or incorporates other events as integral components, and simultaneously, every event is encompassed by other events of which it forms an essential part. In other words, an event is a part of certain wholes and at the same time a whole extending over certain parts. The events that cannot be analyzed into smaller events, that is, the "atomic" events, are the actual entities or actual occasions that became central in Whitehead's later writings. Events

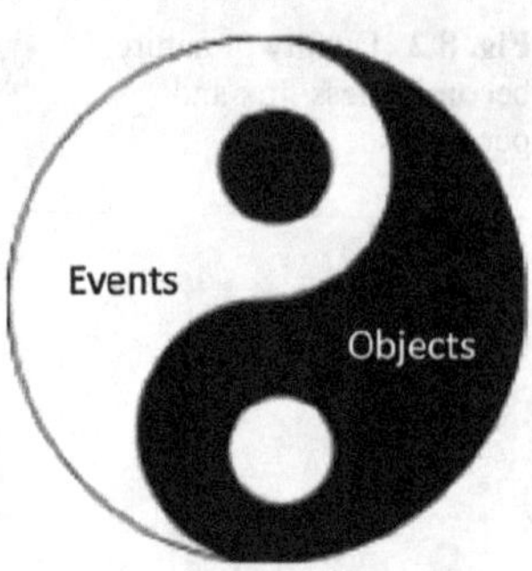

Fig. 8.3 Events and objects

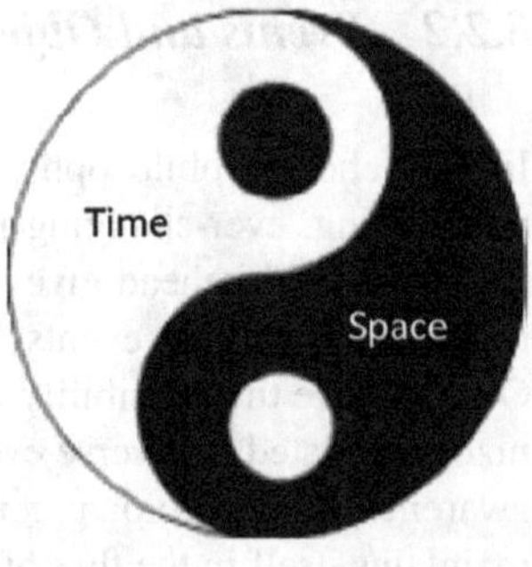

Fig. 8.4 Extension: space and time (Spatial and temporal relations)

are connected by the relations of "extension." An event is just how it is related and nothing else. It is a unity with a spatio-temporal extension which is of the essence of its being. Time and space are relations of extension between events. The relation of extension exhibits events both as actual and as involving the becomingness of nature. The actuality of events comes from spatial relations. The becomingness of events come from the temporal relations. We can consider the spatial and temporal relations, or space and time, as a pair of *Yin-Yang* in which the temporal relation or time is *Yang*, the spatial relation or space is *Yin*, and the spatio-temporal extension as a whole is *Taiji* (Fig. 8.4).

8.3 The Discussion of *Yin-Yang* in Whitehead's Later Writings

Whitehead's later writings focus mainly on metaphysics and cosmology. Major works include *Science and the Modern World* (1925), *Process and Reality* (1929), *Adventures of Ideas* (1933), among others. As Whitehead states in the preface of *Adventures of Ideas*, "The three books are an endeavour to express a way of understanding the nature of things, and to point out how that way of thinking is illustrated by a survey of the mutations of human experience. Each book can be read separately; but they supplement each other's omissions or compressions." (Whitehead 1961 [1933], vii)

Adventures of Ideas is in fact a study of the concept of civilization with an emphasis on the importance of adventure and a few chapters on cosmology and philosophy. *Science and the Modern World* can be considered as an introductory version of *Process and Reality*.

In *Process and Reality*, Whitehead presents his philosophy of organism as a speculative scheme consisting of four sets of categories: the category of the ultimate, eight categories of existence, twenty-seven categories of explanations and nine categoreal obligations. According to Whitehead, "Every entity should be a specific instance of one category of existence, every explanation should be a specific instance of categories of explanation, and every obligation should be a specific instance of categoreal obligations. The Category of the Ultimate expresses the general principle presupposed in the three more special categories." (Whitehead 1978 [1929], 20).

After examining the text of *Process and Reality*, the following five important pairs of *Yin-Yang* can be identified: many and one in the category of the ultimate; actual entities and eternal objects in the categories of existence; mentality and physicality of actual entity; the primordial and the consequent nature of God; God and the world in the final interpretation.

8.3.1 Many and One

In Whitehead's categoreal scheme, the category of the ultimate consists of three ultimate notions: "creativity," "many," and "one." "Creativity" is the universal of universals characterizing the ultimate matter of fact. Creativity is also the principle of novelty. The terms "many" and "one" presuppose each other. "Many" conveys the notion of "disjunctive diversity," and "one" represents conjunctive unity. Creativity is the ultimate principle by which "many become one and are increased by one." (Ibid., 21) At the same time, we may also say that one becomes many and is embodied by the many. This basically is saying that in the universe everything impacts everything else. This is a fundamentally relational metaphysic. In every moment, you and every other being inherit everything that has ever happened, choose how you will express and become a new self. And creativity is the driving force. An analysis of the concept of creativity in Whitehead makes clear that there cannot be three separable independent aspects of the category of the ultimate. There should be only one ultimate, the ultimate of creativity, which describes the becoming of one out of the many and the becoming of the many out of the one. The "*Yin-Yang Taiji* diagram" vividly presents the above relationship among creativity, many, and one. In the *Taiji* diagram, there are also three notions: *Taiji* or the supreme ultimate, *Yin*, and *Yang*. *Taiji* is the fundamental principle behind everything in the universe, so it can correspond to creativity in Whitehead's category of the ultimate. *Yin* and *Yang* are two inseparable aspects of the *Taiji*, just as many and one are two inseparable aspects of creativity. Many become one and one becomes many, just like the constant movement of *Yin* and *Yang* in the *Taiji* diagram. Now the question is: which is *Yin* and which is *Yang* in the duality of many and one? To answer this question, we need to consider the defining characteristics of *Yin* and

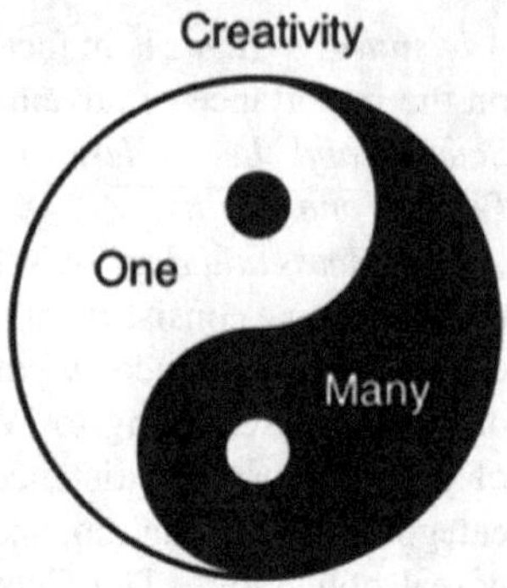

Fig. 8.5 Category of the ultimate

Yang and then compare them to the many and one. Notice that *Yang* is creative or active, while *Yin* is receptive or passive. In the process of many becoming one, one is the one actual occasion and many are the many entities within the complex unity. Among the many entities, there are both actual entities and eternal objects. They serve as the data apprehended by the one actual occasion that is evolving and becoming. In other words, the one apprehends the disjunctive many into a conjunctive unity. It is clear that one should be mapped to *Yang* and many to *Yin* as one is active and many are passive. Therefore, the *Taiji* diagram as shown in Fig. 8.5 can model the category of the ultimate.

8.3.2 Actual Entities and Eternal Objects

In Whitehead's philosophical scheme, there are eight categories of existence. Every entity in the universe should be a specific instance of one category of existence. In *Process and Reality*, the eight categories of existence are presented in the following list:

1. Actual entities (also termed actual occasions), or final realities, or Res Verae,
2. Prehensions, or concrete facts of relatedness,
3. Nexūs (plural of Nexus), or public matters of fact,
4. Subjective forms, or private matters of fact,
5. Eternal objects, or pure potentials for the specific determination of fact, or forms of definiteness,
6. Propositions, or matters of fact in potential determination, or impure potentials for the specific determination of matters of fact, or theories,
7. Multiplicities, or pure disjunctions of diverse entities,
8. Contrasts, or modes of synthesis of entities in one prehension, or patterned entities.

In Whitehead's process philosophy, actual entities are the final and the most concrete realities of which the world is made up:

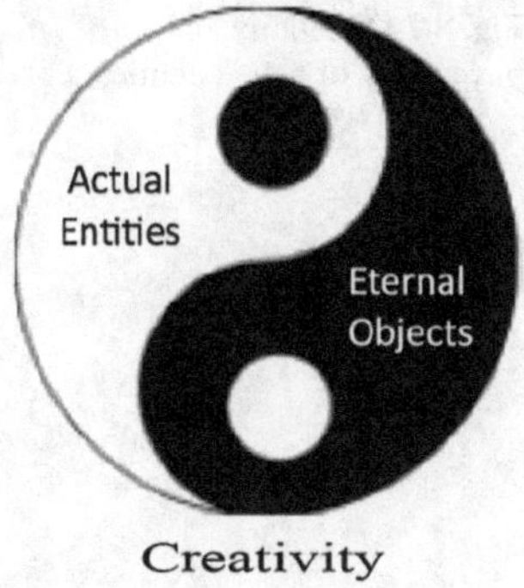

Fig. 8.6 Actual entities and eternal objects

> There is no going behind actual entities to find anything more real…The final real things are all alike, actual entities; and these actual entities are drops of experiences, complex and interdependent. They differ among themselves: God is an actual entity, and so is the most trivial puff of existence in far-off empty space. (Ibid., 18)

By contrast, eternal objects are pure potentialities and the most abstract entities. Actual entities and eternal objects are the two most important categories of existence and are opposite to each other. To describe this relationship, Whitehead writes: "Among these eight categories of existence, actual entities and eternal objects stand out with a certain extreme finality. The other types of existence have a certain intermediate finality." (Ibid., 22) The 19th category of explanation also states, "That the fundamental types of entities are actual entities and eternal objects; and the other types of entities only express how all entities of the two fundamental types are in community with each other, in the actual world." (Ibid., 25).

Therefore, actual entities and eternal objects can be considered as the "two modes" (两仪) that embody the *Taiji*, the category of the ultimate. Actual entities are concrete particulars and should be seen as *Yin*; eternal objects are abstract universals and should be seen as *Yang* (see Fig. 8.6).

8.3.3 Mentality and Physicality

It is generally known that Descartes divided the universe into three main substances: the human mind as the thinking substance, matter as the extended substance, and God as the creator and the sustainer of the first two types. Whitehead rejected Descartes' concept of substance as "an existent thing which requires nothing but itself in order to exist." According to Whitehead, all actual entities are interdependent. Nothing can exist in isolation. To exist in the Whiteheadian sense is to become part of a complex web of relationships and thereby to self-actualize through participating in an organic network. An actual entity in its ultimate analysis is a "becoming." In the becoming of an actual entity, there are two types of entities entering into the novel synthesis: other actual entities and eternal objects. We can also say that the

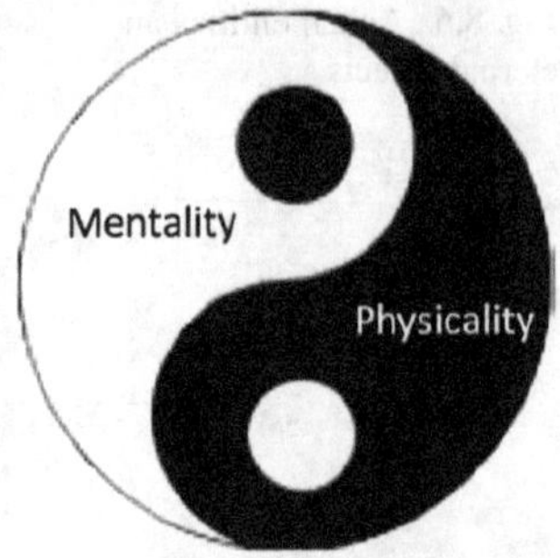

Fig. 8.7 Mentality and physicality of actual entities

new actual entities prehend other actual entities and eternal objects. Respectively, there are two types of prehensions: "physical prehensions" or prehensions of actual entities, and "conceptual prehensions" or prehensions of eternal objects. Prehensions are also called feelings. Therefore, there are two types of feelings: physical feeling and conceptual feeling. Consequently, every actual entity is said to have a physical pole and a mental pole: "Each actuality is essentially bipolar, physical and mental." (Ibid., 108) The mentality and physicality of an actual entity can be considered as another pair of *Yin* and *Yang* where mentality is *Yang* and physicality is *Yin* (Fig. 8.7). This allows Whitehead's process philosophy to overcome the mind–body Cartesian dualism.

8.3.4 The Primordial and Consequent Nature of God

Whitehead rejects the traditional Christian notion of a static God. Instead, his concept of God emphasizes the idea that the divine entity is inseparable from the ongoing creative process of the universe. He is not prior to but with all creation. He is the beginning and the end. He is a process and "analogously to all actual entities, the nature of God is dipolar. He has a primordial nature and a consequent nature. The primordial nature is conceptual, the consequent nature is the weaving of God's physical feelings upon his primordial concepts." (Ibid., 345) We can consider the primordial and the consequent nature of God to be another pair of *Yin-Yang* (Fig. 8.8).

8.3.5 God and the World

In Whitehead's cosmological construction, God and the world are "the contrasted opposites in terms of which Creativity achieves its supreme task of transforming disjoined multiplicity, with its diversities in opposition, into concrescent unity, with its diversities in contrast." In the final part of *Process and Reality*, Whitehead states

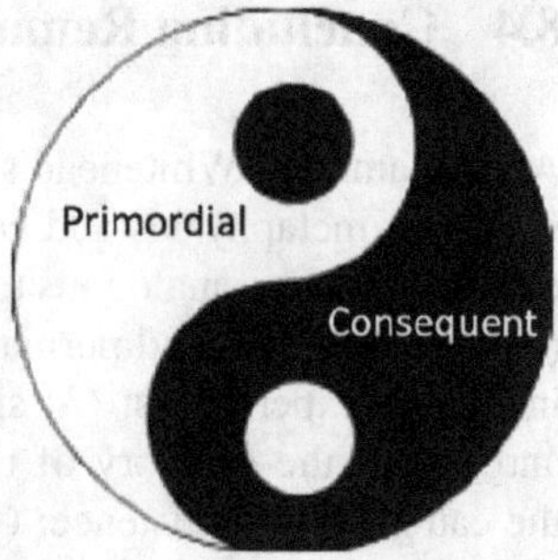

Fig. 8.8 Primordial and the consequent nature of God

that "The final summary can only be expressed in terms of a group of antitheses, whose apparent self-contradiction depends on neglect of the diverse categories of existence. In each antithesis, there is a shift of meaning which converts the opposition into a contrast." (Fig. 8.9).

> *It is as true to say that God is permanent and the World fluent, as that the World is permanent and God is fluent.*
>
> *It is as true to say that God is one and the World many, as the world is one and God many.*
>
> *It is as true to say that, in comparison with the World, God is actual eminently, as that, in comparison with God, the World is actual eminently.*
>
> *It is as true to say that the World is immanent in God, as that God is immanent in the World.*
>
> *It is as true to say that God transcends the World, as that the World transcends God.*
>
> *It is as true to say that God creates the World, as that the World creates God. (Ibid., 346–349)*

Thus, in every respect God and the world are intertwined and interdependently in co-creating the universe in their processes. Therefore, we can consider God and the world to be another pair of *Yin-Yang* in *Process and Reality*.

Fig. 8.9 God and the world

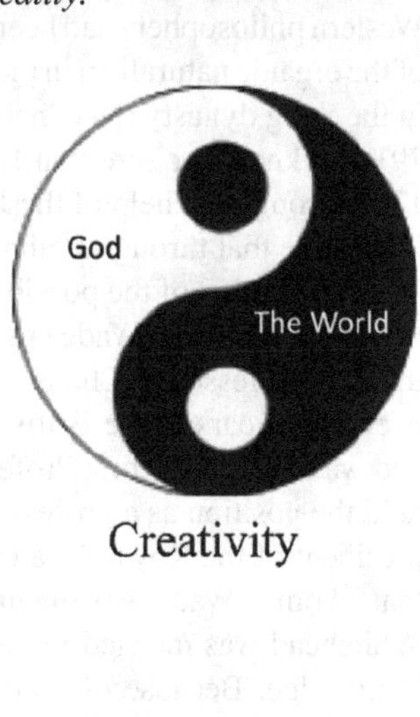

8.4 Concluding Remarks

After examining Whitehead's earlier works on the philosophy of nature and his later works on metaphysics and cosmology, we have identified a total of eight pairs of concepts that are analogous to the binary notion of *Yin-Yang* in Chinese philosophy: (1) becomingness and permanence in the duality of nature; (2) events and objects in human experiences; (3) spatial and temporal relations of extension; (4) many and one of the category of the ultimate; (5) actual entities and eternal objects of the categories of existence; (6) mentality and physicality of actual entities; (7) the primordial and the consequent nature of God; (8) God and the world in the final interpretation. These findings strongly support Whitehead's assertion that process philosophy is similar to Chinese philosophy. More specifically, they show the commonality between process philosophy and the *Book of Changes*. These findings will be beneficial to specialists in comparative philosophy. On one hand, Chinese philosophers may find a way to develop a deeper understanding of Whitehead's process philosophy, and reversely, use that understanding to deepen their analysis of the development of Chinese philosophy. On the other hand, Western philosophers may find the organic and holistic Chinese ways of thinking useful to their understanding of polarities in process philosophy as over against the dualistic model of thought so common in the West. From a broader perspective, Whitehead's process philosophy and Chinese philosophy also form a pair of *Yin-Yang* supplementing and enriching each other to achieve harmony—a global harmony—at a higher level.

Given the striking resemblance between Whitehead's process philosophy and the *Yin-Yang* way of thinking in the *Book of Changes*, and the fact that these two systems were separated by nearly 3,000 years, we cannot help but ask where this resemblance comes from. Had Whitehead ever read the *Book of Changes* and learned the *Yin-Yang* way of thinking? Joseph Needham has repeatedly emphasized that through Leibniz Western philosophers had been informed by Chinese philosophy, particularly in terms of the organic naturalism in the *Book of Changes* and in Neo-Confucianism developed in the Song dynasty (Needham 1962, 168; Liu 2001, 439–451; Schönfeld 2006, 67–79). We know for sure that Leibniz (1646–1716) had read the *Book of Changes* in 1700 through the help of the Jesuit Joachim Bouvet (1656–1730) (Leibniz 1962). Is it possible that through Leibniz Whitehead received the ideas of *Yin-Yang*?

Another clue of the possible Chinese influence over Whitehead might be through Sir Thomas Francis Wade (1818–1895), who was a British diplomat, a sinologist and the first professor of Chinese at Cambridge University. After retiring from working over forty years in the British embassies in China, he returned to England in 1883 and was elected the first Professor of Chinese at the University of Cambridge. Wade held the position as a professor until his death in Cambridge at 77. He served as the president of the Royal Asiatic Society from 1887 to 1890. A fact seldom noticed is that Thomas Wade was the uncle of Whitehead's wife, Evelyn Wade (1866–1961). Whitehead was married in 1890. He had a five-year overlap with Thomas Wade at Cambridge. Because of their close relationship, they might have had an in-depth personal interaction on Chinese culture. Is it possible that through Thomas Wade

Whitehead received the ideas of *Yin-Yang*? Or did Whitehead actually develop the *Yin-Yang* way of thinking independently by himself? These might be interesting questions for further study and investigation.

References

Chen, Shih-Chuan. 2002 [1973]. *Whitehead and The Book of Changes. First International Conference on Whitehead and China*, Beijing, Beijing Normal University: https://www.thomehfang.com/suncrates/chencreat.html

Cheng, Chung-Ying. 1979. Categories of creativity in whitehead and neo-confucianism. *Journal of Chinese Philosophy* 6 (3): 251–274.

Cobb, John. 1979. Post conference reflections on Yin and Yang. *Journal of Chinese Philosophy* 6 (4): 421–426.

Fang, Thomé H. 1980. The World and the Individual in Chinese Metaphysics. In *Creativity in Man and Nature*. Taipei: Linking.

Leibniz, Gottfried Wilhelm. 1962. *Explication de l'Arithmetique Binaire*. Mathematische Schriften. Vol. 7. Ed. C. Gerhardt. Hildesheim: G. Olms.

Liu, Yu. 2001. From Christian Platonism to organism: The two Chinas of Leibniz. *International Philosophical Quarterly* 41 (4): 439–451.

Needham, Joseph. 1962. *Science and Civilisation in China*. Cambridge: Cambridge University Press.

Schönfeld, Martin. 2006. From Confucius to Kant: The question of information transfer. *Journal of Chinese Philosophy* 33 (1): 67–81.

Whitehead, Alfred North. 1919. *An Enquiry Concerning the Principles of Natural Knowledge*. Cambridge: Cambridge University Press.

Whitehead, Alfred North. 1920. *The Concept of Nature*. Cambridge: Cambridge University Press.

Whitehead, Alfred North. 1978 [1929]. *Process and Reality*. Corrected ed. New York: Free Press.

Whitehead, Alfred North. 1961 [1933]. *Adventures of Ideas*. New York: Free Press.

Part III
Innovative Interpretations

Chapter 9
Mythic Narratives in the *Zhouyi* and the *Guicangyi*

Jón Egill Eyþórsson

Abstract The following paper aims to unveil connections between pre-Qin Chinese Mythology and two ancient mantic texts, the well-known *Zhouyi* 周易 on the one hand and the lesser-known *Guicangyi* 歸藏易 on the other. The bronze age text of the *Zhouyi* 周易, being the core text of the *Yijing* 易經, is conspicuously lacking in mythic elements. In fact, this seems counterintuitive, given the text's mantic and shamanic background and the epoch of composition. This lack of mythic character is somewhat lenified by both the extant and recently unearthed fragments of the alternative Guicang text, a text that shares the hexagram structure of the *Zhouyi* but presents a text strikingly different and significantly mythic. Several narrative strands in the *Zhouyi* were reconstructed by Wang Guowei 王國維, Gu Jiegang 顧頡剛, Gao Heng 高亨, and others in the first half of the twentieth century. Some of these have unmistakable links with China's richest repositories of myth, such as the *Shanhaijing* 山海經 and *Chuci Tianwen* 楚辭天問 while most of them are grounded in attestable history. The *Guicangyi*'s textual transmission and history is a rather complicated affair, but for our present purposes, we can refer to two main sources. The first of those is a compendious collection of various fragments of lost books, one of the earliest chapters of which collects the most extant references to the disputed *Guicangyi*. At the time, the text's authenticity was highly disputed. The second source served to settle this century-old dispute in the wake of an archeological discovery in 1983 that included almost 400 slips of bamboo with writing, demonstrated to be remnants of the same text. Among the mythological and historical elements investigated here are: Chinese dragons, the semi-historical or legendary King Hai 王亥 of pre-dynastic Shang 商, Gaozong 高宗 (i.e., Wuding 武丁), Diyi 帝乙, Jizi 箕子, Kang Hou 康侯 (i.e., Ji Feng 姬封), Gun 鯀, Yu 禹, the maiden of Tushan 塗山女and Qi lord of Xia 夏后啓.

Keywords *Zhouyi* · *Guicangyi* · Mythology · Cosmogony · Narratives

---

J. E. Eyþórsson (✉)
Academy of Korean Studies, Seongnam, Republic of Korea
e-mail: jeythorsson@gmail.com
URL: https://grad.aks.ac.kr/index.do

G. Sigurðsson and T. Hon (eds.), *Contemporary Interpretations and Readings of the Yijing*, Chinese Culture 15, https://doi.org/10.1007/978-981-96-0609-2_9

9.1 Introduction

This paper presents some tentative findings in an ongoing quest to unveil connections between pre-Qin Chinese mythology and *Yijing*, the *Book of Changes*. Aspects of the *Zhouyi* 周易 will be investigated in the light of mythological narratives, mostly recounting the findings of distinguished scholars in the field. This paper outlines mythic and legendary narratives that appear to be hinted at in several obscure passages of the *Zhouyi*.

There are in fact many difficulties in this endeavor. As is generally acknowledged in the field, Chinese mythology is fragmentary and lacking in structure. This is likely attributable to the fact that there appears to have been no compiler of myths in ancient China, such as Homer for Greek myth and Snorri Sturluson for Norse myth.

Another obvious difficulty is that the *Zhouyi* itself is conspicuously lacking in obvious mythic references, a fact that is almost counterintuitive, given the mantic and shamanic background and epoch of composition. This lack of mythic character is somewhat lenified by both the extant and recently unearthed fragments of the alternative *Guicang* 歸藏 text.

The idea that in the complex symbolism of the *Yijing* there might be concealed a system of mythic symbolism, somewhat akin to the alleged Hermetic symbols of the Occidental Tarot, has been with me ever since I commenced my studies in Sinology. It is not lost on me that this borders on pseudo-science, however, I have always thought it prudent to entertain such ideas in favor of dismissing them, and in light of my academically unaffiliated status feel I can impudently indulge in this passion.

9.2 The Mythic Landscape

The cosmological topography that can be deduced from the fragmented sources of Chinese myth is fairly complete in basics, albeit necessarily fluid. This is because different conceptions of the cosmos within the Chinese civilization have many universal things in common, while their connectedness one to another is unclear and disputable. For example, the cosmological model represented deities such as Di Jun 帝俊 and Xi He 羲和 does not conflict with that of the "Four Auspicious Beasts" *Sishou* 四獸, but it appears that the *Sishou* cosmology is younger by far and the two have little or no historical overlap. Incidentally, both models overlap nicely with parts of the *Yijing*.

This cosmological model represented by Di Jun and Xi He would appear to have roots going at least as far back as the Shang dynasty (Allan 1991).

This conception is of course much more primal and predates the three astronomically oriented models described in the second century CE by Cai Yong 蔡邕,[1] though

[1] Cai Yong's original astronomical treatise is lost but it is quoted in the *Zhoubi Suanjing*《周髀算經》and the "Treatise on Astronomy" of the *Jinshu*《晉書・天文志》. Both texts contain the almost excact basic description: "Heaven resembles a canopy and the Earth an overturned dish" 天似蓋

it appears to have least conflict with the Domed Heaven (*gaitian* 蓋天) model. A most conspicuous expression of it is in *The Book of Documents* (*Shangshu* 尚書), where it is related that the Divine Emperor / Thearch Yao (Di Yao 帝堯) dispatched astronomers or surveyors to systemize a calendar.[2] Another expression would be in the *Book of Rites* (*Li Ji* 禮記, Yue Ling 月令 chapter). "The Treatise on Heavenly Patterns" (Tianwenxun 天文訓) of the *Huainanzi* 淮南子 is an example of a very clear early articulation. It is not clear when exactly it was first articulated in academic terms as a mythic cosmological model, but it was almost certainly recognized and accepted as such by the intelligentsia of the late Qing dynasty.

I believe this model is perhaps best described, in modern scholastic context, by Ye Shuxian 葉舒憲, and in what follows is a summary of his description. (Ye 1992, 12–18).

In the center of a square earth under a rounded dome of Heaven the Jian tree 建木 or Mt. Kunlun 崐崘山 is an *axis mundi* and formerly a passage between the earth and celestial realms. The planes of earth and sky are tilted a result of the battle between the gods Gonggong 共工 and Zhuanxu 顓頊, and subsequent "fixing" by the goddess Nüwa 女媧. This myth clearly purports to explain both the clockwise paths of celestial objects across the sky and the fact that in China, rivers generally flow south-eastward into an eastern ocean.

The four main compass points on this landscape are defined by the sun's vernal and autumnal equinoxes as well as the summer and winter solstices. Thus, Spring and East, Summer and South, Autumn and West, and Winter and North are equated. The sun rising in the east equated with the return of vitality to nature in spring, the sun at its meridian height in summer equated with noon, the sunset in the west with dusk, autumn, and harvest, and the ensuing night with the cold of winter. In this way, time (seasons and hours) and space (directions) are equated.

These spatiotemporal points (*shikong* 時空) cohere with the Post-natal Trigrams 後天八卦圖 and the Five Phases (*wuxing* 五行). In the vernal east and southeast, we have the trigrams *Zhen* 震 ☳ and *Xun* 巽 ☴, both represented by the Wood Phase. In the Summer, south and southwest, the trigrams *Li* 離 ☲ and *Kun* 坤 ☷, are represented by the Fire and Earth phases, respectively. In autumn, west and northwest *Dui* 兌 ☱ and *Qian* 乾 ☰ are both represented by the Metal Phase. North and northwest are *Kan* 坎 ☵ and *Gen* 艮 ☶, Water and Earth Phase, respectively. The apparent imbalance of assigning two phases to South/Summer and North/Winter is an intuitive way of assigning five phases to four seasons/cardinal directions. On reflection, the nourishing and fertile attribute of *Kun* and the stillness and introspective character of *Gen* may be seen to compensate well and restore an adequate sense of balance to the model.[3]

笠地法覆槃. Unless specified, references to Chinese classics are all taken from the *Chinese Text Project* (2006–2024): www.ctext.org.

[2] Xi He appears as a solar deity in the *Shanhaijing* 山海經 and the *Chuci Tianwen* 天問 but in the *Shangshu Yaodian* 尚書堯典 the name of the goddess appears to be euhemerized as the four shamans Xi Zhong 羲仲, Xi Shu 羲叔, He Zhong 和仲 and He Shu 和叔, who appear to have been astronomers and surveyors. This is neither counterintuitive nor unexpected in mythic thought.

[3] See, for example, *bagua* 八卦 arrangements and cosmology in Moore (1989).

In the mythic fragments, the east (dawn, spring) is called Tang Valley (Tanggu 湯谷or 暘谷) the location of the Sacred Mulberry tree (*fusang* 扶桑). In its branches, the ten suns perch awaiting their turn to ascend and sojourn across the sky. These ten suns are the sons of the sky god Di Jun and his consort the goddess Xi He. And here Xi He is said to bathe the suns before their ascent into the heavens. This setting also involves the myth of Yi the Archer (Hou Yi 后羿), and the eventual demise of nine out of ten suns. The god of the east is Goumang句芒.

The suns, normally by turns, ascend from this place to the zenith (midday, summer, and south), giving light and heat to the earth. The god of this quarter is Zhurong祝融.

Then the suns descend into the Wei Valley (Weigu 昧谷). A complementary western valley (evening, autumn), sometimes called Meng Valley (Menggu 蒙谷). Also close to this western extremity of the earth is a deep body of water called Moulting Abyss (Yuyuan 羽渊, also虞渊) and a similarly named mountain, Yushan 羽山, the location of the brutal sacrifice of the god Gun 鮌. This is also, presumably, where Di Jun's other wife, Chang Yi 常儀, who also appears as the goddess Heng E 姮娥 (Chang E 嫦娥), bathes the twelve moons she gave birth to. The god of autumn and the west is Rushou 蓐收, sometimes identified with King Hai 王亥.[4]

From there the assumed path of the suns, perhaps entered through the Moulting abyss, lies through the underworld, the so-called Yellow Springs (Huangquan 黃泉), a dark and watery place, associated with the north, nighttime, and winter, and ruled by the god Yuqiang 禺彊 (god of northern sea, underworld—psychopompos in the Mawangdui silk manuscripts). And a journey through the dark underworld necessarily concludes with a new dawn.

In this mythic landscape, we also have the mysterious goddess known as Xi Wang Mu 西王母 (usually translated as Queen Mother of the West) and her less conspicuous eastern counterpart Dong Wang Gong 東王公. Xi Wang Mu is a major figure in later Taoist pantheons, but here we are mostly concerned with how she appears in the *Shanhaijing* 山海經 and other Pre-Qin sources. In the *Shanghaijing*, she is described in the following way:

> 又西三百五十里,曰玉山,是西王母所居也。西王母其狀如人,豹尾虎齒而善嘯,蓬髮戴勝,是司天之厲及五殘。(Yuan 1993, 59)
>
> Three hundred and fifty leagues to the west, there is Jade Mountain. It is the abode of Xi Wang Mu. She is human in appearance but with a panther's tail, tiger's teeth and howls a lot. Her messy hair is crowned with a wreath of jades and flowers. She oversees the strictness of heaven and the five ailments.

Later literature, especially religious Taoist works, describes her in a much less ferocious way. She is, however, clearly a goddess of the west, fall, evening, old age

---

[4] *Chunqiu Zuozhuan*: "In the time of Shaohao, there were four men, called Chong, Gai, Xiu, and Xi, able to regulate [the kingdoms of] metal, wood, and water. Chong was made Goumang, Gai made Rushou, and Xiu and Xi made Xuanming. For ages those families did not fail in their duties, but completed the merit of Qiongsang (Shaohao)." (Legge 2000, vol. V, 731) (《左傳·昭公二十九年》: "少皞氏有四叔:曰重,曰該,曰修,曰熙,實能金木及水。使重爲句芒,該爲蓐收,修及熙爲玄冥。世不失職,遂濟窮桑。") Gai 該 refers to Wang Hai 王亥, as in *Heavenly Questions of the Songs of Chu* (*Chuci Tianwen* 楚辭天問), discussed in more detailed below.

and death, and by extension sacrifice and harvest. In other parts of the *Shanhaijing* she is said to reside in a cave in Mt. Kun Lun, surrounded by all the myriad creatures, sometimes specifically nine-tailed foxes and three-legged crows, and subsiding on birds.

Her counterpart Dong Wang Gong 東王公 is much less frequently mentioned in the earliest sources, in fact, it appears that he is first mentioned by that name in the first century BCE *Shen Yi Jing* 神異經, which is barely within the purview of this study. But if we take it that he is in fact the very same Dong Jun 東君 Lord of the East celebrated in "The Nine Songs" (Jiu ge) 九歌 of the *Songs of Chu* (*Chu Ci* 楚辭) then the assumption that Xi Wang Mu had a counterpart in the east from early on seems entirely reasonable. His symbolism concerns the East, the Wood phase of the five phases (*wuxing* 五行), and spring.[5]

9.3 Dragons in the *Zhouyi*

Chinese dragons are undoubtedly one of the first things to spring to mind when considering Chinese mythology and they are indeed a relatively prominent feature in the *Yijing*, both the Bronze-age *Zhouyi* and the Confucian commentaries (*Ten Wings*). Although ancient China's oldest proto dictionary, the *Erya* 爾雅, does not mention dragons apart from the context of flags, the *Shuowen Jiezi* 說文解字, defines the character *long* 龍 with the following gloss:

> 鱗蟲之長。能幽,能明,能細,能巨,能短,能長;春分而登天,秋分而潛淵。
>
> The foremost among scaly creatures. It can be obscure or evident, miniscule or immense, short or long. At the spring equinox it climbs into the sky, at autumn equinox it dives into deep waters. (*Shuowen Jiezi*《說文解字》龍項)

The *Da Dai Li Ji* 大戴禮記 has this to say on the subject: 羣書要語鱗蟲三百六十而龍為之長.

"Various texts say there are 360 (kinds of) scaly reptiles and chief there among are dragons." (*Da Dai Li Ji*) And the Encyclopedia *Guang Ya* 廣雅 lists the following sub-species in its taxonomy of dragons:

> 有鱗曰蛟龍有翼曰應龍有角曰虬龍無角曰螭未升天曰蟠龍
>
> Scaly ones are called Jiao Long and winged ones are known as Ying Long. The horned variety is called Qiu Long and those without horns Li Long. Those who have not ascended into the sky are called Pan Long. (*Guang Ya*)

Although many sinologists like to stress the difference between the western dragon and that mythic creature particular to the Sinosphere, this description here doesn't seem all that different; this indeed seems to be a magical serpent. It can certainly not be disputed that Chinese dragons appear much more benign than their Western

[5] Another very interesting facet of the pair is that they may have evolved into the well-known but much later myth about the Weaving Maid and Cowherd. An overlap with the beginning of the *Zhuangzi*'s first chapter (Xiaoyaoyou 逍遙遊篇) is also hard to dispute.

counterparts, but the present author is equally wary of dismissing the subtle similarities. Chinese dragons are not always auspicious and Western dragons often possess great wisdom. Both seem to represent at times impersonal forces of nature and, at other times, aspects of the unconscious.

Dragons abound in Chinese mythology. This may be especially true of later popular myths and legends but also holds true for the *Shanhaijing* and the *Guicang Yi* that we will examine in a later section. Appearances of dragons and the various forms these take have been examined in various studies, but I feel that we are still far from understanding what sort of spiritual and symbolic meaning they had for the living shamanism of the era under examination. For example, they appear sometimes as "steeds," other times as omens, and yet others as diviners apparently capable of speech and cognition.

In a well known passage in *Zuo's Commentary on the Spring and Autumn Annals*, the raising and breeding of dragons are discussed alongside elements of mythic nature. (*Zuozhuan*, 昭公29 年) And in the *Records of the Historian* (*Shiji* 史記), Confucius is reported to have called Laozi a dragon, apparently utterly awestruck after meeting the old philosopher. It also appears that many mythical and legendary persons sometimes appear as dragons or are dragons who can assume human form. This could be true of Gun 鯀, Yu 禹, and the Yellow Thearch (*Huangdi* 黃帝). The leviathan described in the opening chapter of the *Zhuangzi* 莊子, *Kun*鯤, transforms into a giant bird, Peng鵬. Doesn't this description evoke an image similar to the dragon of the *Qian* hexagram, first slumbering in the deep waters and then ascending high into the sky? The Chinese dragons are by no means simple creatures and doubtless, their symbolic import has transmogrified countless times and in many ways over the centuries.

In light of the *Zhouyi*'s general lack of unambiguously mythic narrative, the first two hexagrams certainly evoke a mythic ambience by virtue of the presence of dragons.

The Judgment and Changing Line text of the first hexagram *Qian*, reads as follows.

䷀ 乾 元亨利貞。

Qian (Sun rising). Supreme Fortune. Sacrifice Received. Profitable Augury.[6]

初九 潛龍勿用。
Sunken Dragon. Do not act.
九二 見龍在田。利見大人。
Sighted: Dragon in a field. Profits to see a big man.
九三 君子終日乾乾。夕惕若厲。无咎。
The noble man is busy all day long, wary at dusk. Danger, No Harm.
九四 或躍在淵。无咎。
Leaps in the deep. No Harm.
九五 飛龍在天。利見大人。
Dragons fly in the sky. Profits to see a big man.

[6] Trans. Minford (2014). The difficulty of choosing a suitable translation is daunting. Since many English translations are available, I have chosen to pick translations suiting the subject matter of each chapter. Conceivably, translations by Rutt (2002) or Field (2015) would be more appropriate here.

上九亢龍有悔。
Dragon gully. Trouble.
用九見羣龍无首。吉。
Sighted: Headless Dragons, a host. Auspicious.

䷁ 坤 上六:戰龍於野,其血玄黃。
Kun (Earth Flow). Six in Top Place. Dragons fight in the wilds. Dark blood, yellow blood.

Edward Shaughnessy has published a study on the dragons of these two most primary hexagrams, which is both fascinating, insightful, and convincing, if not conclusive. His astromythological study demonstrates effectively how the dragon imagery of the hexagram texts refers to the dragon quarter (in ancient Chinese astronomy, the seven lunar lodges of the eastern quadrant) ascending and descending, over and under the horizon. His study covers seasonal and calendrical import of the dragon as a symbol of fertility and spring, delving also into possible contiguity with the Yellow Thearch's 黃帝 Cycle of Myths, namely those concerning his crusade against Chiyou 蚩尤 (Shaughnessy 1997, 197–219).

9.4 Mythic Narratives in the *Zhouyi*

This section relates selections from an article published in 1929 by Gu Jiegang 顧頡剛 (1990 [1929]) where he seeks to reconstruct some narratives in the *Zhouyi*, some of which are acknowledged to belong to the realm of ancient myth while also grounded in history. Gu's purpose with this paper is more focused on establishing a timeframe for the development and authorship of the various strata of the text, less so with rediscovering myths.

In the present author's opinion, a criterion for classifying myths into different cultural eras is needed. Clearly, a great deal of Chinese myths is euhemerized history and the demarcation between the world of gods and mortals is somewhat less clear than in the major Occidental mythologies. When it comes to narratives that are clearly in historical time and involving persons that almost certainly existed, we must carefully consider to what extent and in what ways mythic narrative has been imprinted upon them by posterity. For the purposes of this paper, clearly, historical figures or narratives will be excluded unless they appear to have been imbued with such mythic significance. For example, one would be wary of treating personages of the late Shang and Zhou history as mythic without good reason. Therefore, the most significant narrative that Gu Jiegang's article deals with is the King Hai myth, for the colorful way in which he is depicted in the *Shanhaijing* suggests that we are dealing with an actual historical person who also had, in religious and mythic context, acquired a deeply symbolic role.

That being said, though there is as yet no clear date for the composition ofthe *Zhouyi*, for the purpose of this discussion the assumption will be that the text is named after the Zhou dynasty and that both King Wen 文王 and the Duke of Zhou 周公 contributed to its composition. The question of inclusion of narratives based on persons or events later than the early Zhou does not concern this discussion and other "myths" about the book based mostly on the "Appended Judgments" (Xici zhuan 繫辭傳) of the *Ten Wings* are taken as such, narratives of mythic import that may or may not reflect an objective historical reality.

Gu Jiegang 顧頡剛, a Republican Era scholar most famous for his nine-volume work *Debates on Ancient History* (*Gushi bian* 古史辨) and for co-founding and leading the Doubting Antiquity School (Yigupai 疑古派) raised several proposals about mythic or legendary narratives in the *Zhouyi* in his 1929 article "Narratives in the Judgments and Line Statements of the *Zhouyi*," (《周易》卦爻辭中的故事) all of which are also addressed in a similar fashion by Gao Heng 高亨 (2010) in his *Modern Notes on the Ancient Book of Changes* (*Zhouyi gujing jinzhu* 周易古經今注) and are cited in most recent academic translations focusing on bronze age culture, such as Richard Rutt (2002), John Minford (2014), Stephen L. Field (2015) and others. He states that this work is largely based on the research of Wang Guowei 王國維.

9.4.1 The Myth of King Hai

The first proposed narrative, that of King Hai 王亥, concerns Hexagram 34 (Da Zhuang 大壯) Line 5 and Hexagram 56 (Lü 旅) Line 6 (top):

> 大壯六五:喪羊于易,無悔。
>
> Da Zhuang (hexagram 34) (6 in) line 5: He loses his sheep in the land of *Yi*. There will be no trouble.[7]
>
> 旅上九:鳥焚其巢,旅人先笑後號咷。喪牛于易,凶。
>
> Lü (hexagram 56) (9 in) the top line: A bird burns up its nest. At first the traveler laughs but afterward he weeps (and moans). He loses his cattle in *Yi*. Misfortune.

Based mainly on several obscure lines from *Heavenly Questions* of the *Songs of Chu* (*Chuci Tianwen* 楚辭天問), a passage in the *Shanhaijing* and Guo Pu's commentary thereon, a passage in the *Bamboo Annals*, Wang Guowei's 王國維 expositions of Oracle-bone texts, as well as a few other extant sources, it is proposed that these lines actually refer to a lost mythic narrative. The import of this proposed narrative, it seems, was unknown to the compilers of the *Ten Wings* as well as later commentators, such as Wang Bi 王弼 and Zhu Xi 朱熹. The proposal relies on conjectures involving possible scribal errors and phonetic loans but appears solid enough to warrant serious consideration and is, in fact, the accepted interpretation in most, perhaps all, twentieth-century scholarship. And authorities in Chinese mythology, such as Yuan Ke 袁珂 (1993, 2015), Anne Birrell (1993), and many more have adopted the proposal.

[7] Quotations from the *Zhouyi* in this section are taken from Field (2015) unless otherwise indicated. Sometimes they are slightly amended.

The *Heavenly Questions* of the *Songs of Chu* are a notoriously obscure text but rich in references to cosmogony and mythologems and consequently very important for studies in Chinese mythology. The part that we are primarily concerned with here comes right after a passage/stanza raising questions about the myth of the birth of the Shang clan founder (first ancestor; earliest ancestor) named Qì or Xiè 契. This miraculous birth story is also significant because of the motif of birds which also occurs frequently in the *Zhouyi* including the line statements here under scrutiny. Therefore, we shall take a look at the relevant stanzas from the *Heavenly Questions*, starting with those of the miraculous birth. As mentioned before, this passage was poorly understood until Wang Guowei 王國維 made the connection with the passages that follow.

The lines from the *Songs of Chu*; *Heavenly Questions*:

簡狄在台嚳何宜	If Lady Jiandi was hidden in a tower, how did Di Ku choose her for a wife?
玄鳥致貽女何喜	When the Dark Bird delivered the gift, why was she delighted?
該秉季德厥父是臧	In good works, Hai took up where Ji, his father and model of virtue, left off
胡終弊於有扈牧夫牛羊	So why did he end up dying in Youhu herding those cows and goats?
干協時舞何以懷之	He danced the shield dance—why did he long for her?
平肋曼膚何以肥之	Whose luscious flesh hid the ripple of her ribs? And how did she fatten herself?
有扈牧豎云何而逢	He was but a herd boy in Youyi—how did he meet her?
擊床先出其命何從	She got out before the attackers reached their bed. From whom had the order come?
恆秉季德焉得夫樸牛	In virtue, Heng took up where his father Ji left off. How did he obtain his brother's draft oxen?
何往營班祿不但還來	Why did he go to administer the rewards instead of merely returning?
昏微遵跡有狄不寧	Twilight Wei was next in line to the throne; Youdi would know no peace then
何繁鳥萃棘負子肆情	How could she abandon her child and yield to passion with so many birds perched in the brambles?
眩弟並淫危害厥兄	And the benighted brother, being as lewd as he was, endangered the older Hai
何變化以作詐後嗣而逢長	How could such changeable and deceitful men produce such glorious and enduring posterity?
	(Sukhu 2017, 100–101)

By contrast, the earliest Songs of Chu commentator Wang Yi 王逸 took these passages to refer to Xiang 相, the fifth king of the historically unverified Xia 夏 dynasty and father of Shao Kang 少康, whose birth may be the basis of another obscure passage in the *Zhouyi* (see below). Zhu Xi simply glossed them as "unclear and the various expositions in disagreement."

The next text that concerns this reconstruction is a lost fragment from the *Bamboo Annals* (*Zhushu jinian* 竹書紀年), quoted in Guo Pu's 郭璞 (274–324 CE) "Commentary on the *Classic of Mountains and Seas*." It reads as follows:

> 有人曰王亥,兩手操鳥,方食其頭。王亥託于有易、河伯僕牛。有易殺王亥,取僕牛。
>
> There is a person called King Hai, grasping birds in his two hands, he is about to eat their heads. King Hai stayed in Youyi, the River Lord raised cattle. (The men of) Youyi killed King Hai and seized the cattle.

Guo Pu's commentary here quotes the Bamboo Annals:

> 殷王子亥賓于有易而淫焉、有易之君緜臣殺而放之、是故殷主甲微假師于河伯以伐有易、滅之遂殺其君緜臣也
>
> A prince of Yin (another name for Shang) called Hai was a guest at Youyi and committed adultery there. The Lord of Youyi, called Mianchen killed him and exposed his corpse. Consequently the (next) ruler of Yin raised troops from the River Lord to attack Youyi. He exterminated them (the Youyi tribe) and subsequently killed its Lord Mianchen.

It is clearly true of both the *Heavenly Questions* and the *Shanhaijing* commentary that one is not presented with a narrative as much as references to a narrative that the reader is assumed to already know—a mnemonic or a catechism perhaps, as David Hawkes (1985, 122–126) has suggested. It is therefore unavoidable to use a degree of guesswork in reconstructing these lost narratives and, unsurprisingly, translations tend to disagree when they are basically reconstructing by filling in gaps.

With the assumption that the character *hài*亥 might have been miscopied, further evidence for this reconstruction emerges. We have already seen how in the *Heavenly Questions* the name is written 該 (gāi). In *Shiben*[8] the name of the originator of cattle husbandry is given as Gāi 胲. This is written *hai zuo fu niu* 胲作服牛, and likely referring to the selfsame King Hai. In the *Lüshi Chunqiu* 呂氏春秋 that cultural achievement is associated with the name Wang Bing 王冰, which Wang Guowei 王國維 and Gu Jiegang believe to be a miscopying of Wang (King) Hai due to similarity of seal script forms.[9]

Let us examine yet another interesting passage with possible relevance to King Hai in the *Shanhaijing*:

> 王子夜之尸,兩手、兩股、胸、首、齒,皆斷異處。
>
> The corpse of Prince Ye, his two arms, two legs (or thighs), a chest, a head and teeth, all have been cut off and are located in different places.

The Japanese geologist and sinologist Ogawa Takuji has proposed that the character *yè* 夜 in this passage is a miscopying of *hài* 亥 (see Fig. 1 for seal script and oracle script forms of these characters). (Yuan 1993, 372–373) Furthermore,

---

[8] *Shiben*《世本》is a second century BCE genealogy of rulers, legendary and historical. The book was lost by the tenth century CE but partially reconstructed from extant quotations by Qing scholars, a process similar to the reconstruction of the *Guicang Changes* 歸藏易.

[9] Apart from the names Gai胲and Wang Bing 王冰, the relevant passages in the *Shiben* and the *Lüshi Chunqiu* are otherwise identical: The formulation in the former is "胲作服牛" and "王冰作服牛" in the latter.

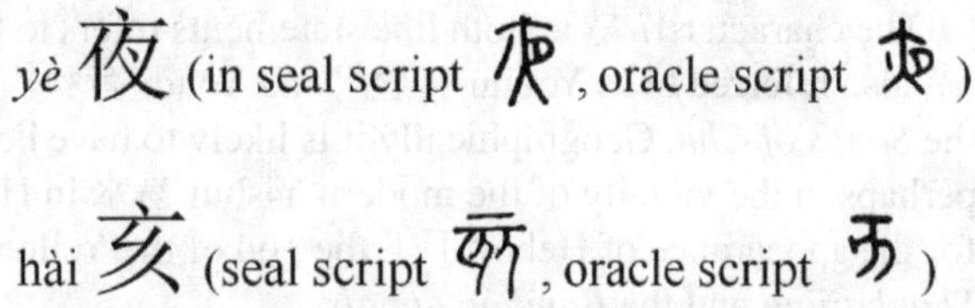

Fig. 1 Seal script and oracle script forms

renowned mythographer Yuan Ke 袁珂 also points out the similarities between this passage and a rather obscure phrase from *Zuo's Commentary on the Spring and Autumn Annals* which goes like this:

> 史趙曰,亥有二首六身,下二如身,是其日數也。
>
> The historiographer Zhao said, "The character hai (see Fig. 1) is composed of two at the head and sixes in the body of it. If you take the two and place it alongside the sixes of the body, you get the number of the man's days." (trans. Legge 2000, vol. V, 552 and 556)

Yuan Ke proposes that this obscure passage may refer not to the glyph *hài* 亥, but to the mythic or historic person King Hai. One might also entertain the possibility that it might refer to both and that King Hai's dismembered corpse was somehow the basis for numerological symbolism. In the *Bamboo Annals* quote from Guo Pu's commentary, it is stated that King Hai's corpse was exposed to the elements, and if we accept that these passages also refer to King Hai, then it would seem that his corpse is also mutilated. By a little stretch of the imagination, one might even propose that this refers to a sort of sacrifice and perhaps a ritual reenactment of the death of *Pangu* 盤古, whose body parts became the various parts of the created earth, like Ýmir in Norse mythology.

The story that emerges from these passages in the *Heavenly Questions* and supplemented by those from the *Bamboo Annals* and *The Classic of Hills and Seas* is that of King Hai, a leader of the pre-dynastic Shang tribe during the legendary Xia 夏 dynasty. He is attributed as the originator of cattle husbandry, the socioeconomic value of which is immense for pastoral cultures (Birrell 1993, 106). He travels to the land of Youyi 有易 and is nobly received by the local chieftain, Mianchen 緜臣. However, some indecorous incident occurs between King Hai and the local chieftain's wife, apparently resulting in the execution of King Hai and the desecration of his corpse and seizing of his cattle assets. The person who killed King Hai was a herdsman of Youyi, and the method of execution was being bludgeoned in bed. King Hai's younger brother Heng 恆 is involved but in what way is not clear. It is eventually King Hai's son Shangjia Wei 上甲微 who restores his father's and their lineage's honor and punishes the Youyi tribe. The import of the story seems to have been that tradition regarded King Hai's transgression as indicative of a moral decline of the Shang state's original virtue, which was again reversed by Shangjia Wei's campaign of revenge.

In any case, we can plot a correspondence of this reconstructed mythic narrative and the relevant line statements of the *Zhouyi* (Gu 1990 [1929], 7–8).

The character *Yi* 易 in both line statements refers to the land and tribe of Youyi 有易, also referred to as Youhu 有扈[10] and Youdi 有狄[11] in the *Heavenly Questions* of the *Songs of Chu*. Geographically it is likely to have been north of the Yellow River, perhaps in the vicinity of the modern Yishui 易水 in Hebei. This could also account for the appearance of Hebo 河伯, the god of the Yellow River, in the quote from the *Shanhaijing* and the *Bamboo annals*.

The name or tag of hexagram 56 is *Lüren* 旅人, usually translated as "The traveler" and according to Gu Jiegang, the traveler 旅人 in the top line of hexagram 56 is King Hai. The hexagram as a whole, including its judgment and line statements, may contain references to the narrative of King Hai (Field 2015, 223–225). If that is the case, it is not clear exactly how the other line statements of hexagram 56 might represent aspects of King Hai and his narrative, but it is interesting to note that the *Heavenly Questions* refer to a cattleherd as *puniu* 樸牛 (usually written 僕牛) or *mushu* 牧豎 (same as *mutong* 牧童 in later parlance), and line statement 2 (六二: 旅即次,懷其資,得童僕貞。) refers to a servant as *tongpu* 童僕, which is also lost, with strikingly similar phonetic elements and a burning house, as opposed to burning bird's nest as in the top line.

"Losing sheep and cattle" 喪羊喪牛 refers to the Youyi tribe seizing of livestock after killing King Hai.

"Birds burn their nests" (*niao fen qi chiao* 鳥焚其巢) refers to King Hai's indecorousness leading to his miserable fate and, moreover, the birds are likely an expression of the bird symbolism strongly associated with the Shang tribe and their symbolic identity.[12] Furthermore, an early form of the glyph *hài* 亥 in oracle-bone inscriptions is frequently accompanied by a bird-element.

"The traveler first laughs but afterwards cries and moans" (*lü ren xian xiao hou hao tao* 旅人先笑後號咷) then refers to the initial welcome that King Hai enjoys and things turning sour with his indecorous behavior.

Furthermore, what may at first appear to be a historical or legendary account of the ancestral linage of the Shang clan that later founded a dynasty, is probably also a part of the mythic landscape, in that the story, though it may have some historicity, was perhaps more important as a mythic narrative. The references to King Hai in *Shanhaijing* seem to fully attest to a sort of primitive religiosity, and further, these appearances occur close to references to Di Jun and other major figures of the mythic landscape.

As for the rest of the line statements for hexagrams 34 and 56, one might ask oneself whether they could also be about King Hai. Many hexagrams' judgments and line texts exhibit clear thematic coherence, such as the ascending dragon of Hexagram 1 and the wild geese of Hexagram 63. Both these hexagrams exhibit some thematic coherence. In the case of hexagram 34, the "Strongman" of the hexagram name is

[10] According to one tradition, this ancient tribe is associated with rebelling against the ascendancy of Qi 啓 of the Xia dynasty. Defeated, its remnants moved to Youyi 有易.

[11] The two glyphs 狄 (Middle Chinese *DEK*) and 易 (Middle Chinese *YEK*) demonstrably belong to the same rhyme group and were used interchangeably through borrowings.

[12] As has been amply demonstrated by Sarah Allan (1991).

referenced in three line statements, and in the case of Hexagram 56, the "Traveler" is mentioned in all but one line statement. Might King Wen be the Strongman and/or the Traveler of these hexagrams? Could the Strongman or the Traveler turn out to be King Heng, the scoundrel brother? Is there a Twin motif? In the case of these two, the idea that a whole hexagram may be grounded in a coherent mythologem is, however appealing, neither evident nor easily demonstrated.

Furthermore, might there be a significant connection between line statements as indicating changing lines and resulting hexagrams? In the case of hexagram 34, line 5 gives the prognostication *wu hui* 无悔 "no regret" and if line 5 is the only changing line the resulting hexagram would be Hexagram 43 (*Guai* 夬) a basically favorable hexagram about being decisive but not rash, which is safe to say is fairly thematically coherent. In the case of the top line of hexagram 56, the resulting hexagram 62 (*Xiao guo* 小過) is, among other things, about meticulous attention to detail, which would be good advice for a traveler, but the prognostication of the hexagram is *xiong* 凶 or "misfortune" and though hardly a glaring contradiction it is hard to see as coherent either. However, I believe most students of the *Yijing* who actually cast would agree that there is no absolute good or bad fortune in any hexagram, all is subjective and relative.

9.4.2 Gao Zong Attacks the Ghostlands

既濟:九三:高宗伐鬼方,三年克之,小人勿用。

Ji Ji (hexagram 63), 9 in line 3. Gao Zong (High Ancestor) attacked the Land of Ghosts and conquered it in three years. The lowborn should not use this omen.

未濟:九四:貞吉,悔亡,震用伐鬼方,三年有賞于大國。

Wei Ji (hexagram 64), 9 in line 4. Omen of good fortune. Problems disappear. *Zhen* used this omen to attack the Land of Ghosts. In three years he was rewarded in the great state.

Both these line statements relate to the Shang King Wu Ding 武丁 whose posthumous name is Gao Zong 高宗. He ruled the Shang state during the second half of the thirteenth century BCE, a time of prosperity and expansion for the dynasty. Gui Fang 鬼方 refers to lands of savage tribes to the northwest of the Shang heartland in modern-day Shanxi, often somewhat casually translated as Ghostland or Demonland which gives the line a bit of an ominous air but is probably simply a derogatory term for troublesome neighbors or perhaps merely a colorful way to describe the folk of strange and distant lands. Viewed in that light, translating in this way is arguably not inappropriate.

According to Gu Jiegang, the historicity of the campaigns against the Gui tribes is well attested by Wang Guowei (Gu 1990 [1929], 8–9). There is, however, little mythic import in this story, although references to both abound and Gu Jiegang believes those references to have held an anecdotal meaning which was later lost. Gu Jiegang believes that number of years is symbolically significant; the three years of the campaign against the Guifang (in one version ten years) and the three years of mourning Gao Zong undertook before assuming the throne signify a long time (and ten years a *very* long time) rather than literally three or ten years.

The glyph *Zhen* 震 in line 4 of hexagram 64 is usually taken to be the name of an otherwise unknown warrior. Identification based on convoluted philological arguments attempts to identify this warrior in various ways, including as King Hai of the previous segment (for in some works the name *He* 核, a phonetic derivative of *Hai* 亥 is associated with the campaign), as pre-dynastic Zhou ruler Ji Li 季歷, and as Wu Ding himself. Though notable, none of these proposals are conclusive.

In the "Decade of Tang" (Tang zhi shen 蕩之什) of the *Book of Odes* (*Shi Jing* 詩經) we find the following stanza:

> 文王曰咨、咨女殷商。如蜩如螗、如沸如羹。
> 小大近喪、人尚乎由行。內奰于中國、覃及鬼方。
>
> King Wen said, "Alas! Alas! you [sovereign of] Yin-shang, [All around you] is like the noise of cicadas, Or like the bubbling of boiling soup.
>
> Affairs, great and small, are approaching to ruin; And still you [and your creatures] go on in this course. Indignation is rife against you here in the Middle kingdom, And extends to the demon regions." (trans. Legge 2000, vol. IV, 508–509)

In this stanza the sovereign being remonstrated against by King Wen is not the one mentioned in the *Zhouyi*, but his descendant the infamous tyrant Zhou 紂, whose infamy was such as to even shock the savages of faraway lands. Also, King Wen and Zhou of the Shang are the major figures in the semi-historical legends of dynastic upheaval that are background to the formation of the text of the *Zhouyi*. Gao Zong on the other hand was venerated in Zhou culture, perhaps to mythic proportions. In *The Book of Documents* (*Shang Shu* 尚書) he is shown as an observer of rites of ancestor veneration, a trait that the Zhou clan and later Confucius and Confucianism clearly valued highly.

Also, in the context of the Guifang tribes, we see references to a marriage and a birth. The following are from the *Fengsu Tongyi* 風俗通義 and the *Da Dai Li Ji* 大戴禮記.

> 楚之先出自帝顓頊,其裔孫曰陸終,娶于鬼方氏,是謂女漬。蓋孕而三年不育,啟其左脅,三人出焉,啟其右脅,三人又出焉。[13]
>
> The ancestors of Chu sprang from the Thearch Zhuan Xu, whose offspring is Lu Zhong, who took a wife from the Guifang tribe. She was called Nü Zi. She was pregnant but for three years did not give birth. Her left flank opened and three "persons" emerged, and her right flank opened and another three emerged.
>
> 陸終氏娶于鬼方氏,鬼方氏之妹謂之女隤,氏產六子;孕而不粥,三年,啟其左脅,六人出焉。[14]
>
> Mr. Lu Zhong took a wife from the Guifang tribe; the girl of the Guifang tribe was known as Nü Tui and she gave birth to six sons. She was pregnant but did not give birth for three years, (then) when her left flank opened and six "persons" came out.

[13] *Fengsu Tongyi*: https://ctext.org/fengsutongyi/huang-ba/zh.

[14] *Da Dai Li Ji*: https://ctext.org/da-dai-li-ji/di-xi/zh.

Although nothing like this is mentioned in the *Zhouyi*, it suggests miraculous circumstances of birth and therefore might be part of a symbolic or religious context for the Guifang tribes.

There is also the fact that these line statements belong to the last pair of hexagrams in the received text of the *Zhouyi*, a matter that has less to do with mythic narrative and more with numerology and symbolism, but an analysis of the hexagram pairs and their connectedness might offer additional insight on the mythic narratives.

In the received text of the *Zhouyi*, the order of the hexagrams, often referred to as King Wen's order, the hexagrams are arranged in pairs in which each pair is most commonly a top–bottom reversal of *yin* and *yang* lines of its mate. This is called *fan gua* 反卦 or "overturned hexagram." This principle of pairing is however only possible for 56 of the 64 hexagrams since the remaining eight would produce themselves if overturned in this way. Therefore, the remaining eight are paired according to a principle called *pan tong gua* 旁通卦 or "laterally linked hexagrams." These four pairs are: Hexagram 1 ䷀ 乾 *Qian* and Hexagram 2 ䷁ 坤 *Kun*; Hexagram 27 ䷚ 頤 *Yi* and Hexagram 28 ䷛ 大過 *Da Guo*; Hexagram 29 ䷜ 坎 *Kan* and Hexagram 30 ䷝ 離 *Li*; Hexagram 61 ䷼ 中孚 *Zhong Fu* and Hexagram 62 ䷽ 小過 *Xiao Guo*, and these eight are by many commentators and practitioners held to have a special significance. There are in addition another eight hexagrams that conform to both principles and as such also stand apart. These hexagrams pairs are: Hexagram 11 ䷊ 泰 *Tai* and Hexagram 12 ䷋ 否 *Bi*; Hexagram 17 ䷐ 隨 *Sui* and Hexagram 18 ䷑ 蠱 *Gu*; Hexagram 53 ䷴ 漸 *Jian* and hexagram 54 ䷵ 歸妹 *Gui Mei*; hexagram 63 ䷾ 既濟 *Ji Ji* and hexagram 64 ䷿ 未濟 *Wei Ji*, collectively called *fei fu sheng jiang jie dui* 飛伏升降皆對 or "the opposites that are flying and hidden, ascending and descending." (Nielsen 2003, 57–58, 62 and 185–188).

The pairing of hexagrams 63 ䷾ 既濟 *Ji Ji* and 64 ䷿ 未濟 *Wei Ji* viewed from the point of view of the constituting trigrams may be interpreted as signifying a setting sun and rising sun, respectively. In the case of hexagram 63 *Ji Ji*, ☲離 *Li*, the trigram most typically signifying fire but also the sun, is underneath ☵ 坎 *Kan*, the trigram of water, the moon, deep and turbulent water, and the sea. In trigram theory, the relationship between upper and lower trigrams of a hexagram, includes the notion of the lower hexagram emerging, a situation akin to the sun "emerging" from an eastern sea and an interpretation supported by the hexagrams tag name, that can be translated as *Already Across / Completed*. Conversely, in the case of hexagram 64 *Wei Ji*, the upper trigram is now ☲ 離 *Li*, the sun and fire, and the lower is ☵ 坎 *Kan*, the deep sea, the sun now having risen above the ocean, a situation also consistent with trigram theory and the tag name *Not Yet Across / Not Completed*. Edward Shaughnessy has also proposed that the relationship of the two hexagrams' tag names may have been seen to signify the decline of the Shang dynasty and the ascent of the Zhou (Shaughnessy 1983, 263–264).

9.4.3 *Di Yi Marries off a Maiden*

> 泰:六五:帝乙歸妹,以祉元吉。
>
> Tai (Hexagram 11) 6 in line 5. Di Yi marries off a daughter, a blessed affair, very auspicious.
>
> 歸妹: 六五:帝乙歸妹,其君之袂,不如其娣之袂良,月幾望,吉。
>
> Gui Mei (Hexagram 54) 6 in line 5. King Di Yi gave his daughter in marriage. The sleeves of her gown will not be as fine as those of her younger sister. The moon is almost full. Good fortune. (trans. Field 2015, 217)

Although Gu Jiegang is convinced there is a lost story here, there really is too little information to work with. He speculates that the story is in all likelihood about political marriages between states during Shang ascendancy. Perhaps the bride in question is King Wen's mother, or perhaps King Wen's first wife but not the mother of his heir, King Wu 武王. In any case, she is a princess or aristocrat of the Shang clan and the Shang king Di Yi 帝乙 was a contemporary of both King Wen and his father King Ji 王季.

S.J. Marshall believes that the attribution to King Wen's wife to be far less plausible than supposing that Di Yi gave his younger sister in marriage to King Ji, King Wen's father, which would make the bride in question his mother, since it is fairly clear from the *Odes* that King Ji was married to a Shang princess and the matter of King Wen's marital situation is unclear (Marshall 2001, 156–158).

9.4.4 *Prince Jizi*

> 明夷:六五:箕子之明夷,利貞。
>
> Ming Yi (Hexagram 36) Jizi's pheasant OR Jizi's imprisonment, advantageous prognostication.

The story of Jizi is well-known and frequently quoted. It is documented in such works as the *Book of Documents* (*Shang Shu* 尚書), *Songs of Chu* (*Chuci* 楚辭), *Hanfeizi* 韓非子, *The Analects of Confucius* (*Lun Yu* 論語) as well as the *Shiji* 史記. His remonstrations with the tyrant Zhou 紂, last king of the Shang dynasty, led to his enslavement and imprisonment. In the Hongfan 洪范 chapter of the *Book of Documents*, Jizi illustrates the five phases (*wuxing* 五行) for King Wu in a passage which I believe may be one of the earliest, if not the earliest, reference to five phases theory in Chinese classics.[15]

[15] *Shangshu, Hongfan* 《尚書》洪範:五行:一曰水,二曰火,三曰木,四曰金,五曰土。水曰潤下,火曰炎上,木曰曲直,金曰從革,土爰稼穡。"… of the five elements. The first is water; the second is fire; the third, wood; the fourth, metal; and the fifth, earth. (The nature of) water is to soak and descend; of fire, to blaze and ascend; of wood, to be crooked and straight; of metal, to yield and change; while (that of) earth is seen in seed-sowing and ingathering." (trans. Legge 2000, vol. III, 325–326).

In a very interesting sidenote based on a much-disputed Korean mytho-historical narrative, Jizi supposedly led his army to regions far to the northwest and founded a dynasty that lasted centuries, the so-called Gija Joseon (箕子 is pronounced Gija 기자 in Korean). The story is recorded in the *Samguk Yusa* 三國遺事 and alluded to in the *Records of the Historian* 史記 as well.

I suspect that this rather belongs to the realm of Confucian moral anecdotes than myth. The interpretation of said lines in the *Zhouyi* is also much in dispute. Some scholars are inclined to reading 箕子 as *qí zǐ* 其子 meaning "his son" or even as *gāi zī* 荄兹, meaning "verdant vegetation."

9.4.5 Kang Hou

> 晉:康侯用錫馬蕃庶,晝日三接。
>
> Jin (Hexagram 35) The Marquis of Kang was given horses. They multiplied. He mated them several times a day (trans. Rutt 2002).

Gu Jiegang identifies the Marquis of Kang with one Ji Feng 姬封, younger brother of King Wu. He was enfeoffed to the state of Kang and thereafter known as Kang Shu 康叔 or less commonly as the Marquis of Kang 康侯. The latter appellation is not seen in ancient books but only in Bronzes, and Gu speculates that earlier commentators may not have made the connection because of this, or they might have thought it impossible that a person living after King Wen's death could be mentioned in the *Zhouyi*. Gu also believes this to have been one of the very first enfeoffments of the Zhou and that the word for the custom (*fengjian* 封建) may have come from his personal name. In any case, the anecdotal story of the Marquis and the horses is lost.

Gu Jiegang raises other points but on the whole his emphasis is not on mythology as much as history, and, being true to the school of thought he represented, he generally does more doubting than rediscovering. He lists many hexagram and line texts that he thinks are likely references to anecdotal narratives but laments that these are but unverifiable tantalizing hints. While expressing hope of further discoveries by excavation, he warns us not to resort to dubious interpretation for the sake of achieving comprehensiveness.

9.5 The *Guicangyi* Myths

Although the silk manuscript of *Mawangdui* 馬王堆 has several very interesting orthographical divergences from the received text, these are mostly phonetic or semantic variants and appear to offer little for our search for alternative and possibly mythic narratives. For example, the trigram tag names for the hexagrams that are doubled trigrams seem to have much more to do with the *gua xiang* 卦象 (natural phenomena trigram attributes) and *gua de* 卦德 (virtue trigram attributes) attributes as described in the Shuogua zhuan 說卦傳 of the *Ten Wings* rather than the tag names of the received text. For example, ☰ 乾 *qian* is 鍵 *jian*, which is very close to the *gua de* attribute of 健, as ☷ 坤 *kun* is 川 *chuan*, akin to 順 *shun*. These raise interesting questions about the semantics and symbolic meaning in relation to the evolution of the trigram concepts.

There is however another archeological discovery of great importance to the field of ancient Chinese religion in general and *Zhouyi* studies in particular. In 1993, peasants in the village Wangjiatai 王家台 in Hubei 湖北 discovered 16 tombs in what used to be the ancient state of Chu 楚 back in the Warring States era. The village is located close to the sites of two ancient Chu capitals and since archeological digs are common in the vicinity, excavations proceeded promptly. One relatively small tomb contained, among other things, heaps of bamboo strips that were remnants of books,[16] the writing style of which was also a major factor in dating the site to the mid-third century BCE.

It turned out that of 813 strips of bamboo, 394 have been definitely identified as belonging to two distinct copies of a divination manual, similar in structure to the *Zhouyi*, in essence an alternative text accompanying a nearly identical hexagram chapter structure. And these can with reasonable certainty be assigned to some 50 traditional hexagrams, albeit most of the bamboo strips are extremely fragmented and in some cases, we have only a hexagram graph or name tag.

Furthermore, the text, fragmented though it is, is clearly the same as the oft-quoted lost text usually called *Guicangyi* 歸藏易 and in fact, this archeological find firmly puts to rest the question of the historical *Guicangyi*'s oft-disputed authenticity. This text has a rather ambiguous history and the whole issue along with everything we can know about the excavated material has been thoroughly and satisfactorily covered by Edward L. Shaughnessy (2014, 141–187). Suffice it to say here that the received fragments were already conspicuously rich in references to mythic, legendary, and semi-historical personages, and the same holds true for the *Guicangyi*. Below, passages from compilations made by various Qing dynasty scholars[17] will be referred to as the "received quotes," while those from the archeological discovery will be referred to as the "*Guicangyi* manuscript."

The form of those hexagram texts is also quite consistently of two main types. All hexagrams begin with a hexagram graph, followed by a hexagram tag name. In the cases of the first most common type (ibid., 152), this is followed by a situation about which someone makes a plastron divination (*pú* 卜), and then appeals to someone, often a shaman, for a milfoil prognostication (variously written as *pū* 攴 or *méi* 枚 in the manuscript, or *shì* 筮 in the received quotes). This is followed by an anecdotal narrative relating the purpose of the hexagram. The second type starts out with a general divinatory prayer for the safety of a state or a charge to a deity for protection,

---

[16] So-called *zhujjian* 竹簡. The books consisted of long strips of bamboo, one side of which contained writing, bound together with leather or silk cords.

[17] The most complete and well known of these is in the *Yuhan shanfang jiyi shu*《玉函山房輯佚書》of Ma Guohan 馬國翰 (1794–1857).

uttered by a historical ruler (ibid., 158). This is followed by a prognostication and a narrative oracle. The third type dispenses with prognostication and delves straight into oracle narratives.

The extant fragments show these trends quite clearly, however, because of the fragmentary and damaged condition of the manuscript as well as the fact that only a transcript in simplified Chinese characters has been published, it is extremely hard to even speculate whether this formula holds true for most or just how many of the hexagram texts.[18]

Let us conclude this discussion of the *Guicangyi* with a few examples of how it relates to the mythic landscape described earlier.

Xia Hou Qi 夏后啓 refers to the legendary first true king of the Xia dynasty, son of Yu the Great. He was miraculously born from a literally petrified pregnant mother when his father cried out at the stone in grief. Now in spite of several references to him in the *Shanhaijing*, a book rich in descriptions and relatively poor in narratives, he comes across as a rather minor deity, since compared to the other godlike personages in the ancient Chinese pantheon, what we are told of his exploits appears limited. We should bear in mind though that the same holds true for Chinese myth in general. Tales of the exploits of gods and heroes are conspicuously few compared to Graeco-Roman or Norse myth.

In the *Guicangyi* however, his prominence feels conspicuous, since we have a total of six hexagrams involving him, which may be a coincidence only, but in any case, we shall commence our discussion of *Guicangyi* mythic references with what could be called the Cycle of Myths revolving around his family, beginning with his grandfather Gun 鯀.

Gun appears to be a minister of Thearch Yao 帝堯 in the semi-historical (but largely mythical) era to which the *Records of the Historian* (*Shiji* 史記) refer as Tang Yu 唐虞, a Golden Age which seems to be the boundary between a mythic time and historical reckoning. At this time, catastrophic floods threatened the civilized realm ruled by Thearch Yao, and he commissioned Gun to take charge of controlling the floods. However, Gun is said to have failed and was punished by death or exile. The following two mentions of Gun's exploits are from the historical *Guicangyi* quotes, both from Guo Pu's commentary on the *Shanhaijing*.

> 滔滔洪水無所止極伯鯀乃以息石息壤以填洪水
>
> So gushing were the floodwaters, with no place to stop the extremes. Elder Gun then used the expanding stone and the expanding soil to stop up the floodwaters.
>
> 鯀死三歲不腐剖之以吳刀化為黃熊
>
> [After Gun died,] for three years [he] did not decompose. They cut him open with a knife from Wu and he transformed into a yellow bear.[19]

The former passage is about Gun's mission to control the floodwaters, and the second is about what happened after his punishment for his alleged failure. How or

[18] Because of unfortunate conditions involving photosensitive fungi, no photographs of the bamboo strips have been released.

[19] The transcripts and translations from the *Guicangyi* are all from Shaughnessy (2014, 174–187).

why he failed is not very clear from the available sources, but what is made clear is that his son, Yu 禹, is charged with finishing his father's work. The birth of Yu is also quite miraculous for he appears to have sprung from Gun's corpse, and since Yu is also reputed to have often taken the shape of a bear in his great work of taming the floodwaters, the yellow bear in the passage in the second passage here may indeed refer to such a transformation. There are in fact alternative narratives about Gun taking a mate and having sons, but a full analysis and account of these as well as the accomplishments of Yu fall outside the scope of this paper.[20]

There is only one passage in the manuscript referring to Yu and somewhat surprisingly, none of the received quotes mention him by name, though some, as the quote above, may be indirectly connected to him. The passage in the manuscript is as follows:

> 曰昔者禹卜食散实而攴占大明占之曰不吉散其 …
>
> … Says: In the past Yu divined about eating the dispersed substance and had the stalks prognosticated by Da Ming, who prognosticated them and said: Not auspicious. Disperse its …

The text is missing its hexagram picture and name tag, but a parallel passage from the 2nd copy of *Guicangyi* in the manuscript, though far more damaged, has both hexagram and tag intact and thus makes it clear that this passage belongs to the hexagram called Jia Ren 家人in the received text of the *Zhouyi* but in the *Guicangyi* goes by a different name: San 散. A possible context for this hexagram text and the stories of Yu can be discerned. The *Heavenly Questions* contains the following stanzas:

禹之力獻功降省下土四方	Yu labored with all his strength. He came down and gazed at the earth below
焉得彼塗山女而通之於台桑	How did he get the Tu-shan girl and lie with her in Tai-sang?
閔妃匹合厥身是繼	His consort became his mate and her body gave forth a child
胡維嗜不同味而快鼂飽	Why did they hunger for the same food, when they had satisfied their hunger for the food of love at dawn? (Birrell 1993, 156)[21]

Though inscrutable as always, what these stanzas of the *Heavenly Questions* illustrate is that Yu was so consumed by his great work that his marriage suffered

[20] A fair but limited account of Gun & Yü is given in Birrell (1993, 146–159) and in the present author's MA thesis (Eyþórsson 2006).

[21] Ch'u Tz'u, Tien wen, SPTK 3.i3b–i4a. Consider Gopal's translation for comparison: "Yu devoted his energy to the task, but, when he came down to inspect all under the sky, how did he happen to meet the daughter of Mud Hill and mate with her under the Towering Mulberries? Though he loved her and made her his wife to continue his family's line, how is it his tastes so differed from most that he was content with but a morning's satisfaction?" In the *Book of Documents*, Yu tells us that after marrying the daughter of the ruler of the Tushan (Mud Hill) state, he stayed with her for only four days so that he could resume the task of stemming the flood. His main purpose in marrying her was to continue the family line. See Legge (2000, vol. 3, 84–85).

greatly for it. It is also said that he often went without eating. Thus, one might reason that "eating dispersed substance or fruit (shi 实 can also mean fruit)" (*shi san shi* 食散实) refers to Yu's neglect of his own nourishment and, by extension, of his wife and household. It also seems quite probable that the situation presented here in the *Guicang Yi* fragments could be thematically related to or be the source of *Zhouyi*'s Jia Ren hexagram.

The story goes that when she was informed that her husband was working in the vicinity, Yu's wife, the Tushan girl, frequently ventured out to bring him food but on one such occasion happened to see him in his bear form. She panicked and ran to Songgao mountain where in her mortification she turned to stone. Yu was certainly not an ideal husband, for when he reached her his first concern was the child that he knew she was carrying, which, according to *Heavenly Questions*, had been conceived that very morning. He cried at the stone "return my son" and the north side of the transformed stone opened up and Qi 啟 was born. Therein also lies the ground for Qi's name, for that ideograph means "open." In light of that, the following fragment of *Guicang Yi* hexagram text hardly needs elucidation.

> 嵩高山啓母在此山化為石而子啓亦登仙
>
> On Mount Songgao, Qi's mother on this mountain was transformed into stone, and her son Qi also ascended to immortality.

A less opaque version of the story of the birth of Qi can be found in a commentary by Yan Shigu 顏師古 (581–645) on the *Han Shu* 漢書, quoting a nonextant passage of the *Huiananzi* 淮南子.

> 禹治鴻水,通轘轅山,化為熊,謂塗山氏曰:"欲餉,聞鼓聲乃來。"禹跳石,誤中鼓。塗山氏往,見禹方作熊,慚而去,至嵩高山下化為石,方生啟。禹曰:"歸我子。"石破北方而啟生。
>
> When Yu was controlling the floodwaters and was making a passage through Mount Huan-yuan, he changed into a bear. He spoke to the Tu-shan girl: "If you want to give me some food, when you hear the sound of a drumbeat, come to me." But Yu leaped on a stone and by mistake drummed on it. The Tu-shan girl came forward, but when she saw Yu in the guise of a bear she was ashamed and fled. She reached the foothills of Mount Sung-kao, when she turned into a stone and bore Qi in her womb. Yu said, "Give me back my son!" The stone then split open on its north flank and Qi was born. (Birrell 1993, 156)[22]

Indeed, as Qi is portrayed in the *Shanhaijing*, he wears what may surely be described as a "shamanly" garb and is renowned for his dealings with the immortal realms. In a chapter of the *Shanhaijing* called "Beyond the Western Sea" it says:

> 大樂之野,夏后啟於此儛九代;乘兩龍,雲蓋三層。左手操翳,右手操環,佩玉璜。在大運山北。一曰大遺之野。
>
> The Wilderness of Bigmusic is where the Lord of the Summer, Open, [that is a literal translation of 夏侯啟] danced the "Nine Successions". He drove two dragons and clouds covered them three layers thick. In his left hand he grasped a feather screen, and in his right hand he held a jade ring. From his belt hung a feather jade half-disc. This Wilderness is north of Mount Bigspin. One author says this happened at the Wilderness of Bigremains. (Birrell 1999)

---

[22] Yan Shigu's commentary on *Han Shu*, Wu-ti chi, referring to a nonextant passage in Huai-nan Tzu, SPPY 6.i7b–i8a.

And later in the chapter titled "Beyond the Great Western Wasteland" it further relates:

> 西南海之外,赤水之南,流沙之西,有人珥兩青蛇,乘兩龍,名曰夏后開。開上三嬪于天,得九辯與九歌以下。此天穆之野,高二千仞,開焉得始歌九招。
>
> Beyond the sea to the southwest, south of Scarlet River and west of Drifting Sands, there is a man called Hsia-hou Kai[23] who wears a green snake in his pierced ears and rides a pair of dragons. Kai went up to Heaven three times as a guest. He received the "Nine Counterpoints" and the "Nine Songs," and he brought them down to earth. This Plain of Heavenly Mu is sixteen thousand feet high, and it was here that Kai first came to sing the "Nine Summons." (Birrell 1993)[24]

This extremely vivid depiction of Qi is echoed in the *Guicangyi*, particularly in Hexagram *Ming Yi*, which, though in a fragmented state in the manuscript, can be supplemented with historical quotations and form a coherent statement.

> 明夷曰昔者夏后启卜乘飞龙以登于天而支占…
>
> Ming Yi "Brightness Obscured" says: In the past Xia Hou Qi divined about flying on a dragon to rise into heaven and had the stalks prognosticated …

And a corresponding passage from the historical quotations reads thus:

> 昔夏后啓筮乘龍以登于天枚占于皋陶皋陶曰吉而必同與神交通以身為帝以王四鄉
>
> In the past Xia Hou Qi divined by milfoil about riding a dragon in order to rise into heaven, and had the stalks prognosticated by Gao Yao. Gao Yao said: Auspicious. Yet it must be the same, communicating with the spirits, with his body being Di, to rule over the four directions.

In this way, expositions of the mythic narrative fragments from the *Guicangyi* hexagram texts, truly seem to reflect the mythic landscape we have described, and furthermore, the language of the *Guicangyi* and the *Shanhaijing* seem to echo one another in such a way that one is justified believing them to be the products of a similar or the same culture and era.

Further expositions of *Guicangyi* excavated text fragments and historical quotes are also quite evidently possible for such figures of the mythic landscape as: Nüwa the creatrix 女媧; Yi the Archer (Hou Yi 后羿); Xi He 羲和 the mother and charioteer of the ten suns; Heng E 姮娥 the lunar deity; and The Royal Mother of the West (Xi Wang Mu 西王母); as well as Wu Xian 巫咸 and other diviners, all of which appear distinctly in the *Guicangyi*. It is, however, sadly, beyond the scope of the present paper.

---

[23] Kai refers to Qi, written with a different character as a consequence of the naming taboo for Emperor Jing of the Han dynasty. Cf. Chen Yuan (1962, 130).

[24] *Shan hai ching*, Ta huang hsi ching, SPPY i6.7b–8a.

9.6 Conclusions

In the present author's opinion, the evidence before us as summarized here, though not conclusive, suggests that a correlation exists between the mythic worldview of pre-Qin China and the *Zhouyi*. We can see how the fragments of myth in the *Zhouyi* may be very subtle and obscured and it is likely that narratives of mythic, legendary, or historic nature embedded into the hexagram and line statements were included or referenced in order to imbue the statements with recognizable symbolic meaning for the divinatory process.

The reconstruction of more mythic remnants and rediscovery of symbolism in the *Zhouyi* may considerably deepen our understanding of this mysterious and continually inspiring and fascinating book.

The *Guicangyi* 歸藏易 materials suggest the existence of a divination manual similar to the *Zhouyi* that is more embedded in mythology. As for the dating of those materials, it would appear that *Zhouyi* is the older of the two or at least probably older than the version of the *Guicangyi* under discussion, but the mythology in question is largely that of the Shang dynasty, giving credence to the *Liji* attribution of the *Guicang* in the *Zhouli* 周禮.[25] There may have been earlier version of the *Guicang* and the mythic symbolism may be that of the Shang, reinterpreted by or for the Zhou dynasty.

The *Zhouyi*, though not exclusively a Confucian text, was canonized by Confucian literati and the Confucian tendency to expunge illogical myths but retain moral stories is a point often assumed about the fragmentation and relative dearth of Chinese myth. It is not unthinkable that mythic elements were avoided and even censored in the compilation of the text.

References

Allan, Sarah. 1991. *The Shape of the Turtle: Myth, Art, and Cosmos in Early China*. Albany, NY: State University of New York Press.

Birrell, Anne. 1993. *Chinese Mythology: An Introduction*. Baltimore: The Johns Hopkins University Press.

Birrell, Anne (tr.). 1999. *The Classic of Mountains and Seas*. Middlesex: Penguin.

Chen Yuan 陳垣. 1962. *Shiwei Julie* 史諱舉例 [Examples of Taboos in History]. Beijing: Zhonghua Book Company (中華書局).

Chinese Text Project. 2006–2024. https://ctext.org.

Eyþórsson, Jón Egill. 2006. *The Myths of Yu the Great and the Wheel of Rangarhverfi* 伯禹之神話傳説群和朗河地區之輪. MA thesis. Hangzhou: Zhejiang University.

Field, Stephen L. (tr.). 2015. *The Duke of Zhou Changes: A Study and Annotated Translation of the Zhouyi* 周易. Wiesbaden: Harrassowitz Verlag.

Gu Jiegang 顧頡剛. 1990 [1929]. "Zhouyi" guayaoci de gushi《周易》卦爻辭中的故事 in *Zhouyi yanjiu lun wenji* 周易研究論文集. Vol. 4. Beijing: Beijing shifan daxue chubanshe.

[25] *Zhouli*, Chunguan Zongbo:《周禮》春官宗伯:掌三易之法,一曰「連山」,二曰「歸藏」,三曰「周易」。其經卦皆八,其別皆六十有四。

Hawkes, David (tr.). 1985. *The Songs of the South: An Ancient Chinese Anthology of Poems by Qu Yuan and other Poets.* Middlesex: Penguin.

Gao Heng 高亨. 2010. *Zhouyi Gujing Jinzhu* 周易古經今注. Taipei: Tsinghua University Press.

Legge, James (tr.). 2000. *The Chinese Classics.* 5 vols. Taipei: SMC Publishing.

Marshall, S.J. 2001. *The Mandate of Heaven: Hidden History in the I Ching.* New York: Columbia University Press.

Minford, John (tr.). 2014. *I Ching: The Essential Translation of the Ancient Chinese Oracle and Book of Wisdom.* New York: Viking Penguin.

Moore, Steve. 1989. *The Trigrams of the Han.* Wellingborough: Aquarian Press.

Nielsen, Bent. 2003. *A Companion to Yi Jing Numerology & Cosmology.* London: RoutledgeCurzon.

Rutt, Richard (tr.). 2002. *The Book of Changes (Zhouyi): A Bronze Age Document Translated with Introduction and Notes.* London: RoutledgeCurzon.

Shaughnessy, Edward L. 2014. *Unearthing the Changes: Recently Discovered Manuscripts of the Yi Jing (I Ching) and Related Texts.* New York: Columbia University Press.

Shaughnessy, Edward L. 1983. *The Composition of the Zhouyi.* PhD dissertation. Stanford: Stanford University.

Shaughnessy, Edward L. 1997. The Composition of "Qian" and "Kun" Hexagrams of the *Zhouyi.* In *Before Confucius: Studies in the Creation of the Chinese Classics.* Albany, NY: State University of New York Press.

Sukhu, Gopal (tr.). 2017. *The Songs of Chu: An Anthology of Ancient Chinese Poetry by Qu Yuan and Others.* New York: Columbia University Press.

Ye Shuxian 葉舒憲. 1992. *Zhongguo Shenhua Zhexue* 中國神話哲學. Beijing: China Social Sciences Press.

Yuan Ke 袁珂. 2015. *Zhongguo Shenhua Dacidian* 中國神話大辭典. Taipei: Huaxia Publishing House.

Yuan Ke 袁珂. 1993. *Shanghaijing Jiaozhu* 山海經校注. Chengdu: Ba Shu Shu she.

Chapter 10
Yijing in Chinese Aesthetics: Shitao's Theory of Individual Creativity and the Holistic Brushstroke

Téa Sernelj

Abstract The article explores the impact of the *Yijing* on the aesthetic theory of the early Qing Dynasty painter Shitao. Based on compelling evidence, it illustrates the close interconnection between Shitao's aesthetic theory and the onto-cosmology of the *Yijing*. He adeptly integrated its concepts into his artistic framework, emphasizing the pivotal role of individual creativity and the preservation of a holistic approach throughout the creative process. In his seminal work, "Remarks on Painting," Shitao presents an exceptionally distinctive theory of Holistic Brushstroke inspired by the teachings of the *Yijing*, *Daodejing*, and Chan (Zen) philosophy. Based on these profound philosophical traditions, he creates a unique and innovative approach to the art of painting that transcends conventional boundaries. This article focuses on the specific parts of Shitao's aesthetic theory that relate directly to the *Yijing*, revealing his alignment with the aesthetics of the literati painters. It illuminates the long tradition within Chinese aesthetics, firmly rooted in the foundations of the *Yijing*, in which the act of creation and artistic expression is seen as a profound reiteration of the cosmic creative force—the *Dao* itself. In this context, the artist becomes a channel through which the universal creative energy flows, producing art that reflects the very essence of existence. Shitao's aesthetic theory, deeply influenced by *Yijing* and *Daodejing*, reflects a harmonious connection between the natural world and the human spirit, emphasizing the interconnectedness of all things that resonate with the rhythm of the cosmos through the interplay of ink and brush.

Keywords *Yijing* · Shitao · *Huayulu* · Aesthetics · Individual creativity · *Daodejing* · *Dao* · Holistic Brushstroke

---

T. Sernelj (✉)
University of Ljubljana, Ljubljana, Slovenia
e-mail: tea.sernelj@ff.uni-lj.si

G. Sigurðsson and T. Hon (eds.), *Contemporary Interpretations and Readings of the Yijing*, Chinese Culture 15, https://doi.org/10.1007/978-981-96-0609-2_10

10.1 Introduction

Shitao 石濤, also known as Zhu Ruoji 朱若極 (1642–1707), was one of the most important painters in the early Qing dynasty's artistic milieu. Embracing the ethos of the Individualist or non-Traditionalist school of painting (*feizhengtong pai* 非正統派), he championed an approach that celebrated the artist's personal encounter with life, drawing inspiration directly from nature, and embracing unrestricted artistic expression. In stark contrast to the Traditionalist school (*zhengtong pai* 正統派), which upheld imitation and emulation of past masters' technical prowess and stylistic conventions, Shitao forged his own path. He created a unique aesthetic theory that not only criticized the Traditionalist painters but also advocated for a renaissance of the aesthetic taste and sensibilities seen in the Wei-Jin (220–589 CE) literati landscape painting. For Shitao, the aesthetics of literati painters embodied the authentic essence of Chinese art and aesthetics.

Shitao's aesthetic theory undoubtedly promoted subjectivity and artistic freedom, and led to innovative forms of expression in art. To understand his aesthetic theory, we will first introduce the basic characteristics of the literati aesthetics and address the problem of creative decline that led to the emergence of Traditionalist painting, which is under critical consideration in Shitao's aesthetic theory of painting.

His seminal work, the *Huayulu* 畫語錄 (*Remarks on Painting*) was written in the last decade of his life and encompasses his entire theoretical and practical knowledge as an artist and philosopher. His *Remarks* eloquently reflect the profound influence of the *Yijing*, Daoism and Chan philosophy on his aesthetic theory and artistic practice. This influence is evident in the masterful blend of binary categories and parallelisms, concepts, and rhetoric that he skillfully employs.

Shitao's aesthetic theory finds its foundation in the concept of "Holistic Brushstroke" or "Unity of Brushstroke" (*Yihua* 一畫), which embodies his ultimate painting method known as "method without method" (*Wufazhi fa* 無法之法) or simply "no method" (*wufa* 無法). A full exploration of these concepts will be provided in the following subsections. However, it is important to reiterate that the *Huayulu* clearly expresses Shitao's deep dissatisfaction and theoretical criticism of the Traditionalist theory of painting. It can also be regarded as a kind of manifesto aimed at preserving and reviving the genuine aesthetic spirit of Chinese art, in contrast to the prevailing mainstream school that had led to a state of creative stagnation.

The theory boldly challenges the "traditionalist" understanding of art, which adheres to strict rules and insists upon imitation of old masters and classical paintings. This approach advocates exact copying (*fang* 仿), correctness (*zheng* 正), and conveying the spirit of antiquity by applying painting techniques from the past (*guyi* 古意) as the ultimate model to be imitated in the present and future, dismissing individual expression as unnecessary and undesirable.

Shitao critiqued such a formalist emphasis on solely pictorial elements, particularly its disregard for nature as the primary wellspring of inspiration (Strassberg 1989, 3), and its failure to recognize the central importance of the individual artist and their creative abilities. He argued for the restoration of an original, spiritual totality in art, symbolized by his central aesthetic concept, the Holistic Brushstroke. Through the Holistic Brushstroke and other related concepts and methods, he advocated a resurgence of natural cosmology in art and underscored the need for the individual artist to reconnect with a Nature deeply rooted in Daoist philosophy (ibid).

His approach to overcoming creative stagnation goes beyond the constraints of historicism and embraces a holistic foundation in art. By tracing the act of painting back to the principles of unity and autonomy, Shitao strives to recover the innate harmony between nature, art, and the heart-mind, as originally formulated by the classical literati painters. This pursuit of a spiritual connection with nature and an attempt to visually represent one's inner self revitalizes painting as an original and unique experience, liberating it from mere imitation of other artists' styles. Shitao's theory exudes a liberating and empowering essence that prevents *Huayulu* from being reduced to a mere commentary on other works of art. Within the Chinese aesthetic tradition, there is no other theory that exhibits such deep literary consciousness and originality of expression, eloquently voicing a distinctively personal perspective.

The aesthetic theory born from Shitao's efforts is unquestionably distinctive, profoundly philosophical, and even poetic in nature. Its significance lies in its reference to the *Yijing* that forms a foundation of his theory of painting, which is rooted in Shitao's onto-cosmological understanding of artistic creativity embodied in the Holistic Brushstroke. This fundamental concept, which is central to his theory, is introduced in the first chapter of the *Huayulu* and explored thoroughly throughout the work, revealing its multiple and multifaceted meanings.

This article focuses primarily on those elements of *Yijing* that were directly addressed by Shitao. Nevertheless, it is important to acknowledge that in aesthetic theory, Shitao predominantly drew from Daoist philosophy, even though he was particularly interested in its engagement with the onto-cosmology[1] of the *Yijing*.

[1] Onto-cosmology is a term coined by Cheng Chung-Ying (1991, 174–175) indicating interconnectedness and inseparability of ontological and cosmological in Chinese philosophy. According to Cheng (ibid.), the ontological refers to that which pertains to the original substance (*benti*) which unifies the meaning of origin (*ben*) and base or substance (*ti*). *Ti* refers to what gives the human body its shape and to the base and centre of human activity. The metaphysical use of *ti* is a metaphysical projection of the experienced reality of human existence. As a verb, *ti* means to personally experience something, and to embody and assimilate a given reality into the given framework of human existence. However, *ti* is not a static but a dynamic concept suggestive of embodiment, integration, and harmonization in the expression and consideration of reality. It is with this *benti* understanding of the ontological that we can speak of the ontologization of the cosmological in Chinese philosophy in which cosmological and ontological consideration of the world are not separated. With other words, ontology reveals itself in cosmology and should be called onto-cosmology. This idea of the dynamic unity of the cosmological and the ontological is well presented in the notion of the *dao* as presented in the Great Appendix of the *Yijing* (ibid.).

10.2 Brief Biography

Shitao, originally named Zhu Ruoji, was born in 1642 in Guilin. He belonged to the eleventh generation of descendants of a grandnephew of one of the founders of the Ming dynasty (1364–1644). Tragically, he was only two years old when the Ming dynasty collapsed. Power struggles between the Ming loyalists and the Manchus resulted in the execution of Shitao's entire family. However, he was spared such gruesome faith through the help of one of their servants, who brought him to Quanzhou in Fujian province (Strassberg 1989, 12–13). When Shitao was around ten years old he was taken to a Chan Buddhist monastery in Wuchang in Hebei province. He began studying calligraphy following renowned Tang master Yan Zhenqing (709–785). Captivated by the master's bold and vigorous brushstrokes, as well as the solid structure of his work, Shitao developed an enduring fondness for these artistic qualities that would last a lifetime.

Later, he received encouragement to explore the style of Dong Qichang. However, upon immersing himself in Dong's paintings, Shitao found himself less than enchanted with the approach. Instead, he made a resolute decision to wholeheartedly embrace the artistic expressions of more ancient models, thus distancing himself from Dong's style altogether (ibid. 14).

By the age of fourteen, Shitao had already earned a reputation as a talented painter of flowers, birds, landscapes, and figures. He received guidance from a retired official who had collaborated with the Manchus, as well as from his ten-years-older fellow monk, Hetao 喝涛 (Drinking Waves), who would become his traveling companion for more than three decades (ibid.). Following in the footsteps of his older fellow Buddhist monk, Zhu Ruoji now adopted the name Shitao 石涛 (Stone Wave) (ibid.). In 1657 when the two monks arrived to Hangzhou, Shitao already declared his affinity to the Individualist path in art and disdained the Traditionalist approach. In a colophon of his painting from that year, he wrote:

> In painting there are the "Northern" and "Southern" schools … do I follow them or do they follow me? Suddenly I grasp my sides and break out in laughter as I say, I use my own method (ibid., 15).

In 1662, Shitao embarked on his Chan training under the guidance of the renowned Chan master Luan Benyuan. Just two years later, he received the transmission of the dharma from his master. However, Shitao was always on the move, and during his extensive journeys, he made frequent visits to Mount Huang in Anhui. This majestic landscape served as a profound wellspring of inspiration and played a pivotal role in shaping his artistic development.

Through his continuous painting of Mount Huang, Shitao diligently refined his techniques and styles, drawing from the legacy of old masters and the artistic traditions of antiquity. Additionally, he honed his own methods, skillfully incorporating allusion, dynamic composition, dramatic ink contrast, and fluid brushwork into his repertoire (ibid.).

Even in his youth, Shitao attracted the attention and support of numerous merchants and patrons in Anhui, who remained steadfast advocates of his art over the years. For a decade, Hetao and Shitao resided in Anhui, a period during which Shitao had the opportunity to connect with prominent Individualist painters and poets from the local Anhui school. This environment encouraged Shitao to further delve into the artistic representation of Mount Huang. As pointed out by Shitao himself (ibid., 17), Mount Huang and the association with the Anhui Individualist circle held paramount significance in his artistic development. They provided him with a unique and powerful natural example, allowing him to reevaluate the unconventional compositions and ink effects of the Individualist approach.

Shitao often spent weeks at a time dwelling in the temples on Mount Huang, immersing himself in its breathtaking vistas, encountering the peculiar rock formations, the twisted and stunted pines, and the enchanting sea of clouds. These experiences bestowed upon him a wealth of landscapes that he would go on to capture in numerous paintings and albums throughout his illustrious career. In his painting philosophy, he unwaveringly stressed the importance of artists learning directly from nature itself.

Shitao made a significant life change in 1680 when he relocated to Nanjing. Nanjing held prominence as both a vital cultural center and a hub for Buddhism. Compared to the provincial town in Anhui where he had previously resided, Nanjing offered artists broader opportunities for patronage and a more diverse artistic milieu.

Over the following decade, Shitao remained in the city but continued to stay in contact with artists from Anhui. During this period, Shitao wholeheartedly dedicated himself to the rigorous practice of meditation, laying the foundation for a career as a Chan master. In October 1690, he ascended to the position of successor at the Single Branch Studio, located in a temple south of the city. There, he embraced a solitary existence, committing himself entirely to the practice of meditation, eventually attaining the esteemed status of a Chan master (ibid., 22, 23).

The relationship between Shitao as a painter and his role as a Chan master reveals an intriguing overlap of artistic and religious objectives. In the Chinese art realm, the concept of a monk-painter was firmly established and harmonized seamlessly with a religious vocation. Both pursuits functioned as mutually reinforcing paths toward spiritual enlightenment. Shitao even went so far as to describe his profession as "painting Chan" (*hua chan* 畫禪).

In a colophon to a painting, he stated:

> Discussing painting is like discussing Chan: what is important is to forget one's knowledge of things and enter into the Primary principle,[2] which is what defines the master. Otherwise, one sinks into dualism, which definitely indicates that one is not an expert (ibid.).

Around 1693, Shitao made the significant choice to renounce his formal position as a Chan master and took on the role of a Daoist priest. He adopted the Daoist name Dadizi 大滌子, which translates to "The Pure One," or, as Chai (2021, 97)

[2] The concept of the Primary Principle can be traced back to Song poetry critic Yan Yu (1180–1235), who stressed the importance of poets experiencing spiritual enlightenment. For Shitao, this concept represented a profound insight into reality that transcended mere knowledge of artistic styles and techniques. Although Shitao embraced Daoism in his *Huayulu*, many of his ideas find their origins in Chan Buddhism or remain highly aligned with its teachings (ibid., 36).

notes, "Master of Great Cleansing," symbolizing the purification of all accumulated worldly impurities. This decision reflected his rejection of the political corruption that had become associated with Buddhism (Coleman 1978, 29). From 1697 until his passing, Shitao resided in Yangzhou. Around 1700, he completed his renowned theory of painting, *Remarks on Painting* (*Huayulu* 畫語錄). A revised version of this text, known as *Manual for Painting* (*Huapu* 畫譜), was published a decade later[3] (ibid.).

10.3 Shitao's Aesthetic Theory

Shitao's fundamental work *Huayulu*, written in the last decade of his life, embodies the wholesome theoretical and practical knowledge that he acquired during his life as a philosopher and an artist. His artistic reflections and practice captured in this exceptional theoretical work are at their core imbued with his experience of Chan Buddhism and Daoism, which is clearly reflected in the concepts and categories he discusses and the rhetoric of the work itself. The theoretical discourse that Shitao conducts through the implementation of binary categories and parallelisms of the *Daodejing* and *Yijing*, Chan concepts and even those of the Song-Ming Neo-Confucianism (*li* 理 and *xin* 心) all resonate harmoniously with his unique aesthetic theory.[4] However, the text predominantly leans toward Daoism. This inclination is not surprising, considering that Shitao identified as a Daoist when he wrote his *Remarks*.[5]

As noted above, Shitao's core aesthetic theory centers around his concept of the Holistic Brushstroke or Oneness of Brushstroke (*yihua* 一畫), which represents his ultimate painting method known as the "method of no method" (*wufa zhi fa* 無法之法), or simply "no method" (*wufa* 無法). While a detailed exploration of these concepts will follow in the next subchapter, it is worth mentioning at this juncture that Shitao's idea of "no method" embodies his strong critique of the Traditionalist theory of painting. His *Remarks on Painting* can also be seen as a manifesto advocating for the preservation and restoration of the genuine spirit of literati painting in opposition

---

[3] For an in-depth study of Shitao's life, see Hay 2001.

[4] Incorporating all three philosophical traditions, Shitao appears to aim at demonstrating their interconnectedness, rather than viewing them as mutually exclusive aspects of Chinese art and aesthetics. For example, when discussing the concept of emptiness, he uses the Buddhist *kong* and Daoist *xu* interchangeably in one sentence in order to express ultimate emptiness.

[5] As David Chai observes (2021, 96), the notion that Shitao's treatise is primarily Daoist does not command unanimous consensus, especially among Chinese scholars. Some contend that the text is entirely Buddhist, albeit with differing opinions on whether it aligns more with the Huayan, Theravada, or Chan traditions. Conversely, others assert that Shitao's treatise exclusively adheres to Daoism, though their interpretations diverge regarding whether he speaks in the spirit of Laozi 老子 and Zhuangzi 莊子, advocates solely the views of Laozi and his *Daodejing* 道德經 or follows the cosmology of the *Yijing* 易經. Additional perspectives suggest that Shitao should be viewed as a Neo-Confucian, given his use of terms such as "principle" (*li* 理) and "heart-mind" (*xin* 心), among others. Finally, there are scholars in China and Taiwan who primarily see him as a syncretist, as he exhibits traits belonging to all aforementioned philosophical traditions (ibid).

to the prevailing mainstream schools of his time, which he believed had led to artistic stagnation.

The Traditionalist school of painting is characterized by strict adherence to rules and the emulation of techniques used by past masters. This approach emphasizes exact copying and transmission of historical painting methods as a model to be followed. Individual artistic expression is discouraged within this framework, as stated by Dong Qichang. Shitao strongly criticized such conception of art, highlighting the profound metaphysical foundations of Classical aesthetic theory.

Shitao's approach seeks to transcend the limitations of historicism by grounding art in a holistic foundation. He aims to reestablish painting on the principles of unity and autonomy, with the goal of recapturing the inherent harmony between nature, art, and the artist's heart-mind. This approach revitalizes painting as a primal, spiritual experience rather than a mere emulation of other artists' styles. The theory promotes a liberating and empowering intention, protesting against the reduction of painting to a mere commentary on other artworks (Strassberg 1978, 3–4).

Shitao's *Remarks on painting*, however, is composed of eighteen relatively short but compact essays or chapters. The initial three explore the notions of the "Holistic Brushstroke" and "method." The following three essays focus on the act of painting itself. Chapters seven to fourteen provide a detailed exploration of these concepts in relation to the symbolism and profound representational power of painting. The final four essays interweave these themes by discussing the paradigmatic person (*zhiren* 至人), the interconnectedness of all things, and the art of mastering life (Chai 2021, 98).

The essays encompass intricate and multifaceted content. However, our focus will be specifically on the sections that directly relate to the *Yijing* and illustrate how Shitao incorporated its onto-cosmology into his aesthetic theory of the Holistic Brushstroke and the process of artistic creation.

Before delving into Shitao's aesthetic theory of painting and his references to the *Yijing*, it is essential to underscore that classical Chinese aesthetic theory is deeply rooted in the onto-cosmology of the *Yijing* and Daoist philosophy. All foundational concepts in Chinese aesthetics, such as the binary category of *Yin* and *Yang*, the vital creative force of *qi*, the notion of image or representation (*xiang* 象), the continuity of change and transformation (*tongbian* 通變), and the *Dao* as the ultimate creative cosmic principle, are thoroughly discussed and analyzed within the realm of human creativity and artistic production. This alignment is unsurprising as artistic production in the Chinese aesthetic tradition is perceived as an inherently cosmogonic act.

In Chinese art theory and aesthetics, the concept of copying reality (Nature) and its entities (*wanwu* 萬物) does not hold any particular aesthetic value. Instead, the artist's aim is to imitate and recreate reality in a manner that appears natural and spontaneous, effectively forming a microcosm of the macrocosm. This achievement relies on both precise observation and a profound understanding of reality on one hand, and the complete fusion of the inner world of the human spirit with the external world (*tianren heyi* 天人合一) on the other. In this context, artistic practice and the creative process in Chinese aesthetics occupy a remarkably important, indeed fundamental, domain. It extends beyond mere mastery of artistic techniques or skills, encompassing the sphere of aesthetic transformation and transcendence. In this sense, the artist's self-cultivation involves emptying the self and harmonizing one's spirit with the cosmic *Dao*. Only on such foundations can an artist create artwork that possesses genuine aesthetic value, capable of conveying a transformative and transcendent experience of life to the viewers.

10.4 *Huayulu* and *Yijing*

The first chapter of the *Huayulu* directly addresses the meaning of the *Yihua* that can be translated as Holistic Brushstroke, oneness or unity of brushstrokes, or even the first (or one) brushstroke.[6] However, these translations are not mutually exclusive; rather, they offer various perspectives on the concept. They all provide descriptive definitions because it is challenging to confine it to a single semantic meaning. Nevertheless, "Holistic Brushstroke" is arguably the most fitting choice, as Shitao's aesthetic theory is rooted in holism, which is the foundational paradigm of Chinese philosophy. The "oneness of brushstroke" is essentially synonymous with the "Holistic Brushstroke," while the "first brushstroke" directly alludes to the artistic performance as a kind of cosmogonic act itself. In the opening lines of the first chapter, we read:

> 太古無法。太樸無散。太樸一散而法立矣。法於何立。立於一畫。一畫者衆有之本。萬象之根。見用於神。藏用於人而皆人不知。所以一畫之法乃自我立。立一畫之法者。蓋以無法生有法。以有法貫衆法也。夫畫者。從於心者也。(Shitao 石濤 1989 [s.d.], ch. 1)
>
> There were no (painting) methods in remote antiquity, for the uncarved block had not yet disintegrated. When it did, methods were established. But what is the basis of any method? They are all based on the Holistic Brushstroke. The Holistic Brushstroke is fundamental to

[6] The concept of *yihua* was not coined by Shitao, but it is an ancient concept in Chinese painting. According to Chai (2021, 98), The earliest recorded use of *yihua* can be traced back to Cui Yuan (78–143 CE), a renowned master of the cursive-script calligraphy style and author of the influential essay "Configuration of Cursive Script" (草書勢). This marked the inception of *yihua* as an aesthetic construct. Soon after, it was accompanied by the emergence of "one-stroke writing" (*yibishu* —筆書), exemplifying the cursive-script calligraphy style of Wang Xianzhi (344–386 CE). Additionally, "one-line drawing" (*yibihua* —筆畫) gained prominence, referring to the painting style pioneered by Lu Tanwei (dates unknown, approximately 485 CE) (ibid.). As Guo Si, the son of the famous Song dynasty landscape painter, Guo Xi, wrote: "Zhang Yanyuan said Wang Xianzhi could do one stroke calligraphy and Lu Tanwei could do one-stroke painting. This does not mean that all characters of an essay or all the lines in a picture of an object can be finished in a single stroke, but rather that, from start to end, the brushwork is consistent and linked together with an unbroken breathing thread." (In: Gao 2018, 78) Throughout successive generations leading up to the era of Shitao, the concept of oneness or holism consistently held a pivotal position within Chinese art. This notion encompassed both a tangible aspect, demonstrated through the fluid motion of the brush and the artist's wrist, as well as a metaphorical dimension, revealing the artist's breath and spirit within their creations. This enduring essence of oneness remained a fundamental cornerstone in the realm of Chinese art.

depicting everything in existence and is the root of all images.[7] It is perceptible spiritually, yet works mysteriously in the human-mind so my contemporaries remain unaware of it. Therefore, I, myself, established a "method" of Holistic Brushstroke. This method is created out of "no method" to string together all other methods. Painting is guided by the heart-mind. (trans. Strassberg 1989, 61[8]).

The opening two lines can be seen as parallelism which connects remote antiquity (*taigu* 太古) with primordial simplicity (*taipu* 太樸), usually translated as the uncarved block. In the *Daodejing*, *pu* is used for the description of the *Dao*. In the Chapter 32 of the *Daodejing* we read:

道常無名。樸雖小, 天下莫能臣也。(*Daodejing*, s.d.: 32)

Dao is constant and cannot be spoken of. Although small, no one can subjugate it.

In the third line, Shitao writes that the principles emerged when primordial unity dispersed, which resonates with Chapter 28 of the *Daodejing*, where it is stated that the formation of material forms emerged after the dispersion of pure simplicity.

樸散則為器。(*Daodejing*, s.d.: 28)

The dispersion of primordial unity forms vessels.

In conceptualization of the concept of *pu* 樸, Chai's comment (2021, 98, 99) is extremely important, pointing out the fact that *pu* was a general term of ancient Chinese philosophy, used in both Daoist and Confucian texts, and that the Daoist concept of *pu* must be understood in a wider context, namely as a description of the natural unperturbedness of things, including the human heart-mind, when left alone. Chai asserts:

[7] *Xiang* serves as a pivotal bridge that traverses the realms of the visible and the invisible, the concrete and the abstract, the actual and the imagined, as well as the interplay between imitation and creation. The establishment of *xiang*, denoted as an "image" or a "symbolic image," as a paramount aesthetic term, found its roots in the profound influence of Wang Bi's epistemological interpretation of the intricate interweaving between linguistic components—words (言 *yan*), symbolic images (象 *xiang*), and meaning (意 *yi*)—within the *Yijing*. While "form" (形 *xing*) encapsulates an object's physical shape, thus worthy of imitation, "*xiang*" represents the construct that must find its place on the canvas of painting. It encapsulates the mental imagery that materializes when one keenly observes tangible forms, skilfully processing their diverse qualities through a meticulous curation involving selection, editing, and rearrangement. As a term intertwined with artistic discourse, "*xiang*" first made its appearance within the literary and painting theories of the Six Dynasties era, subsequently maturing into a profound aesthetic concept during the Tang dynasty (Kang 2022, 33). From Wang Bi's commentaries on the *Yijing*, we see that both, words and images, are tools of transmitting the spirit that are inherently limited. What is important is that despite these limitations, we strive to express the infinity of the essence (*benti*) of things: 盡意莫若象, 盡象莫若言, 言者所以明象, 得像忘言, 象者所以以存意, 得意忘象. "Nothing can express a meaning more fully than an image. Nothing can express an image more fully than words. It is the words that make the image clear. When this happens, the words are forgotten. The image is the place where there is meaning. When meaning is achieved, the image is forgotten." (Wang Bi, in: Li Zehou 2003, 87).

[8] Unless otherwise noted, the translations of Chinese texts are mine.

What Shitao is doing with this opening line is not making a cosmogonic claim but retracing the roots of image thinking. To think in images is not only how the Chinese language arose as pictograms but as the first "written" text (the *Yijing*) too (ibid.).[9]

In the following lines, Shitao explains that the principles (or methods) are founded in the Holistic Brushstroke which is the origin of everything and the root of all images. Here, we find a reference to the *Yijing:*

是故, 易有太極, 是生兩儀, 兩儀生四象, 四象生八卦, 八卦定吉凶, 吉凶生大業。是故, 法象莫大乎天地, 變通莫大乎四時。

(*Yijing*, s.d., "Xici" 1: 11).

Therefore, in (the system of) the Yi there is Grand Terminus, which produced the two elementary forms. Those two forms produced the four images, which again produced the eight trigrams. The eight trigrams served to determine the good and evil (issues of events), and from this determination was produced the (successful prosecution of the) great business (of life). Therefore, of all things that furnish models and visible figures there are none greater than Heaven and Earth; of things that change and extend an influence (on others) there are none greater than the four seasons (trans. by Legge).

As Strassberg (1989, 39) posits, the Holistic Brushstroke is linked to the generative role of the legendary Sage king Fuxi who was often credited with drawing the first stroke from which the elements of reality emerged through a sequence of parturitions, i.e., the eight hexagrams representing the natural forms (Heaven, Earth, mountain, water, fire, lake, thunder, wind).

Shi Junchang (1618–1683), a writer and a friend of Shitao, restated this view:

The numbers all begin with one. When "one" is obtained, then the Two Primal Forces (*Yin* and *Yang*), the Four Images, and the Eight Trigrams become set. Altogether, the three-hundred and eighty-four commentaries on the lines of the Hexagrams all derive from this "one." Thus, ever since Fuxi drew the first line, and revealed the *Changes* to humankind, there was nothing more that needed to be said. This is what is meant by "in obtaining one (得一), the ten thousand things are completed" (ibid).

The transposition of *Yijing's* cosmology into Shitao's onto-aesthetics of the Holistic Brushstroke evidently holds an important role especially in the process of artistic creation.

Chinese art historian Wen C. Fong (1930–2018) describes the physical act of applying brush to paper as being parallel to spontaneous creation as the way the universe acts. He states: "the blank page is the undifferentiated oneness of the universe before creation; the first stroke, born of the union of brush and ink, establishes on the paper a primary relationship between *Yin* and *Yang*, and each additional stroke creates new *Yin-Yang* relationships, until the whole is reunited into the harmonious oneness that is *Dao*" (Gao 2018, 11).

---

[9] However, in the context of Shitao's critique of the Traditionalist theory of painting, Strassberg (1989, 38) claims that primordial simplicity in the remote antiquity refers to simple existence unburdened by complex institutions, rules, social distinctions, and dualistic thinking. Shitao used it as a reference to signify an innocent state of aesthetic consciousness in contrast to the history of art with its canonization of methods (or principles), its rival ideologies and disunity. In his theory, Shitao seeks to recover the innocent (*pu*) state of the great tradition of Chinese painting.

Similarly, Strassberg asserts (1989, 39) that the Holistic Brushstroke in painting is capable of creating a landscape as a microcosm of the universe. The blank paper can be regarded as an original, undefined cosmic state which Shitao calls "Primordial state of the universe" (*hundun*), after a Daoist creation myth. Applying the first stroke to the surface recapitulates the decisive moment of bringing things into being and setting into motion the forms of Nature, and thus endows the artwork with the spiritual coherence of the universe.

The same onto-cosmological statement is presented in chapters 42 and 25 of the *Daodejing*:

> 道生一,一生二,二生三,三生萬物。萬物負陰而抱陽,沖氣以為和。(*Daodejing*, s.d.: 42).
>
> *Dao* gives birth to one, one to two, two to three, and three to myriad entities. Myriad entities, bearing *Yin* and embracing *Yang*, form a unified harmony through the fusing of these vital forces.
>
> 人法地,地法天,天法道,道法自然。(*Daodejing*, s.d.: 25).
>
> Humanity models itself after the Earth, the Earth models itself after Heaven; Heaven models itself after the *Dao*, and the *Dao* models itself after its own naturalness.

When applied to the empty surface, the Holistic Brushstroke as the interplay between ink and brush (*Yin* and *Yang*) generates subsequent strokes producing the scene that is harmonious and full of vitality. However, as Shitao states, when pure simplicity dispersed, the methods were established and the Holistic Brushstroke which is the root of all images and all things maintains its holism as no method (*wufa*). Which means that it does not carry within itself the dispersion of the holistic state, but rather maintains the primordial state of pure simplicity of the *Dao* throughout the creative process. It derives from effortless or unintentional action (*wuwei*) which can be seen as a paradox because the creative process is itself an action. However, it aims at maintaining the naturalness or spontaneity of the creative process which reflects the creative mode of the *Dao* itself.

We shall now move to the Perfect Method (*Liaofa*了法[10]), embodying the cosmological principles of *Qian* and *Kun*:

> 規矩者。方圓之極則也。天地者。規矩之運行也。世知有規矩。而不知夫乾施坤轉之義。此天地之縛人於法。人之役法於蒙。。。一畫明。則障不在目。而畫可從心。畫從心而障自遠矣。夫畫者。行天地萬物者也。舍筆墨其何以形之哉。(Shitao 石濤 1989 [s.d.], ch. 2)
>
> Compass and ruler measure perfect circles and squares. Heaven and Earth move in the patterns marked by compasses and rulers. While people know about these tools, few understand the activity of the Creative and Receptive forces of the Universe. Such a conception of Heaven and Earth traps one in rules, keeping one in ignorance … when Holistic Brushstroke is understood, then inhibitions vanish from sight and painting can proceed naturally

---

[10] *Liaofa* has been translated by Strassberg as "Enlightenment into method" (1989, 63), by Coleman as "Liberation from methods" (1978, 117), and by Wang (2007, 19) as "The general law over regulations." All three translations refer to the content of the chapter, i.e., to Shitao's conception of the method. However, if we follow the etymological meaning of the term, we have to remember that *le*了 means to complete, to finish, to make perfect. Hence, I have translated the title of the second chapter as "The Perfect Method".

> (from the heart-mind). When painting proceeds naturally, inhibitions fade away by themselves. Painting represents the forms of Heaven, Earth and all things. How else could they be depicted but with brush and ink? (trans. Strassberg 1989, 63)

Compasses and square sets were used in ancient Chinese painting as the instruments for drawing lines—rulers for straight lines and compasses for circles and curves. In the Tang dynasty, the famous painter critic and historian Zhang Yangyuan (ca. 815–907) discussed the traditional division made between "real" paintings and "dead" paintings. The latter referred to paintings made by instruments, whereas real paintings were made freehand. Zhang asserted:

> Now, if one makes use of marking line and ruler, the result will be a dead painting. But if one guards the spirit and concentrates upon a single thing, the result will be a real painting. Is not even plain plaster better than a wall of dead painting? Yet even one stroke of real painting will show its breath of life. (Gao 2018, 4).

In the passage above from the second chapter, Shitao obviously refers to this distinction and criticizes the Traditionalists' rigidity in following methods and rules that lead to the creation of so-called dead paintings because they were not aware of the true creativity behind the real paintings, i.e., deriving from the creative source (*Dao*) represented by *Qian* and *Kun* (*Yang* and *Yin*).

Shitao's reference to the *Yijing* (i.e., to *Qian* and *Kun*) brings forth his onto-aesthetics of the Holistic Brushstroke. As we can see from this passage of the text, the act of painting, i.e., the interplay of the ink and brush led by the painter must derive from the harmonious relationship between Heaven, Earth, and human followed by the spirit of the ultimate creativity of the *Dao*.

Qian represents Heaven and the Way (*Dao*), symbolizing the origin of life and the diversity of existence. It is described as a transformative force, guiding each thing to attain its inherent nature. Through the interplay of *Yin* and *Yang*, *Qian* facilitates the manifestation of all things and embodies the creative essence of the cosmos. It imparts dynamic growth to all forms of life, revealing the inherent creativity of the universe (Li and Kuang 2012, 180–181).

Kun, on the other hand, represents Earth and symbolizes the birth of all life. It endows physical form (*xing*) to living beings and operates through the principles of strength and softness (*gang/rou*). It acts as the supporting force that allows things to flourish under the guidance of heaven's bestowal. The virtue of Earth, which serves as the foundation of life, fulfills three vital functions: it carries forward the messages of life, gives birth to and nourishes life, and facilitates the development and fulfillment of life (ibid.).

Qian initiates the grand beginnings of existence, while *Kun* brings them to completion. Together, they embody the ontological and cosmological underpinnings of life. The virtue of Heaven and Earth is described as the bestower of life, ensuring its continuity and existence. The transformation of *Yin* and *Yang* harmoniously unfolds the rhythms and messages of life, permeating the cosmos with ceaseless creation and generation (ibid.).

In the next lines of the second chapter, we read:

古今法障不了, 由一畫之理不明。一畫明, 則障不在目而畫可從心。畫從心而障自遠矣。。。法無障, 障無法。法自畫生, 障自畫退。法障不參。而乾旋坤轉之義得矣, 畫道彰矣, 一畫了矣。(Shitao 石濤 1989 [s.d.], ch. 2)

Throughout time, the reason that people have not liberated themselves from the inhibitions of methods is that the natural order (*li*) inherent in the Holistic Brushstroke has not been properly understood. When it is understood, then inhibitions vanish from sight and the painting can follow the heart-mind.[11] If painting follows the heart-mind then the inhibitions fade away by themselves… True method (e.g., the Holistic Brushstroke) is without inhibitions, just as inhibitions destroy true method. True method arises from the act of painting, while it is through the act of painting that inhibitions are banished. When the method can be separated from inhibitions, then the activity of creative and receptive forces (*Qian* and *Kun*) can be grasped. *Dao* of painting will shine forth and enlightenment gained into the Holistic Brushstroke (tr. Strassberg 1989, 63).

Shitao's holistic method derives from the absence of all methods and ultimately represents the method or operation of the *Dao* itself. Hence, the Holistic Brushstroke has the ability to reflect the entire universe on a microcosmic scale precisely because of its ability to represent the innermost nature (or structure) (*li* 理) of all things.

Holistic Brushstroke can be understood as the first and initial act that pervades the painting process from the beginning till the end. It is done in one vital breath which means that the scene or landscape that is to be presented in the painting as a microcosm of the macrocosm is already structured in the artist's heart-mind. It gives liveliness to the painting in the sense that it is a recreation of reality which is the result of spiritual synchronicity of the artist with the external world. For Shitao, the realization of the Holistic Brushstroke is attained through the complementarity of the ink and brush. The interplay of ink and brush, however, is a cosmic union of the two poles, i.e., the *Yin* and *Yang* which form a pair responsible for arranging all aspects of reality and their universal transformations or changes. This is reflected in Shitao's reference to the meaning of *Qian* and *Kun* in the *Yijing*.

The operation of the holistic method is hence rooted in the naturalness and spontaneity of *Dao* (*daofa ziran* 道法自然). Using the principle of the oneness of *Yin* and *Yang*, *Dao* harmonizes all things by allowing these natural elements to self-regulate (*zhi* 治). Similarly, Shitao argues that the Holistic Brushstroke, rooted in primal simplicity, governs the myriad strokes that emanate from it. This regulation occurs as the brush and ink freely alternate their positions of dominance and inferiority, much like the dynamic interplay of *Yin* and *Yang*, without disrupting the overall harmony of the artwork (Chai 2021, 103).

The third chapter brings forward the idea of transformation and continuity of change (*tongbian*) from the *Yijing* and discusses it in the framework of the creative process. However, in the first lines of the chapter, Shitao delves into the issue of transformation and change, emphasizing that the knowledge of past masters (or antiquity) should merely serve as a tool for the painter:

古者。試之具也。化者。試其具而弗為也。(Shitao 石濤 1989 [s.d.], ch. 3).

[11] According to Coleman (1978, 44), the heart-mind refers to intuitive mind and its penetrating power is sensitive to the moral and aesthetic without being limited to rational, analytical or discursive thought.

Works by the ancients are the means to knowledge. Those who transform know these sources of inspiration; yet they are not trapped by them (trans. Coleman 1978, 118).

Shitao perceives the artist's role as one that goes beyond mere utilization of past knowledge and firmly advocates the necessity of transforming that knowledge to express one's unique individuality and create innovative artworks that stem from the artist's heart-mind.

至人無法。無法而法。乃為至法。凡事有經必有權。有法必有化。。夫畫天下變通之大法也。山川形勢之精英也。古今造物之陶冶也。陰陽氣度之流行也。借筆墨以寫天下萬物。而陶泳乎我也。今人不明乎此。。(Shitao 石濤 1989 [s.d.], ch. 3)

The perfect man has no method. No method is the method which is the perfect method. All things have both, a constant aspect and one which responds to circumstances; similarly, any method must be capable of transformation… Painting is the greatest method for representing the world in the process of transformation and interaction, for capturing the essential beauty of landscapes' dynamic forms, the eternal creativity of creation, the succession of day and night and of the seasons. With brush and ink, I can describe everything between Heaven and Earth, for all this is molded by myself. People nowadays don't seem to understand this… (trans. Strassberg 1989, 64).

For Shitao, only the Holistic Brushstroke (i.e., the Perfect Method) can represent the dynamic process of change in the world through the art of painting. However, he emphasizes the importance of the artist's agency (i.e., the manifestation of one's capacity to act) in the process of creative production. This agency refers to the autonomy of the artist that derives from one's aesthetic experience of the world and is represented in the artwork. As we can see from this passage, Shitao directly correlates onto-aesthetics of the Holistic Brushstroke with the paradigm of transformation and continuity of change as presented in the *Yijing*:

闔戶謂之坤; 闢戶謂之乾; 一闔一闢謂之變; 往來不窮謂之通。(*Yijing*, "Xici" I: 11)

A door's being shut may be called [analogous to] *Kun* 坤, and its opening, *Qian* 乾. Opening succeeding shutting may be comprehended as an [event] of *bian* (change); getting through a process of [one] opening to shutting to another may be called *tong* (the constant course of [things or events]) (trans. Tian 2019, 16).

As Tian posits (2019, 16), *biantong or tongbian* involves four significant ideas. First, everything (or event) in the world correlates with another. Second, the manifold and diverse relationships of things (or events) to any other things (or events) are a matter of interconnectedness, and can be viewed as following the same basic pattern as *Yin* and *Yang*, namely, the interaction and interdependence of complementary opposition. Third, it is this basic pattern of *Yin* and *Yang* that ceaselessly brings everything (or event) in the world into constant change or movement. Fourth, everything is in a continuous process of change.

In this passage, however, both *bian* and *tong* are analogically related to the two events of the door's opening and being shut, depicting the process of transitioning between these states. *Bian* pertains to a becoming that arises from difference, while *tong* signifies a becoming based on continuity—a seamless progression from one event to another. This observation implies the existence of a continuum in the process of becoming. If there were no continuum bridging the gap between these events, the concept of becoming would be rendered meaningless. Conversely, without variation between these states, any notion of becoming would also lose its significance[12] (ibid).

On the basis of this conception, Shitao's last sentence of the third chapter in which he again emphasizes the importance of the self becomes even more interesting and complex. He writes as follows:

> 知有古而不知有我知也。我之為我。自有我在。。。我於古何師而不化之有。(Shitao 石濤 1989 [s.d.], ch. 3)
>
> One may know of the existence of the ancient, but not realize that they have the existence of their own. I exist as myself. I am within myself... In the face of the ancient, how could I have learned form it without transforming it) (trans. Strassberg 1989, 64).

As previously mentioned, Shitao criticizes the conservative painters who blindly follow the regulations and methods of painting because they are ignorant of the great oneness of arts behind them. While it is essential for a painter to be knowledgeable about these methods and regulations, it becomes imperative, when aspiring to create art in harmony with the *Dao*, to seamlessly incorporate them to the point where they appear spontaneous and innate—embodying the concept of *wuwei*, or effortless action—and do not hinder the artist's free expression. Only by achieving this level of integration can an artist authentically convey their individuality and innovative artistic expressions.

In the fifth chapter, Shitao discusses the complementary dialectics of the brush and ink by using different examples of binary categories borrowed from the *Yijing*. As we have already seen, brush and ink are representation of *Yin* and *Yang* or *Qian* and *Kun*, i.e., the creative and receptive principles in the act of painting. However, in the context of the interplay of brush and ink, Shitao introduces the concept of *mengyang* from the *Yijing*.

> 。。墨之濺筆也以靈。筆之運墨也以神。墨非蒙養不靈。筆非生活不神。能受蒙養之靈而不解生活之神。是有墨無筆也。能受生活之神而不變蒙養之靈。是有筆無墨也。(Shitao 石濤 1989 [s.d.], ch. 5)
>
> Ink is splashed onto the brush using the soul but ink is moved by the brush using the spirit. Ink without nourishing potentiality will be soulless, while the brush without vital impetus will be spiritless. The painter who receives the soul of nourishing potential but does not understand the vital impetus of spirit will possess ink but not the brush. The painter who receives the vital impetus of spirit yet does not change the soul of nourishing potential will possess the brush but not ink (tr. Chai 2021, 104).

It is generally agreed among scholars that Shitao borrowed the concept of *mengyang* (蒙養) from the *Yijing*, i.e., from the hexagram *meng* which says:

---

[12] As Tian points out (2019, 16), *bian-tong* 變通 is also seen reversed, i.e., as *tong-bian* 通變, which means "knowing *bian*," whereby *tong* has changed from meaning "the opening succeeding the being shut" and "the passing from one of these states to the other endlessly" to "comprehending changes and doing in accordingly changing manners" and "what to carry out and what to operate with." This indicates that *bian-tong* extends its analogical relations into *tong-bian; tong-bian* is to comprehend *bian-tong*, to comprehend is thus a continuum and to do a process of getting through to *bian* and *tong*. Or to put it briefly, to think and do correlatively as the world does.

"蒙以養正, 聖功也." (*Yijing*, 4:1).

The work of the sage is to cultivate rightness from the basis of chaos.[13] (trans. Chai 2021, 105).

Shitao explained this concept on the colophon added to his painting from 1703:

> In writing out paintings, it is necessary to understand the nourishment of potentiality (*mengyang*). Potentiality derives from the absence of method (*fa*) in antiquity; nourishment derives from the lack of differentiation in the primordial chaos. From lack of differentiation comes nourishment; from the absence of *fa* comes potentiality. Before the paper receives the ink, first reflect upon the ink's potentiality; and once you start activating the brush, examine the brush's nourishment. You yourself can develop the potentiality to complete the work of the Ancients; you yourself can visualize transformation and become free of *fa*. When transformation is visualized and *fa* abolished, the painting naturally conforms to the Way of nourishing potentiality (In: Chai 2021, 105).

From this, we can discern a connection to both the first and second chapters of the *Huayulu* shedding clearer light on the meaning of the Holistic Brushstroke. *Meng* refers to the uncarved block, or the state of pure simplicity (prior to dispersion) while *yang* symbolizes the future emergent. In the context of Shitao's painting process, splashing ink onto the brush symbolizes the painter's mindset, reflecting a deeper metaphorical connection. As the painter's spirit merges with the inherent simplicity of the *Dao*, they not only draw inspiration from it but also unleash the hidden potentiality residing within the ink that saturates their brush. This harmonious union allows the painter to be nourished by the *Dao* while simultaneously nurturing the latent creative power within their artistic tools (ibid).

However, Shitao also brings forth two complementarities, namely *shenghuo* 生活 (life revealing strokes) and *mengyang* (nourishing potentiality). In order to succeed in achieving the *Dao* of painting, the painter must unite both complementary elements.

As Strassberg points out (1989, 54), Shitao correlates brush and ink with other aesthetic notions, such as spirit and soul (神/靈), nourishing potential and vitality (蒙養/生活). This goes beyond the mere technical meaning of brush and ink, creating a profound vertical structure composed of alternating binary elements that symbolize the harmony of *Yin* and *Yang*, ultimately representing wholeness. Moreover, he employs a horizontal structure of syntactical transferences, allowing him to articulate his views on the issues raised by earlier theorists regarding "ink quality without brushmanship" and "brushmanship without ink quality"[14] (ibid.).

For Shitao, these problems stem from the artist's failure to recognize the inherent intelligence and energy within brush and ink. Consequently, he implies a pervasive spiritual quality associated with the Holistic Brushstroke, which unifies three levels: materials, consciousness, and experience (ibid). In the next lines of the fifth chapter, we read:

---

[13] Chaos or *meng* refers to the state of primal simplicity before the dispersion and differentiation of things, the so-called *taipu* state (see the first chapter of the *Huayulu*). In general use, *meng* refers to uncultivated or ignorant state.

[14] Jing Hao (c. 855–915) was the first to discuss this issue in his work *A Notes on the Art of Brushwork* (*Bifaji* 筆法記).

山川萬物之具體。有反有正。有偏有側。有聚有散。有近有遠。有內有外。。有虛有實。。此生活之大端也。故山川萬物之薦靈於人。因人操此蒙養生活之權。苟非其然焉能使筆墨之下。有胎有骨。有開有合。有體有用。有形有勢。。。一一盡其靈而足其神。(Shitao 石濤 1989 [s.d.], ch. 5)

The forms of landscape and all myriad things can be represented from the back or front, vertical or horizontal, gathered or dispersed, near or far … empty or solid … These are all main aspects of liveliness (or lively potentiality). Thus, because landscape and myriad things offer and reveal their soul to man, one grasps the power of nourishing potentiality and vitality. If this was not so, how could one's brush and ink represent the "flesh" and "bone structure" of the phenomena, the openness and closedness, substance and function, forms and momentum (power) … without all this, how can one enable brush and ink to fully reveal the spirituality of things?

In this passage from the fifth chapter, Shitao discusses various ways of depicting landscape through the use of numerous binary categories, such as substance and function (*ti/yong* 体用), internal and external (*nei/wai* 内外), form and momentum (*xing/shi* 形势), and more. However, within the context of this article, the most relevant binary category is that of opening and closing (*kai* 開/*he* 合) because it aligns with the principle of movement observed in *Kun* (*Yin*) and *Qian* (*Yang*), which leads to continuous change and transformation, as defined in the *Yijing*.

Shitao's aesthetic principle of *kai/he* involves the precise execution of brush movement, which should be grounded in the harmonious interplay of *Yin* and *Yang*. *Kai* or openness of the brush, initiates and activates the brushstroke's motion, aligning with *Qian* or *Yang*. On the other hand, *he* or closedness, corresponds to *Kun* or *Yin*, completing the brushstroke and generating the momentum for the inception of a new brushstroke movement.

Rowley (In: Coleman 1978, 58–59) gives an interesting explanation of the conceptual pair *kai/he*. He asserts that *kai* refers to expanding and *he* to gathering up. In the painting process, however, when you expand you should think about gathering up and there will be a structure; when you gather up you should think of expanding and then you will have inexpressible effortlessness and an air of inexhaustible spirit. In using brush and laying out the composition, there is not one moment when you can depart from the process of *kai-he*, for otherwise the composition will fly apart through the explosive tendency of creativity and the structural unity of the whole will be lost; when you gather parts (*he*), you should think of the vital force which gave them birth (*kai*) or else the result will be dead mechanical adjustment and the whole will have missed the life breath of the spirit.

Harmoniously coordinated movement (kai/he) between *Yin* and *Yang* produces continuity of change and transformation and represents the movement of the *Dao* itself which is comprehended by the spirit. As written in the *Yijing*:

一陰一陽之謂道。。。通變之謂事, 陰陽不測之謂神。(*Yijing*, "Xici" I: 5).

The successive movement of *Yin* and *Yang* is called the *Dao*. The comprehension of the continuous change (of *Yin* and *Yang*) is what we call how to approach in managing the affairs. That which is unfathomable in the movement of *Yin* and *Yang* is called the spirit.

Shitao uses *kai-he* for describing the continuous movement of *Yin* and *Yang* in the process of painting. In order to capture the essence and true nature of the landscape, the artist must be mindful of achieving a harmonious balance between these two elements. The significance of these aspects is extensively explored in chapter seven, titled "*Yinyun*" (Clouds and Mists), a term borrowed from the *Yijing*. It has been translated as "Harmonious Atmosphere" by Coleman (1978, 66) and as "Fusion" by Strassberg (1989, 71). It is within this chapter that Shitao's metaphysics of the Holistic Brushstroke is most vividly articulated.

> 筆與墨會。是為絪緼 。絪緼不分。是為混沌。闢混沌者。捨一畫而誰耶。。自一以分萬。自萬以治一。化一而成絪緼。天下之能事畢矣。(Shitao 石濤 1989 [s.d.], ch. 7)
>
> When brush and ink come together, this is known as clouds and mist (harmonious atmosphere). When clouds and mist do not separate, this is known as undifferentiated wholeness. What, apart from the Holistic Brushstroke, can unlock undifferentiated wholeness? (trans. by Chai 2021, 106) … From oneness, distinguish the myriad things; through myriad things attain the oneness. By transforming oneness into harmonious atmosphere, everything in the world can be completed (tr. Strassberg 1989, 71).[15]

As mentioned above, Shitao borrowed *yinyun* from the *Yijing*, in part two of the "Commentary on the Appended Phrases," we read:

> 天地絪緼, 萬物化醇。(*Yijing*, "Xici" II:5).
>
> When Heaven and Earth mix like clouds and mist, the myriad things transform and mature. (tr. Chai 2021, 106).

The literal meaning of *yinyun* is clouds and mists and refers to generative forces of Heaven and Earth, since the original meaning of *yinyun* indicated the parting of the primal breath (*yuanqi* 元氣) obscuring Heaven from Earth. We can thus understand it as the parting of the primordial clouds and mist, allowing sunlight to reach the ground (ibid.).

This mistiness, however, is the profound spiritual atmosphere generated by *mengyang* which reflects the wholeness of the universe (or *Dao*) through the fusion of Heaven and Earth.

In painting, Shitao relates *yinyun* to the harmonious unity of brush and ink. The undifferentiated state of the *yinyun* refers to primordial unity or *pu* and only Holistic Brushstroke is able to maintain the oneness and simplicity of the *pu* through its intervention (or action). *Yinyun* can be understood as the *Taiji*, or the ultimate unity of two complementary poles that represents the movement of *Dao* through the vital breath energy of *qi*. When applied to the art of painting, the harmonious unity of brush and ink (*yinyun*) produces myriad forms, but the Holistic Brushstroke is of paramount importance when seeking to portray the emanation of diversities from their original *Dao*-state.

As Chai aptly asserts (2021, 106), the true essence of artistic expression comes to life when *yinyun* becomes an integral part of the painter's creative repertoire. It is at this point that the ink gains the essential vitality of spirit, and the brush acquires the

[15] Coleman translated this last sentence as "Transform oneness into harmonious atmosphere and this is indeed the highest achievement of art in the world" (Coleman 1978, 124). Although Strassberg's translation is more accurate regarding the original text, Coleman's illuminates the fundamental meaning of Shitao's Holistic Brushstroke.

nurturing potential of the soul. The profound depths achieved through the interplay of clouds and mist result from the seamless fusion of brush and ink in perfect harmony.

Moreover, the manifestation of *yinyun* within a Holistic Brushstroke appears remarkably organic and spontaneous, as if the artistic process flows effortlessly. When imbued with spirit and soul, the brush and ink transcend their static nature, becoming agents of self-sculpting that leave no visible traces on the canvas. It is in this state that the painter, selflessly guiding the ink and skillfully wielding the brush, embodies the method of no method, embracing the philosophy of the Holistic Brushstroke.

10.5 Conclusion

Through an examination of Shitao's aesthetic theory of painting, it becomes evident that it draws significant inspiration from the ontological cosmology found in the *Yijing* and *Daodejing*. While Shitao certainly builds upon the aesthetic theories of his predecessors, specifically the artistic perspectives of literati artists that had developed since the Wei-Jin period, his work, *Remarks on Painting*, stands out as undeniably unique. This uniqueness is especially pronounced during a period marked by a prevailing spirit of conservatism and creative stagnation in China. Shitao's work initiates a discussion on the foundational principles of Chinese aesthetic theory, rooted in Daoist philosophy and, naturally, the cornerstone of Chinese philosophy as a whole, the *Yijing*.

The integration of *Yijing's* onto-cosmology into the realm of artistic production, particularly within the creative process, holds a central and profound significance in Shitao's work. It serves as an aesthetic theory addressing how to produce an artwork that embodies the creative principles of nature or the *Dao*. Moreover, it delves into the idea that these principles can only find expression through the hands of an artist who, through the expression of their own individual experience, continually recreates all existence and the world as its most discrete manifestation. This individualistic approach, as Shitao advocates, does not arise from a rejection of tradition in the sense of respecting and drawing inspiration from the works of masters. Rather, it underscores the belief that artistic creation must originate from the individual artist themselves rather than relying solely on imitation of the prevailing painting masters—a favored practice of the time. Shitao's emphasis on the uniqueness and individuality of the artist emerges as an essential condition for meaningful creativity and innovation. Such creativity must be rooted in the artist's own unique experience of existence including both their innermost heart-mind and the external world that surrounds them.

As illustrated in the article, Shitao's aesthetic theory is fundamentally rooted in Daoist philosophy and metaphysics, with a particular focus on the onto-cosmology found in the *Yijing*. Through an analysis of seven out of the eighteen essays comprising his work, it becomes clear that Shitao's theory embraces a holistic approach that effectively maps Chinese onto-cosmology onto the realm of aesthetic theory.

In my view, the paramount significance of Shitao's Holistic Brushstroke lies in its embodiment of the belief that the artistic process itself should emanate from the cosmic creative principle (*Dao*) in its purest form. This, in turn, requires both an enlightened insight into the deepest reality of all existence, and a profound internalization of the experience that arises from the merging of the human with the cosmos.

Shitao's theory of the Holistic Brushstroke serves as a compelling illustration of the paradigm of transcendence within immanence, as articulated in the *Yijing*:

> 形而上者謂之道, 形而下者謂之器。(*Yijing*, "Xici" I:12).
>
> What is above forms is called the *Dao*. What is below forms is called the vessel.

The Holistic Brushstroke finds its origin in the *Dao* and serves as its tangible expression, ultimately materializing itself in the process of artistic creation. Once more, this highlights another aim of Shitao's aesthetic theory, an objective unattainable through copying, but only through the creative process of pointing to the image of *Dao* itself.

Acknowledgements The author acknowledges the financial support from the Slovenian Research and Innovation Agency (ARIS) in the framework of the research project (J6-50202). The Confucian Revival and its Impact on Contemporary East Asian Societies through the Lens of the Relation between the Individual and Society and the Chiang Ching-kuo Foundation for International scholarly exchange in the scope of the research grant (RG001-N-23) for the project entitled The problem of freedom, humanism and the human subject in intercultural perspective: Europe and Taiwan.

References

Chai, David. 2021. Shitao and the enlightening experience of painting. *Dialogue and Universalism* 31 (3): 93–112.

Cheng, Chung-Ying. 1991. Chinese metaphysics as Non-metaphysics: Confucian and Daoist insights into the nature of reality. In *Understand the Chinese Mind: The Philsophical Roots.* Ed. Robert E. Allison. New York: Oxford University Press.

Coleman, Earle. 1978. *Philosophy of Painting by Shih-Tao: A Translation and Exposition of his Hua-P'u.* The Hague: Mouton Publishers.

Daodejing 道德經. s.d. In *Chinese Text Project*: https://ctext.org/dao-de-jing.

Gao, Jianping. 2018. *Aesthetics and Art, Traditional and Contemporary China in a Comparative Perspective.* Berlin: Foreign Language Teaching and Research Publishing and Springer Verlag.

Hay, Johnathan. 2001. *Shitao: Painting and Modernity in Early Qing China.* Cambridge: Cambridge University Press.

Kang, Yoewool. 2022. Zhen as the ideal of landscape painting. *Sungkyun Journal of East Asian Studies* 22 (1): 27–47.

Li, Shuhua, and Zhao Kuang. 2012. Natural philosophy of "Zhouyi" and life practice. *Frontiers of Philosophy in China* 7 (2): 179–190.

Shitao 石濤. 1989 [s.d.]. *Huayulu* 畫語錄. In *Enlightening Remarks on Painting by Shitao.* Tr. Richard Strassberg. Pasadena, CA: Pacific Asia Museum Monographs.

Strassberg, Richard. 1989. *Enlightening Remarks on Painting by Shitao.* Pasadena, CA: Pacific Asia Museum Monographs.

Tian, Chenshan. 2019. Mao Zedong, Sinization of Marxism, and traditional Chinese thought culture. *Asian Studies* 7 (1): 13–37.
Wang, Hongyin. 2007. 注译与石涛画论研究 [*Shitao: Arts of Painting and his other Works*]. Beijing: Beijing Tushuguan Chubanshe.
Yijing 易經, s.d. In *Chinese Text Project*: https://ctext.org/book-of-changes/yi-jing.
Zehou, Li. 2003. *Meixue San Shu* 美学三书. Tianjin: Tianjin Shehui Kexue Yuan Chubanshe.

Chapter 11
Three Paradigm Shifts: *Yijing* Studies in North America, 1980–2020

Kar Bo Wong

Abstract Since the 1960s, *The I Ching or Yijing* by Richard Wilhelm and Cary F. Baynes has been a standard translation of the Chinese classic *Yijing*. To many readers in the Anglophone world, the Wilhelm-Baynes translation successfully renders the *Yijing* into a "book of wisdom" that addresses contemporary issues such as alienation, family structure, gender roles, and social inequality. Nonetheless, since the mid-1970s, scholars have been dissatisfied with this "book of wisdom" approach that suppresses the authentic voice of the *Yijing* text. Rather than looking for contemporary relevance, they have turned their attention to the different layers of the *Yijing* text and the different commentarial traditions to render the text. This article examines the origin and development of this "historical turn" that decidedly transforms the image of *Yijing* in the Anglophone world. The article begins with a discussion of the social-intellectual milieu of the 1960s that gave rise to North American scholars' interest in discovering China's historical path. Then, it compares three distinctive approaches to historicizing the *Yijing*: (1) uncovering the complexity of the original text based on recent archeological discoveries (e.g., Edward Shaughnessy and Richard Kuhn); (2) comparing the different commentarial methods of interpreting the *Yijing* text (e.g., Kidder Smith, Richard John Lynn, Joseph Adler, Tze-ki Hon, and Harrington); and (3) tracing the travels of the *Yijing* around the world (e.g., Richard Smith). The article argues that although different in many regards, these three approaches highlight the importance of *Yijing* in times of crisis, whether personal, national, or global.

Keywords Book of wisdom · Historical turn · Global *Yijing* · *Yi* in history

K. B. Wong (✉)
BNU-HKBU United International College, Zhuhai, China
e-mail: sarakbwong@uic.edu.cn

G. Sigurðsson and T. Hon (eds.), *Contemporary Interpretations and Readings of the Yijing*, Chinese Culture 15, https://doi.org/10.1007/978-981-96-0609-2_11

11.1 Introduction

Yijing (or *I Ching*, the *Book of Change*), one of the oldest Chinese classics, has traditionally been a divination manual and a philosophical work inspiring endless dialog among authors, readers, and diviners navigating life's crossroads. Its influence extends far beyond China and continues to inspire people around the globe (Ng 2021).

Western academic research on the *Yijing* has been extensive and diverse, especially in North America during the twentieth century. The dissemination of the *Yijing* began in Germany with the 1924 translation by Richard Wilhelm. This German translation piqued the interest of Swiss psychiatrist and psychoanalyst Carl Gustav Jung (1875–1961). Jung encouraged his student, Cary F. Baynes, to retranslate Wilhelm's work into English, which was completed in 1950. This new translation made the *Yijing* more accessible to a wider Western audience. The Wilhelm-Baynes translation served as a cultural bridge and interpretive lens for understanding human life. Its publication attained iconic status during the turbulent 1960s, appealing to a diverse audience seeking timeless, universal wisdom. This approach to reading the *Yijing*, derived from Wilhelm's work, is often referred to as the "book of wisdom" approach by later researchers (Lynn 1994, 7; Cheng Yi 2019, 1), suggesting that the *Yijing* can provide valuable insights and guidance to all, regardless of their individual backgrounds or circumstances.

The Wilhelm-Baynes translation of the *Yijing* has enjoyed widespread success, with many English-speaking readers mistakenly perceiving it as a faithful rendition of the original text. In reality, it draws heavily from the *Zhouyi Zhezhong* (*Balanced Compendium on the Zhou Changes*), a work compiled during the Qing dynasty that combined commentaries from the Song dynasty scholars Cheng Yi and Zhu Xi, alongside other minor commentaries. Completed in 1715 under the editorial guidance of Li Guangdi, this compilation held authoritative status during Wilhelm's time in Qingdao, China from 1899 to 1920. During his visit, Wilhelm worked closely with the esteemed Chinese scholar Lao Naixuan (1843–1921), who provided invaluable guidance in the translation process. Richard Wilhelm believed *Zhouyi Zhezhong* was "a very good edition" (Wilhelm and Baynes 1967, lxi) of understanding the *Yijing* for "it presents the text and the wings separately and includes the best commentaries of all periods" (Ibid, lxi). His translation aims to "present not only the text but also digests of the most important Chinese commentaries" (Ibid, lxi). Moreover, he integrated his own understanding of the work into this free translation. In summary, Wilhelm-Baynes' translation differs significantly from the original text and the received text of *Yijing*. The received text of *Yijing* refers to the version that has been traditionally accepted.

Initially, the *Yijing* was a manual used for divination and prediction. The received text of *Yijing* is composed of three primary layers. The first layer consists of 8 trigrams, which are symbols and signs created by the Chinese mythical Sage Fuxi, i.e., ☰, ☱, ☲, ☳, ☴, ☵, ☶, ☷.

The second layer is the reduplicate of the 8 trigrams, i.e., the 64 hexagrams, along with the oracles text recorded by the first Sage King Wen and his son Duke of Zhou of the Zhou Dynasty (1122–256 BCE).

The third layer includes seven commentaries on the first two layers, which were possibly written during the Spring and Autumn period (770–476 BCE) and Warring States period (476–221 BCE) of China; although these commentaries are group authored at different times, they are traditionally ascribed to Confucius as author. These Confucian commentaries have transformed the *Yijing* from an oracle text into a philosophical Confucian text. Later, these Confucian commentaries were edited into ten parts, attached to the original text and became the received text in the Han Dynasty. These commentaries are known as the *Ten Wings*; they aim to aid readers in understanding the text better by providing additional insights into the symbols, signs, and text.

While the *Ten Wings* may assist readers in gaining a better understanding of its contents, the basic text, containing the original oracles, is ambiguous and open to varied interpretations by each diviner or reader herself. Furthermore, the seven essays keep inspiring readers to conduct further philosophical discussions. Due to the elusive nature of both the basic text and the *Ten Wings*, readers are likely to generate their unique perspectives and understandings of *Yijing*, treating the *Yijing* as an open and subjective piece of writing, and thus forming the exegetical traditions of *Yijing* studies.

Clarifying the distinction between the Wilhelm-Baynes translation and three-layer structure of the *Yijing*. We will now explore how the Wilhelm-Baynes translation gained recognition for its philosophical insight and wisdom in the English-speaking world. Its popularity rose, especially among the hippie counterculture movement of the 1960s. This was a time when many young people, frustrated by the Vietnam War and the prevailing norms of their Western society, were seeking alternative perspectives and philosophies. The Eastern classic text of the *Yijing* provided a source of contemplation and a means to critically reflect on their own Western culture. In this context, the Wilhelm-Byanes *Yijing* became a tool for self-reflection and a mirror for many to examine their own lifestyle, offering insights that diverge from conventional Western philosophies. Famous figures like Bob Dylan got inspiration from just reading the *Yijing*. As such, the *Yijing* acts as a philosophical foil, proffering a rejuvenating perspective on life, society, and the individual's role within the vast tapestry of existence.

The Wilhelm-Baynes translation remained a standard edition of *Yijing* until 1970s and the situation started to shift. Applying Thomas Kuhn's "paradigm shift" concept (Kuhn 1962) , I will elucidate the shift of Anglophone scholarship on *Yijing* in North America from 1980 to 2020. Kuhn's framework offers insights into the dramatic transformations and shifts in perspectives and methodologies reshaping this field.

11.2 Paradigm Shift from Book of Wisdom Approach

The reception of the Wilhem-Baynes *Yijing* began to shift starting from 1970s. While Wilhelm's translation found resonance with the broader public, particularly within the counterculture hippie movement of the 1960s, it fell short when subjected to rigorous academic examination. The academia realized that Richard Wilhelm's translation of the *Yijing* is lack of fidelity to the original text. Academics pointed out that Wilhelm interpretive lens, heavily influenced by the *Zhouyi Zhezhong*, failed to acknowledge the historical and cultural changes of the *Yijing* studies. This period marked the beginning of a more critical and nuanced understanding of the *Yijing* in North American scholarship, setting the stage for the paradigm shift that was to come in the following decades. In response to the "book of wisdom" approach established by Richard Wilhelm, North American scholars have since adopted three interrelated approaches to study this classic text.

By the 1970s, scholars had identified significant discrepancies between the Wilhelm-Baynes versions and the multiple excavated versions of the original text. This sparked a renewed interest in exploring alternative methodologies for understanding the *Yijing*, marking a new era of academic research on this ancient text. The first approach, i.e., the foundationalist approach, delves into the origin and early development of the compositions of the *Yijing* in its "original context," they mainly rely on the excavated texts of *Yijing*, focusing on the period before the *Yijing* was brought into a philosophical framework by Confucians.

Thus, since the 1980s, a historical approach for studying the *Yijing* has been adopted by scholars. This approach strives to comprehend the specific historical and cultural contexts within which it was received and developed after the era of Confucius, and how its interpretations evolved across different dynasties. To frame their research, scholars have proposed three alternative approaches, each with a unique emphasis on "historical context" and "cultural context." This second approach mainly focuses on the Song Dynasty, a period of significant change and intellectual ferment, during which the *Yijing* was used by the literati as a guide to navigate the shifting sociopolitical landscape, and multiple commentaries burst out in this period.

Starting from 1999, a third approach traces the path of the *Yijing*'s dissemination both within China and globally, examining how individuals across various cultures have referred to the Book to address their unique circumstances. These approaches have yielded valuable insights into the *Yijing*, enhancing our understanding of its historical significance and the diverse ways in which it has been interpreted and applied over centuries.

11.3 First Approach: In Search of the Original Meaning of the *Yijing*

The foundationalist approach involves conducting archeological and philological examinations of texts to highlight the original and historical complexity of the *Yijing*. Distinguished scholars who have significantly contributed to this approach include Edward L. Shaughnessy, Richard Alan Kunst, and Richard Rutt (1925–2011). Shaughnessy's seminal work was his 1983 Ph.D. dissertation, titled *The Composition of the "Zhouyi."* Kunst's contribution was his 1985 Ph.D. dissertation named *The Original "Yijing": A Text, Phonetic Transcription, Translation, and Indexes, With Sample Glosses.* Rutt, on the other hand, is known for his 2002 translation, *The Yijing (Zhouyi): A Bronze Age Document.*

Among the three scholars, Shaughnessy is especially prolific. Since the mid-1980s, he has produced several influential works explaining the layers of meaning in the discovered texts. One of his notable contributions is *Unearthing the Changes: Recently Discovered Manuscripts of and Relating to the* Yi Jing (Shaughnessy 2014), where he translated three significant excavated manuscripts related to the *Yijing*, namely, the Shanghai Museum manuscript of *Zhouyi*, the Wangjiatai Guicang fragments, and the Fuyang manuscript of *Zhouyi*. His most recent comprehensive study, *The Origin and Early Development of the* Zhou Changes (Shaughnessy 2022), is an updated and revised version of his doctoral dissertation. In this work, he has cohesively and comprehensively integrated all his previous findings. Among the three scholars, Shaughnessy stands out as the most seasoned researcher in the field of the *Yijing*, having devoted nearly four decades to its study.

Together, all three scholars concurred that the traditional "book of wisdom" approach in North America was inadequate for unveiling the original message of the text. Consequently, they turned to the disciplines of archeology and philology to gain a deeper understanding of this ancient work. This "historical turn" aimed to uncover the original meanings of the *Yijing* when it was compiled and redacted during the Western Zhou period (1100–771 BCE).

The scholars criticized the "book of wisdom" approach for its inability to unearth the original or primitive content of the *Yijing*. This new approach, proposed by the trio of scholars, could be termed as the "Historical turn to the *Yijing*." These scholars found common base in the "Doubting Antiquity School" (Yigupai), particularly in the works of scholars like Gu Jiegang (1893–1980), Gao Heng (1900–1986), and Li Jingchi (1902–1975), who were active from the 1920s onwards. These Chinese scholars offered a unique interpretation of the *Yijing*, viewing it not as a philosophical treatise but as a valuable archeological artifact that reveals specific historical aspects of the Zhou era. To gain insights from the "Doubting Antiquity School" (Yigupai), Richard Kunst even traveled to China in 1980. He personally interviewed Gao Heng at Peking University and, in 1983, visited the students of Li Jingchi in Guangzhou. The perspectives of these Chinese scholars served as inspiration for the three Western proponents of the historical context approach.

Shaughnessy, currently still active in Chinese scholarship, should serve as the linchpin of the three. Shaughnessy's research suggests that the *Yijing* was authored by various individuals at different times, implying that there is no singular original version or prototype to rely upon. His work primarily focuses on the composition and development of the *Yijing* during the Zhou Dynasty. Archeological findings have unearthed multiple versions of the text, each providing a unique interpretation and revealing the text's evolution over time. The original meaning of the text can only be discerned by analyzing the excavated texts based on their language, philology, and the context in which they were written. Shaughnessy underscores the importance of considering the historical context of the texts and dismisses any interpretation that overlooks it.

He draws a clear distinction between the original text and the subsequent commentarial interpretations of the *Yijing* that emerged during the late Zhou Dynasty. According to Shaughnessy, the original text served primarily as a guide for divination, the context for all early versions of the *Yijing*. Divination was a means for individuals to express their intent for specific actions, irrespective of their moral implications. Each divination is unique.

However, the *Ten Wings* that interpreted the text shifted focus from divination to the conveyance of philosophical and moral beliefs. Shaughnessy's main argument opposes the Wilhelm-Baynes translation and the entire exegetical tradition of the *Yijing* that dates back to the *Ten Wings* and Confucius. He examined the authorship of "Shuogua Zhuan" ("Commentary Discussing the Trigrams"), the "Wenyan Zhuan" ("Commentary on the Words and Sayings"), the "Tuan Zhuan" ("Commentary on the Judgments"), and the "Xici Zhuan" ("Commentary on the Appended Statements"), his conclusion is that these four texts have transformed "the ancient divination text into the classic *Yijing*" (Shaughnessy 2022, 497). Although these four texts are not written by Confucius, he speculated that these four texts are written "by people who took their intellectual inspiration from Confucius" (Shaughnessy 2022, 497). He largely dismisses the philosophical exegetical tradition of the *Yijing* unless it supports his principal argument. His argument is that while the unearthed texts may appear similar to each other, each divination reflects a unique intention of the individual seeking a "medium" from the *Yijing*.

Before consulting the spirits, the individual had already made a decision but chosen not to express their intention directly. Instead, they used divination and related rituals to communicate their intentions and actions. These rituals served as a conduit for the individual to express their desires to others. Scholars using the historical approach rejected the notion that the *Yijing* text is based on universal or immutable moral principles. For these scholars, the *Yijing* should serve as a "medium" for expressing constantly changing intentions, not as a timeless book of unchanging wisdom. The meaning of the text changes with each divination ritual, reflecting the underlying intention of the individual.

The first hexagram judgment of the first hexagram *Qian* 乾, comprised of the four characters *Yuan* 元, *Heng* 亨, *Li* 利, and *Zhen* 贞, serves as an excellent illustration. According to Baynes' rendition, it translates to "THE CREATIVE works sublime success, Furthering through perseverance" (Wilhelm and Baynes 1967, 4). However, the three scholars advocating the foundationalist approach translate the same four characters differently:

"Primary receipt: beneficial to divine" (Shaughnessy 1983, 120).

"Grand treat. A favorable determination" (Kunst 1985, 241).

"Supreme offering. Favourable augury" (Rutt 2002, 224).

Baynes' translation relies on an allegorical interpretation, whereas the foundationalist triad employs a literal interpretation and historical–critical method. Their methodology delves into the historical context in which the basic text of the *Yijing* was written, encompassing the study of the culture, history, and languages of the *Yijing*'s original authors and audience. They interpret the first hexagram line as part of the divination rituals; the spirits receive a treat from the intentional person, and the individual receives an outcome supportive of their determination from the spirits.

Another instance is the translation of the first line judgment of the first hexagram. Baynes' rendition is as follows: "Nine at the beginning means: Hidden dragon. Do not act" (Wilhelm and Baynes 1967, 7). Her interpretation, which provides the metaphorical meaning of the hidden dragon in Chinese culture, is as follows:

> In China, the dragon has a meaning altogether different from that given it in the Western world. The dragon is a symbol of the electrically charged, dynamic, arousing force that manifests itself in the thunderstorm. In winter this energy withdraws into the earth; in the early summer it becomes active again, appearing in the sky as thunder and lightning. As a result, the creative forces on earth begin to stir again.
>
> Here this creative force is still hidden beneath the earth and therefore has no effect. In terms of human affairs, this symbolizes a great man who is still unrecognized. Nonetheless, he remains true to himself. He does not allow himself to be influenced by outward success or failure, but confident in his strength, he bides his time. Hence, it is wise for the man who consults the oracle and draws this line to wait in the calm strength of patience. The time will fulfill itself. One need not fear lest strong will should not prevail; the main thing is not to expend one's powers prematurely in an attempt to obtain by force something for which the time is not yet ripe (Wilhelm and Baynes 1967, 7).

The foundationalists, on the other hand, have different translations, which are as follows:

> First Nine: Submerging dragon. Don't use (Shaughnessy 2022, 410).
>
> A submerged dragon. Don't use (the outcome of this determination) (Kunst 1985, 241).
>
> Base (9): A dragon lies beneath the lake. No action take (Rutt 2002, 224).

Shaughnessy argued that "it would be reasonable that the dragon or dragons of *Qian* 'Vigorous' hexagram should also be sought in nature rather than within human society" (Shaughnessy 2022, 413) and he offered a lot of evidence to show the audience that the six dragons refer to the "Dragon constellation," he identifies:

> the dragon of *Qian* "Vigorous" hexagram with the Dragon constellation of China's night sky, it is then a simple matter to correlate the various lines with the Dragon's movement across the night sky throughout the year. The First Nine line, "Submerging dragon," refers to the winter season when, at dusk (which is when astronomical sightings were taken), the Dragon constellation was still out of sight beneath the eastern horizon, in what in Chinese mythology was regarded as the watery depths. In explanations of the *Zhou Changes* correlating the hexagrams and lines with months of the year, this line was always correlated with the zi

month, the month containing the winter solstice, more or less equivalent to December or early January (Shaughnessy 2022, 413–417).

For the foundationalists, "dragons" denote a factual, real object in the natural world. Conversely, Wilhelm prefers the interpretation of the "dragon" as a symbol of growing energy, providing moral guidance for individuals' actions. What the foundationalists emphasize is that the "polysemy" of *Yijing*-related texts is contingent upon people's "intentions" in their divinatory context.

These foundationalist scholars place their emphasis on the basic text of the *Yijing*, rather than the received text or the Chinese commentarial tradition. They stand in opposition to the Confucian interpretation of the *Yijing*. Despite this, the Chinese commentarial tradition of the *Yijing* remains largely uncharted territory in Western academia, prompting other scholars to explore alternative methodologies.

11.4 Second Approach: The Commentarial Tradition of the *Yijing*

The second approach shifts its focus from the basic text to the diverse interpretations that emerged and thrived within a rapidly evolving sociopolitical landscape. Each interpretation presents a unique way of reading the *Yijing*, suggesting that individuals have their own distinct voices when navigating life's uncertainties. In particular, scholars delve into how the *Yijing* was allegorically interpreted by literati of the Song Dynasty to express their worldviews and their practical schemes for the reformation of the Song society, exploring the text's practical applications in society instead of its mere existence on a bookshelf.

Since 1990, scholarly work following this second approach has begun to appear. A significant contribution is *Sung Dynasty Uses of the I Ching* (Smith et al. 1990), which scrutinizes the commentaries of four Song scholars—Su Shi (1037–1101), Shao Yong (1012–1077), Cheng Yi, and Zhu Xi. This book aims to highlight the distinct personalities and originality of these four Song scholars, who did not merely propagate universal wisdom but sparked competing ideas about the cosmos and societal change. The result is a collection of commentaries as unique as their authors, each representing a distinct style of thinking and creating their own wisdom.

While Cheng Yi and Zhu Xi may seem to share similar ideas, their interpretations of the *Yijing* are far from identical and should be treated respectively. However, further elaboration is needed on the differences between Cheng Yi's and Zhu Xi's commentaries.

It wasn't until 1994 that Richard John Lynn offered a seminal translation of the *Yijing* commentary by Wang Bi (226–249 CE). His choice is crucial because Wang Bi was considered orthodox in the Tang and Song dynasties before Cheng-Zhu orthodoxy took hold. Early Song literati began to diverge from Wang Bi's commentary. However, in Western scholarship, there had been no translation of Wang Bi's commentary on the *Yijing*, let alone a narrative of how Song literati began to deviate from Wang Bi.

Lynn's translation is the first and only translation of Wang Bi's commentary to date, providing Western readers with a valuable reference. It is important to note that every translation inevitably involves interpreting the basic text of the *Yijing*, and Lynn's strategy was to translate this text in line with Wang Bi's commentary.

Wang Bi's commentary possesses certain characteristics: firstly, Wang Bi is widely considered as one of the founders of Neo-Daoism (Xuanxue, or "Learning in the Profound"), and his commentary, a crucial work of the Wei Dynasty, became orthodox in the Tang Dynasty, supplemented by Kong Yingda's subcommentaries. This differs from the Confucian text of the *Yijing*. Secondly, it diverges from Pre-Qin texts or Song Dynasty interpretations, showcasing the diversity of exegetical traditions across different dynasties.

What is particularly noteworthy is Lynn's meticulous comparisons between the commentaries of Wang Bi, Kong Yingda, Cheng Yi, Zhu Xi, and others, which he details in the footnotes of each hexagram of the *Yijing*. For instance, his translation of Wang Bi's commentary on the top *Yang* line of Hexagram 4 Meng (Juvenile Ignorance) reads as follows:

> Here, one is located at the end point of Meng. Occupying the top position with strength, he can strike at and drive away Juvenile Ignorance and so alleviate their [the *yin* lines'] darkness. Thus the text says: "Strike at Juvenile Ignorance." Juvenile Ignorance wishes to be alleviated, and Top *Yang* itself wishes to strike at it and drive it away. As this meets the wishes of those above and those below [all the *yin* lines], none fails to comply. If one were to provide protection for them, then all would attach themselves to him, but to try to take them over by force would make them all rebel. Thus, the text says: "It is not fitting to engage in harassment; it is fitting to guard against harassment" (Lynn 1994, 163).

In a footnote, Lynn elaborates on the differences between Cheng Yi's and Wang Bi's interpretations, but also the similarities between Zhu Xi's and Wang Bi's views:

> Cheng Yi interprets this passage differently. He thinks that Top *Yang* represents Juvenile Ignorance at its worst and strongest, at the point where it leads one to banditry and rebellion. Thus, one must strike hard at it. In the light of his commentary, the text would mean: "Attack the Juvenile Ignorant. It is not fitting that he engage in banditry. It is fitting to prevent such banditry." Zhu Xi's commentary, however, seems to agree with that of Wang Bi: one should strike at Juvenile Ignorance but avoid excessive force. He also adds the remark: "All one can do is guard against enticements to evil from without, so that the Juvenile Ignorant can perfect his truth and purity." As such, Zhu provides a more specific gloss on "guard against harassment" than does Wang Bi (or Kong Yingda) (Ibid., 164–165).

This seminal work underscores the differences and individual creativity of each commentator and has earned high praise. Richard Smith lauds it, saying,

> Although no single translation can suffice for all purposes, Lynn's translation is the best one available in terms of its breadth of coverage, consistency of terminology, scholarly rigor, and ease of access. Moreover, although it is based on Wang Bi's third-century redaction of the text, Lynn provides a great many footnotes that reveal other understandings, particularly, but not exclusively, those of Song Dynasty commentators such as Cheng Yi and Zhu Xi (Smith 2008, xviii).

Through Lynn's quotations or summaries of *Zhouyi Zhezhong*, English readers can now discern the similarities and differences among the commentaries of Wang Bi, Kong Yingda, Cheng Yi, Zhu Xi, and others, all from Lynn's perspective. Additionally, in 1997, Richard John Lynn wrote a book review on *Song Dynasty Uses of the I Ching*. Here, he encapsulated the methodology of scholars who focus on *Yijing* commentaries, asserting that "the Classic of Changes exists in as many versions as there are commentaries on it: its text is so dense and opaque that its meaning depends on how commentaries interpret it" (Lynn 1997). This statement marks a paradigm shift from the first approach, suggesting that the focus has shifted from the received text of the *Yijing* to the diverse interpretations within the exegetical traditions.

However, certain elements remain elusive, such as the complete translations of Cheng Yi's and Zhu Xi's commentaries. English readers need assistance to access the primary source texts from these two thinkers. It is evident that, even after all these years, people primarily understand their thoughts through secondary sources rather than primary ones. Their original meanings represent a significant research gap, largely due to the complexity and difficulty of interpreting their works.

Another fascinating point is the opposition to Wilhelm's translation, even though Cheng Yi and Zhu Xi remain central to Song research. Scholars persist in their efforts to understand their thoughts need to move beyond this Cheng-Zhu school-centric approach. A third issue is that readers require a guiding lens to comprehend the Song *Yijing* exegetes and their extensive commentaries. These are the challenges that scholars will wrestle with over the next two decades.

In 2005, Tze-ki Hon published his seminal work, *The Yijing and Chinese Politics: Classical Commentary and Literati Activism in the Northern Song Period, 960–1127* (Hon 2005). This book provides English readers with a much broader and deeper understanding of *Yijing* studies during the Song Dynasty, deviating from the Cheng-Zhu-centric perspective. His methodology demonstrates that not only are Cheng Yi and Zhu Xi not identical, but the chronological development and synchronous comparison of each individual *Yijing* scholar during the Song Dynasty are intricately intertwined.

In his book, Hon divides the Northern Song period into three stages: early Northern Song (960–1022), mid-Northern Song (1023–1085), and late Northern Song (1086–1127). In each of these periods, he selects a group of synchronic commentaries and compares them. For instance, in the early Northern Song, he compares Hu Yuan's (993–1059) *Zhouyi kouyi* [*The orally transmitted meanings of the Yi from the Zhou Dynasty*] with Li Gou (1009–1059) and Ouyang Xiu (1007–1072). In the mid-Northern Song, he compares Zhang Zai's *Hengqu Yishuo* [An explanation of the meanings of Yi (by a reader from Hengqu)] with Sima Guang (1019–1086) and Shao Yong. In the late Northern Song, he compares Cheng Yi with Su Shi.

Hon underscores that when the Northern Song literati confronted the crises of their era, they sought solace in the *Yijing*, embedding their *Yijing* studies not only in the resulting commentaries but also in their personal lives and sociopolitical endeavors. In one respect, their commentaries function as historical resources, illuminating the social, political, intellectual, and spiritual dimensions of individual Song literati's lives.

According to Hon, a defining characteristic of the Song literati is their dynamism: they were activists, eager to tackle their nation's challenges and propose innovative strategies for societal transformation. This was accomplished not solely through direct political engagement but also through intellectual discourse and lifestyle choices. Additionally, in response to a rapidly evolving society, they infused their thoughts on societal reform into their commentaries, thereby catalyzing debates. When recontextualized within their social and historical milieu, the Song *Yijing* commentaries form a discursive space where their words mirror their actions.

Moreover, since no plan is everlasting, their thoughts were in a state of constant evolution. Consequently, their surviving commentaries can only capture certain facets of their thought processes and actions. Hon has recently expanded on this concept, positing that as long as they are reacting to the sociopolitical landscape, every moment will engender a unique intention from the literati and a fresh interpretation of the *Yijing*. Furthermore, each new commentator will generate their own interpretation at every given moment. This reflects the essence of the *Yijing*: the potential for interpretation is ceaseless and boundless.

Joseph A. Adler, a distinguished and prolific scholar, has made significant strides in the study of the *Yijing* during the Song Dynasty. Over four decades, Adler immersed himself in an in-depth analysis of Zhu Xi's works pertaining to the *Yijing*. His research shed light on Zhu Xi's religious practices and revealed how Zhu Xi's personal spiritual crises and his solutions profoundly shaped the philosophical foundations of the Cheng-Zhu School.

Among Adler's key contributions is his co-authorship of *Sung Dynasty Uses of the I Ching*, a work that explores the intricate persona of Zhu Xi. Zhu Xi is celebrated not only as a disciplined, rational philosopher of the *Dao* but also as a religious figure who committed himself to spiritual development and guided others on their spiritual paths. The harmony or discord between these two aspects of Zhu Xi—the rationalist and the religious man—is contingent upon our interpretation of his thoughts, particularly in relation to critical terms from the *Yijing*, such as *Taiji*.

In 1999, Adler advocated for the translation of *Taiji* as "Supreme Polarity," rather than the traditional "Supreme Ultimate." This proposal shaped his 2002 translation of Zhu Xi's *Zhouyi Qimeng* [*Introduction to the Study of the Classic of Change*], where he highlighted *Taiji*'s dual nature—activity and stillness—thereby emphasizing the religious facet of Zhu Xi's approach, especially his practice of the dynamic and tranquil states of the mind or heart.

Adler further expanded on this in his next work, *Reconstructing the Confucian Dao: Zhu Xi's Appropriation of Zhou Dunyi* (2014). Here, Adler charted the intellectual path from Zhou Dunyi to Zhu Xi and clarified their understanding of *Taiji*, the most foundational concept of the *Yijing*. A pivotal argument in this book is Adler's insistence on translating *Taiji* as "Supreme Polarity" instead of the conventional "Supreme Ultimate." This translation underscores the crucial *yin-yang* duality in Zhu Xi's interpretation of the *Yi* and his personal spiritual practice, which focuses on the mind/heart or *qi* within the individual, rather than a supreme unity from the heavens. The *yin-yang* duality symbolizes the interchangeable states of activity and stillness, mirroring Zhu Xi's spiritual practice of balancing the "still and active phases of the mind/heart" (Adler 2014, 201). Adler's work emphasizes that Zhu Xi's amalgamation of previous philosophical thought is deeply rooted in his personal spiritual experiences of cultivating the mind/heart, rather than being purely theoretical conjectures.

North American scholars have recognized the importance of providing comprehensive and original resources for Cheng Yi's and Zhu Xi's works. This understanding led to two significant translations: Cheng Yi's *The Yi River Commentary on the Yijing*, translated by L. Michael Harrington, and the 2020 first complete English translation of Zhu Xi's remarkable work *Zhouyi Benyi* [The Original Meaning of the *Yijing*: Commentary on the Scripture of Change] by Adler. These translations allow Western scholars to better discern the differences between these two original thinkers. Consequently, *Zhouyi Zhezhong* is distinguished for the first time in Western languages, and the two individual commentaries are presented in their authentic and complete forms.

Both Lynn and Harrington bring a similar approach to their translations of the foundational text of the *Yijing*. Harrington decidedly aligns with the consensus of prior scholars, adopting the historical approach. To highlight the distinctiveness of Cheng Yi's commentary, he undertook a "verbatim translation." He expressed disagreement with many traditional English translations, particularly those by James Legge and Baynes, as these translations are primarily based on the *Zhouyi Zhezhong*. As Harrington asserts in his translation,

> The translation of a commentary on the *Yijing* demands a new translation of the Book itself. Some of the characters in the original text may be given different meanings, and some portions of the original text may be given different sentence structures, depending on the interpretive decisions of the commentator (Cheng Yi 2019, xii).

However, several differences emerge when we compare the two commentaries of Zhu Xi and Cheng Yi. The most significant distinction lies in their respective approaches to the two prevailing traditions of *Yijing* exegesis in Chinese history: the School of Images and Numbers (*xiangshu* 象數), which gained prominence starting in the Han Dynasty, and the School of Meanings and Principles (*yili* 義理), represented by Wang Bi.

Cheng Yi, a staunch adherent of the School of Meanings and Principles, infused his commentary with as much of his Confucian philosophical ideas as possible. He placed the utmost value on the words of the text and displayed little interest in the ritual of divination. On the other hand, Zhu Xi's commentary on the *Yijing* represents a synthesis of the divination manual, the School of Images and Numbers, and the School of Meanings and Principles. Zhu Xi believed that anyone could use the *Yijing* as a tool for self-cultivation toward sagehood, facilitated by the rituals of divination. In this light, the differences between the two translations become a reflection of the diverse interpretive traditions within *Yijing* studies.

Adler aligns with Zhu Xi in the belief that each individual is in a unique situation at a different stage on their path to sagehood. Consequently, the basic text of the *Yijing*, which is considered the first layer of the received text and attributed to Fu Xi, does not provide explicit directions to the seeker. Instead, it serves as a medium through which the seeker must discover their own answers and navigate their own path during divination.

Adler refers to this as Zhu Xi's "minimalist commentary" (Zhu Xi 2020, 20). He notes that.

> For the most part Zhu Xi does not spell out all the moral philosophical implications of the text. As a result, his commentary is briefer than the commentaries of Wang Bi and Cheng Yi. And that means that the scriptural text itself must remain as gnomic, or runic, as it really is. In other words, I have resisted the impulse to make sense of the text where that sense is not evident. The text is jumbled, fragmentary, cryptic, and exceedingly obscure, and for the most part I have left it that way (Zhu Xi 2020, 19).

This approach respects the inherent ambiguity and complexity of the *Yijing*, allowing the text to retain its mysterious and cryptic nature. Adler's translation and commentary do not attempt to impose a definitive interpretation, but rather, they facilitate the reader's personal exploration and understanding of the text. This approach is in line with the tradition of *Yijing* studies, which emphasizes the text's role as a tool for personal reflection and divination.

Three decades after the publication of *Sung Dynasty Uses of Yijing* in 1990, North American scholarship has, for the first time, produced complete English translations of Cheng Yi's and Zhu Xi's commentaries. Does this mark the culmination of research related to the Cheng-Zhu School's engagement with the *Yijing*? Or is it merely the starting point for further exploration? It is important to note that these translations pose a challenge for the average reader. None of them are without flaws, as translation is, in essence, another form of interpretation. Together with Lynn's translation, these three versions have laid a fresh foundation for Western scholars to broaden their research scope and delve deeper into *Yijing* studies. Nevertheless, the research gap remains conspicuous; for instance, translations of works by Hu Yuan (993–1059), Zhang Zai (1020–1077), Su Shi, or Sima Guang's school are still needed.

As for the *Zhouyi Zhezhong* itself, while it primarily draws upon Zhu Xi's and Cheng Yi's commentaries, it also includes commentaries from the Han Dynasty (202 BCE–220 CE) and other periods.

11.5 Third Approach: Global Circulation

At first glance, the initial two approaches appear diametrically opposed. The first zeroes in on the origin and early development of the *Yijing*, challenging the Confucianization of the text, while the second centers on the Confucian commentaries on the *Yijing* during the Song Dynasty. However, the third approach harmonizes these seemingly contradictory perspectives by threading them together under the umbrella concepts of "diversity" and "openness."

This third approach, exemplified by Richard Smith, situates the study of the *Yijing* in a broader context, transitioning from a domestic Chinese history to a global historical narrative. This approach, much like its predecessors, also counters the "book of wisdom" perspective. Smith asserts, "This is especially the case because the widespread Western notion of a timeless and universal *Yijing*—an idea encouraged by the influential German missionary-translator Richard Wilhelm—is not only inadequate but also misleading" (Smith 2008, xi).

The Chinese commentary tradition on the *Yijing* is expansive and profound, akin to a vast ocean. The translations and studies discussed thus far only represent a minuscule fraction. For example, studies on the Han Dynasty's *Yijing* remained largely unexplored in Western scholarship until Bent Nielsen's book *A Companion to Yi Jing Numerology and Cosmology* (2003) surfaced as an excellent resource on the School of Images and Numbers approach. However, this book did not delve into the intricacies of Han *Yijing* studies, let alone the enormous impact and global reception of the *Yijing*.

Smith, trained as a specialist on the Qing Dynasty (1644–1912) scholars, initiated his research through the lens of Qing *Yijing* scholars. These scholars, representing the final phase of ancient Chinese *Yijing* studies, summarized and evaluated the evolution of the *Yijing*. Through this perspective, Smith acquired a more comprehensive understanding of the *Yijing*. Smith extended his research beyond Qing *Yijing* studies, aiming to outline the entire evolution of *Yijing* studies from their inception to the present, from domestic expansion to international reception. In an effort to dispel the influence of Baynes' translation in the Western world, Richard Smith acknowledged and built upon the research findings of the two preceding academic groups, whereby he introduced this third approach. He expanded the research scope beyond the birth of the *Yijing* or the Song Dynasty *Yijing* study, integrating them into the overall development of the history of *Yijing* studies. He launched this project by first delivering lectures in 1999. Subsequently, he consolidated his findings into his seminal work, *Fathoming the Cosmos and Ordering the World: The Yijing (*I Ching*, or* Classic of Changes*) and Its Evolution in China* (2008). Later, he extended the scope of his work to a global context, culminating in *The* I Ching*: A Biography* (2012).

The writing style of *Fathoming the Cosmos and Ordering the World* aligns with the tradition of "the history of *Yijing* studies易學史" in Chinese scholarship. To date, it remains the sole representation of this genre in Western scholarship. The book traces the domestic evolution of the *Yijing* and its interpretation across various Chinese dynasties, spanning from the birth of the Zhou Dynasty, through the Han Dynasty, the Six Dynasties, the Tang Dynasty, the Song Dynasty, the Yuan and Ming Dynasties, the Qing Dynasty, to modern China up until the 1980s.

In each chapter, Smith underscores the "openness" and "diversity" of *Yijing* scholarship, elaborating on how it innovatively evolved within each specific historical and cultural context. This approach effectively illustrates how a historian views the history of *Yijing* studies. For instance, in Chinese academia, the *Yijing* studies of the Yuan Dynasty have often been overlooked, as Yuan scholars were eclipsed by their Song Dynasty counterparts. However, Smith recognized and highlighted the unique value of the *Yijing* studies conducted during the Yuan Dynasty.

What sets Smith apart from traditional Chinese scholarship on the "history of *Yijing* studies" is his attention to the international exchange of ideas between Chinese and Western intellectuals. For example, he details the interactions between

Ming scholars and Christian missionaries concerning the *Yijing*, as well as Joachim Bouvet's (1656–1730) work on *Yijing* studies. Such information is often absent in conventional Chinese scholarship, which typically segregates these international exchanges from the domestic narrative of *Yijing*'s history.

While traditional studies outline how the *Yijing* evolved within the Chinese context through various dynasties, Smith's work also incorporates the global and transcultural exchanges that shaped the text. By extending the domestic history into a transnational narrative, Smith shows that the *Yijing* is not merely a classic of China, but a classic of the world.

Smith's approach to the "history of *Yijing*" is unique in Chinese scholarship. Chinese researchers on the *Yijing* generally focus on domestic studies, often due to language barriers. The integration of domestic and international research is a formidable task, and most Chinese scholars tend to compartmentalize research into distinct domains handled by different scholars. Therefore, Smith's successful bridging of domestic and international studies is a significant achievement.

As a historian, Smith objectively critiques James Legge's (1815–1897) translation of the *Yijing* and his cultural biases as a Jesuit scholar. Smith states,

> Legge had no love of China and no respect for the *Yijing*. Indeed, he described it as "a farrago of emblematic representations." Although admitting that the Changes was "an important monument of architecture," he characterized it as "very bizarre in its conception and execution." Legge's highly literal translation followed the prevailing neo-Confucian orthodoxy of the Qing Dynasty, as reflected in the Balanced Compendium on the Zhou Changes. His goal was to produce a translation that made it possible for him to downplay aspects of the *Yijing* he deemed unimportant, such as its imagery and numerology, and to underscore themes he considered essential—not least the obviously mistaken idea that passages in the Explaining the Trigrams commentary refer to the Judeo-Christian God (Smith 2012, 184–185).

Smith, therefore, provides a critical perspective on Legge's approach, highlighting the latter's lack of appreciation for the cultural context and nuances of the *Yijing*.

"Diversity" and "eclecticism" are key concepts in comprehending Richard Smith's two seminal works. In his earlier work, he demonstrated how the *Yijing* inspired varied interpretations from different readers across China's historical contexts. In his later work, he traced how the *Yijing* was accepted, adapted, and appropriated within different nations and cultural traditions in East Asia and the West. It is not a case of one timeless wisdom encountering various people; instead, one classic text has the allure to captivate individuals from different countries, possessing the flexibility to meld with its readers.

Beyond the "history of *Yijing* studies," Smith also emphasizes the multidisciplinary nature of *Yijing* studies. The *Yijing* is not just a historical artifact; it is a cultural encyclopedia that permeates various aspects of Chinese culture and beyond, influencing fields such as architecture, art, science, and language.

However, Smith's research is not exhaustive. While he aims to portray the "globalization" of the *Yijing*, his primary focus is on how the *Yijing* circulated in East Asia and the anglophone world. Still, the *Yijing* has sparked a series of academic responses worldwide. Smith's work has inspired more scholars around the globe to expand on the concept of the "Global *Yijing*." In 2021, two works built upon Smith's research: *The Other Yijing: The Yijing in Chinese History, Politics, and Everyday Life*, edited by Tze Ki Hon (Hon 2021), offered more details about the *Yijing*'s influence, and *The Making of the Global Yijing in the Modern World*, edited by Benjamin Wai-ming Ng, explored cross-cultural interpretations and interactions of the *Yijing*. In the twenty-first century, the "Global *Yijing*" has emerged as a new trend attracting scholarly attention.

11.6 Conclusion

This review article traces the evolution and reception of *Yijing* studies in North America from 1980 to 2020. The field has undergone a significant transformation, shifting from the "book of wisdom" perspective, primarily shaped by the Wilhelm-Baynes translation, to a "historical approach" championed by three interrelated scholarly groups.

Richard Wilhelm's translation of the *Yijing* has had a profound and enduring impact on English scholarship. Since its English publication over eight decades ago, it has served as a seminal text for Western readers and scholars interested in Chinese philosophy and culture. Wilhelm's translation introduced the *Yijing* to a wider audience, igniting a wave of interest in the text and its teachings. This fascination has resulted in over four decades of meticulous research and analysis, leading to remarkable contributions in the field of *Yijing* studies. Despite ongoing debates regarding the accuracy and interpretation of Wilhelm's translation, its influence is undeniable. It has acted as a catalyst for the expansion of *Yijing* studies in the English-speaking world and continues to inspire scholars and readers alike.

Under the umbrella of the "historical approach," three distinct but interconnected methodologies have evolved, each striving to contextualize the *Yijing*. The common assumption among these methodologies is that there is no "original *Yijing*" or definitive first edition. Even if such an edition were to be discovered, it would simply reflect the intentions of a particular group of people at a specific time. The *Yijing* is inherently multifaceted, its text and interpretations perpetually expanding and uniquely accessible to each reader at their specific moment of engagement. All three methodologies prioritize the historical context and the intentions of the *Yijing*'s diviners, interpreters, and readers, but each focuses on different areas of inquiry, creating a clear division of labor within *Yijing* studies. Collectively, these three branches provide a comprehensive historical framework for *Yijing* studies.

The *Yijing* has enriched lives across China, East Asia, and the West. Its enduring significance lies in its ongoing ability to guide individuals worldwide as they navigate life's challenges and our constantly evolving world. The latest trend in the field is the focus on the "Global *Yijing*." This shift in perspective signifies a new paradigm in the twenty-first century, attracting an increasing number of scholars worldwide to contribute to this emerging discourse.

These contributions have not only deepened our understanding of the *Yijing* and its philosophical implications but have also paved the way for future research. Scholars continue to delve into the text's rich layers of meaning, its historical context, and its influence on various aspects of Chinese and global culture.

References

Adler, J.A. 2014. *Reconstructing the Confucian Dao: Zhu Xi's appropriation of Zhou Dunyi*. Albany, NY: State University of New York Press.

Cheng Yi. 2019. *The Yi river commentary on the book of changes*. Translated by L. Michael Harrington. New Haven, CT: Yale University Press.

Hon, T. 2005. *The* Yijing *and Chinese politics: Classical commentary and literati activism in the northern song period, 960–1127*. Albany, NY: State University of New York Press.

Hon, T. 2021. *The other* Yijing*: The book of changes in Chinese history, politics, and everyday life*. Leiden: Brill.

Kuhn Thomas. 1962. *The structure of scientific revolutions*. Chicago: University of Chicago Press.

Kunst, Richard Alan. 1985. *The original "Yijing": A text, phonetic transcription, translation, and indexes, with sample glosses*, Ph.D. diss: University of California, Berkeley.

Lynn, R.J. (Trans.). 1994. *The classic of changes: A new translation of the I Ching as interpreted by Wang Bi*. New York: Columbia University Press.

Ng, Benjamin Wai-ming (Ed.). 2021. *The making of the global Yijing in the modern world: Cross-cultural interpretations and interactions*. Singapore: Springer.

Rutt, R. 1996. *The book of changes (Zhouyi): A bronze age document translated with introduction and notes*. Durham EastAsia Series 1. Richmond, Surrey: Curzon Press.

Shaughnessy, Edward L. 1983. *The composition of the "Zhouyi"*, Ph.D. diss: Standford University.

Shaughnessy, Edward L. 2014. *Unearthing the changes: recently discovered manuscripts of the Yi Jing (I Ching) and related texts*. Columbia: University Press.

Shaughnessy, Edward L. 2022. *The origin and early development of the* Zhou changes. Leiden and Boston: Brill.

Smith, R.J. 2008. *Fathoming the cosmos and ordering the world: The Yijing (I Ching, or classic of changes) and its evolution in China*. Charlottesville, VA: University of Virginia Press.

Smith, R.J. 2012. *The I Ching: A biography*. Princeton, NJ: Princeton University Press.

Smith Jr, Kidder, Peter K. Bol, Joseph A. Adler, and Don J. Wyatt. 1990. *Sung dynasty uses of the I Ching*. Princeton, NJ: Princeton University Press.

Wilhelm, Richard and Cary F. Baynes (Trans.). 1967. *The I Ching or book of changes*. Princeton, NJ: Princeton University Press.

Zhu Xi. 2020. *The original meaning of the Yijing: Commentary on the scripture of change*. Trans. Ed. Joseph A. Adler. New York: Columbia University Press.

Chapter 12
Yijing and Feminism: The Scandinavian Interpretations of the *Book of Changes*

Bjørn Åge Blix

Abstract This chapter compares three Scandinavian versions of the *Book of Changes* to examine how Danish, Norwegian, and Swedish authors have interpreted the classic for gender equality. It focuses on the *Changes* of Margaret J. Pearson who is known for her challenges against the Western interpretation of the *Changes* as male-centric. Pearson's interpretation of the *Changes* serves as the basis for my comparison of three Scandinavian renditions, each from Denmark, Norway, and Sweden. My comparison suggests that the three Scandinavian authors interpreted the *Changes* from the perspective of gender equality, but they differ starkly in their approaches and arguments. Whereas the Danish author Jens Windeleff alters important terms and highlights the feminine, the Swedish author, Kristine Tranmark Kossman, merely altered some terms to make them gender neutral. In comparison, the Norwegian author, Eva Skodvin, utilizes the *Changes* to accuse Western culture of being "yang-centric" (prioritizing masculine values). In the process, Skodvin highlights, like Windeleff, the importance of *yin* values (feminine values) for both genders and uses the *yin-yang* dichotomy to become a primordial concept propagating gender equality. Through this comparison, this article presents a complex feminist interpretation of the *Changes* interpretation and argues that the three Scandinavian authors are creative and thoughtful in interpreting the Chinese classic to deal with gender issues in contemporary society.

Keywords *Book of Changes* · Gender equality · *Yin-Yang* · Scandinavia · Travel of texts

B. Å. Blix (✉)
Hunan University, Changsha, China
e-mail: blix1990@hotmail.com

G. Sigurðsson and T. Hon (eds.), *Contemporary Interpretations and Readings of the Yijing*, Chinese Culture 15, https://doi.org/10.1007/978-981-96-0609-2_12

12.1 Introduction

Venerated as the oldest classical text of China, the *Book of Changes* (hereafter *Changes*) has aroused curiosity around the world for centuries. In China, the text relates to almost everything Chinese from cultural, historical, spiritual, and philosophical, to being a scientific text with poetic features and medicinal guidelines. When transported out of China, the *Changes* continued its far-reaching significance by inspiring Gottfried Wilhelm von Leibniz's binary numbers (Ryan 1996), Nils Bohr's physics (Adler 2022, 149–150), Carl G. Jung's depth psychology (Robinson 2018), and John Cage's *Music of Changes* (Smith 2012, 204–205). Recently, it has been shown that the *Changes* did not only inspire individuals but have also shaped itself in its interpretations by social and political movements like Western counterculture (Redmond 2021). My question is then, has the Chinese classic been adapted to movements like feminism? It is well known that Pearson's (2011) translation of the *Changes* was meant to correct gender imbalance in the established anglophone reception of the classic. But have other Western interpretations dealt with the patriarchal tone of the *Changes*? Considering that Cary F. Baynes, who rendered Richard Wilhelm's *I Ging* (1924) into English, decided to preserve terms like "the superior man (*junzi* 君子)" and "the great man (*daren* 大人)" in her rendition (Wilhelm and Baynes 1967, 8), it is legitimate to ask: Have other European translators of the *Changes* viewed the patriarchy of the *Changes* differently?

To answer these questions, this chapter examines the reception of the *Changes* in Scandinavia by comparing the renditions by Jens Windeleff of Denmark (first published in 1973), Kristine Tranmark Kossman of Sweden (first published in 1981), and Eva Skodvin of Norway (first published in 1988). Since the 1960s, Denmark, Norway, and Sweden have implemented progressive gender equality policies and are by many considered among the most gender-equal countries in the world (Nielsen 2014, 187). Due to these Scandinavian countries' progression on gender equality, this chapter will juxtapose the renditions of the three aforementioned Scandinavian authors with the famous rendition of Baynes and Pearson's to discuss the relationship of the *Changes* with feminism.

Windeleff, Kossman, and Skodvin are the first to render the classic into Danish, Swedish, and Norwegian, respectively. Compared with how the influential English tradition of James Legge (first published in 1882) and the German tradition of Richard Wilhelm (first published in 1924) needed to consider Chinese culture when translating their *Changes*, the three Scandinavians did not account for the patriarchal development of the classic in China. Instead, they base their renditions on the English version by Christopher Markert first published in 1986 (cf. Markert and Skodvin 2001), and the German version by Richard Wilhelm from 1924 (cf. Wilhelm and Windeleff 1973; Wilhelm and Kossman 1991). As pioneers, Windeleff, Kossman, and Skodvin had ample opportunities to decide how the classic should be formulated in their native languages. Availing themselves of this freedom of interpretation, Windeleff and Kossman made deliberate attempts at improving Wilhelm's outline of women by translating "*der Edle*" (with masculine article "der" in German), rendered "the superior man" (*junzi* 君子) by Baynes (Wilhelm and Baynes 1967, 8), into "*det ædle mennesket* (the noble human)" (Wilhelm and Windeleff 1973, 34) and "*den upphöjde* (the heightened)" (Wilhelm and Kossman 1991, 31). In comparison, Skodvin decided to translate Markert's transcreation of James Legge's translation (1899) of the *Changes* which strongly emphasizes gender equality and accuses Western culture of *yang*-centrism (Markert and Skodvin 2001, 35). As a result, the *Changes* has never been considered a patriarchal text in Scandinavia like it has been received in the anglophone world before Pearson's translation.

In the following sections, I will briefly discuss how the *Changes* can be read as a text about gender equality. This discussion will start with a brief introduction of the *Changes* and some core sources from Chinese intellectual history before moving on to the classic's development in the West, beginning with the popular rendition by Baynes (Wilhelm and Baynes 1967) and ending with Pearson's more recent translation (2011). Next, I will discuss Windeleff and Skodvin's renditions in more detail due to their focus on the feminine aspect and the gender equality message contained in the binary *yin-yang* model. Then, I will discuss how Windeleff and Kossman dealt with the important Chinese terms *junzi* 君子 and *daren* 大人. In the conclusion, I assess whether Windeleff, Kossman, and Skodvin rendered the *Changes* for feminist purposes like Pearson.

12.2 The Textual Layers of the *Changes*

The *Changes* is considered the most ancient classic from China's rich corpus of texts. It is believed to have been written over a period of thousand or more years by legendary Chinese figures starting with Fu Xi's 伏羲 64 hexagram images (Hon 2019). These hexagrams were later provided with titles and short texts by the treasured leaders of the Zhou Dynasty (周代, ca. 1050–221 BCE), King Wen 文王 and the Duke of Zhou 周公 (Wu 2021, 41–42). Subsequently, several philosophical discussions, known as the *Ten Wings* 十翼, are believed to have been added by Confucius 孔夫子, resulting in the multilayered and multifaceted work titled the *Yijing* 易经 in Chinese or *Changes* in the West. Now, there is no concrete evidence about the relationship between these important Chinese figures and the texts in the *Changes*. However, it is generally accepted that pieces of the *Changes* were written in the Spring and Autumn period, some parts before that period, and some parts written after (Zhang 2019, 10), maybe as late as in the Han Dynasty (*Han Dai* 漢代, 202 BCE—9 CE, 25–220 CE) (Rongen 2006, 248).

In its earliest form of hexagram images, it can be argued that the broken lines represent female or feminine values while the unbroken line represents male and masculine values. As such, the commonly placed first two hexagrams in the *Changes*, ䷀ *Qian* 乾 and ䷁ *Kun* 坤, are considered divine-like perfect representatives of the two gendered forces of creation while the remaining 62 hexagrams are different synergies of *Qian*-and *Kun's* coactions. Based on the images alone, there is no reason to arrange them hierarchically by granting either of these forces a superior status.

While the complex meanings and importance of these two hexagrams are still being discovered, their simple gendered version whereby *Qian* is male and *Kun* is female should likewise not be portrayed in a hierarchical fashion because both genders are equally important in the creation and survival of humans and humanity. If anything, women should be on top of that hierarchy because, as research has shown about ancient cultures, women were kept close at home and safe due to their importance regarding childbearing and child rearing (Bonvillain 2007, 9–10). Men, on the other hand, are best considered as the disposable gender since, to put it simply, a fertile man can provide dozens of new humans while a fertile woman can normally only provide one at a time. As a result, men would be the natural choice to go on dangerous hunting trips and do more strenuous labor (Ibid., 8). If we accept that Fu Xi made the hexagrams and that he was the first individual in China to lead the ancient hunting and agricultural society into a form of early civilization, it is reasonable to assume that males and females had their roles in society for survival and collaborative purposes without a structured hierarchy.

Even in the earliest texts of the *Changes*, the *Changes* of the Zhou Dynasty, or *Zhouyi* 周易, the character for female (*nü* 女) is only mentioned nine times and the character for male (*nan* 男) is entirely absent. While there are other terms like *fu* 夫 and *fuqi* 夫妻, which might directly, indirectly, or inclusively refer to a male, there are not any obvious patriarchal frameworks attached to these characters in the earliest texts of the *Changes*. Quite the contrary, several of the *Zhouyi* texts discuss women as healthy and strong, persevering, and several passages highlight their importance for happy marriages and their contribution as child bearers. For instance, in a recent English translation of the *Changes* by Redmond (2017, 247), the only hexagram displaying the character for woman 女 twice in its initial line, hexagram 44 *Gou* 姤, is translated as "Though the woman is robust, do not choose this woman." Redmond writes about the initial line, "[Hexagram 44's initial line] may be the most misunderstood line in the entire *I Ching*, having been translated as meaning that *because* the woman is strong, she should not be taken as a wife (or concubine, or servant)" (Ibid., 248). Redmond's argument is that strong women should not be taken as wives because they fulfilled important roles in their family. In other words, despite being an ideal spouse for marriage, a woman should not be removed from her birth family because of her important contribution to it. Redmond writes:

> In traditional China, life expectancy for women was only into the mid-twenties and death in childbirth was frequent, making health a major factor in suitability for marriage. In addition, food preparation and housework were physically challenging, making robust or strong women desirable as members of the household (Ibid.).

While the robust women of the *Changes* are primarily discussed in relation to marriage and their contribution to the household, this should not be considered patriarchal. Rather, it means that she is someone very important and treasured by the members of the household. Another interpretation of the robust woman in the *Changes* is that she is a fierce and powerful warrior, like Lady Fu Hao 婦好 of the Shang Dynasty (商代, ca. 1600–1046 BCE) (Redmond and Hon 2014, 90), and thus she should not be confined to the roles of marriage since her contribution on the battlefield is too important. How, then, did the roles and status of men and women become patriarchal in China's history based upon the *Changes*?

It is likely due to the roles and values assigned to men and women in the *Ten Wings* discussions of the *Changes* and China's development as a civilization that the classic enters its patriarchal trajectory. The *Ten Wings* consists of the texts "Wenyan" 文言, "Tuan" 彖, "Xiang" 象, "Xici" 繫辭, "Shuogua" 說卦, "Zagua" 雜卦, and "Xugua" 序卦. These seven texts are considered ten because "Tuan," "Xiang," and "Xici" are commonly separated into two, thereby bringing the total up to ten. Regarding the patriarchal development of the *Changes*, perhaps the most important statement is found in the "Tuan," where we are told that for families, women's proper position is inside while men's proper position is outside (Rongen 2006, 160). However, this should not be understood as patriarchal because 2000–2500 years ago, when the *Tuan* was probably written, "inside" should be perceived as a place of safety, comfort, warmth, with food and drink. "Outside," on the other hand, should be understood as the space containing the hardships that come with things like war, weather, and manual labor. The problem of this inside-outside separation, however, changes alongside a country's development as a civilization whereby the role of "inside" is relatively unchanged or becomes even more simpler and easier for those inside, and the outside role is enhanced through educational, political, social, and entertaining opportunities. Arguably, due to the development of what is inside and what is outside the home, the different texts of the *Changes*, which originally highlighted, treasured, and protected women, became subjected to patriarchal discourses.

It was during the Han Dynasty that the ideas of the *Changes* received many influential patriarchal outlines by philosophers (Hinsch 2006, 97). Previously, the text mainly served as a prominent divination manual (Camman 1991, 576), and although parts of the *Ten Wings* are patriarchal by contemporary standards, the deliberate subjugation of women through the philosophy of the *Changes* did not rise to prominence until the influential writings of Han Dynasty's Dong Zhongshu 董仲舒 (Wang 2005, 209). Dong is recognized as one of the most influential Confucian scholars in Chinese history as he is credited to have established Confucianism as the Imperial state doctrine (Fung 1976, 191). Due to his influence and philosophical reinvention of the *yin-yang* 阴阳 dichotomy to become hierarchical in connection with gender, it resulted in a powerful subjugation of women. Since Dong, the idea of *yin* as "feminine," as well as how the *yang*-men should raise and treat them, became increasingly discussed to the disadvantage of the female gender. It arguably reached its peak a thousand years after Dong's writings in the Song Dynasty (宋代, 960–1279) when foot binding became endorsed by Neo-Confucian philosophers and the *Changes'* idea of wife, daughters, and sisters became further developed by Cheng Yi 程頤 to emphasize the superiority of the husband, sons, and brothers (Ess 2010, 64–70). With some simplification, the doctrines that subjugated women in historical China remained prominent until Mao Zedong 毛泽东 and the revolutions of the Chinese Communist Party re-established the Chinese social and political order. Although aspects of the philosophical culture since the Han and Song Dynasties may still remain in China's social sphere, women's position and role in society have improved immensely. That being said, the early globalization of the *Changes*, however, was mentored by Confucian masters from the Qing Dynasty (清代, 1644–1911). These traditional philosophers were central in making the Western translations by the most famous names in the early circulation of the global *Changes*—James Legge, Richard Wilhelm, and Cary F. Baynes—who published their translations in the years 1882, 1924, and 1950, respectively.

12.3 Cary F. Baynes' Rendition of the *Changes*

Although not commonly recognized as such, Cary F. Baynes' rendering of Wilhelm's *Changes* was an important step in the early development of the *Changes* as a feminist classic in the West. The reason is not so much that it can be considered a feminist text, but because of its immense popularity during the United States counter-cultural movement (Redmond 2021) and how that movement braided into feminist movements (Gatlin 1987, 97). As a text that introduced new and intriguing spiritual and philosophical ideas, Baynes' *Changes* received immense popularity for its useful guidance on individuals' self-discovery and psychological improvement. A particularly important contribution of Baynes' *Changes* to the anglophone world was its re-evaluation of *yin-yang*, a binary concept previously gendered in Rev. Canon Thomas McClatchie's 1876 translation of the *Changes* and neglected by Legge. In Legge's translation, which was the most dominant English translation until Baynes' rendition received popularity, the *yin-yang* dichotomy is described as an odd idea which is not worthy of attention. Legge writes:

> I confess my sympathy with P. Regis, when he condenses the fifth ["Wing"] into small space, holding that the 8th and following paragraphs are not worthy to be translated. "They contain," he says, "nothing but mere enumeration of things, some which may be called *Yang*, and others *Yin*, without any other cause for so thinking being given" (Legge 1899, ch. 3).[1]

Legge seems to have discarded *yin-yang* for the same reason as McClatchie, namely because they both assumed the terms were basic primitive words which separated males and females. This misconception of the Chinese *yin-yang* dichotomy was important for Wilhelm to correct when he translated the *Changes* into German. Likewise for Baynes, in her rendering of Wilhelm's *I Ging*, *yin-yang* became reinvented for anglophone readers as a complex idea of how everything in the world is in a constant complementary coaction, including men and women. Previously, *yin-yang* had been semantically related to other terms where *yin* and female were associated with words like winter, night, and below, while *yang* and male became related to words like summer, day, ruler, and above (Graham 1986, 27–28). To amend the previous anglophone misunderstanding of *yin-yang*, Baynes argues:

[1] The P. Regis translation to which Legge refers in the citation is the first translation of the *Changes* into a Western language by Jesuit scholars. The translation project started in 1707 but was not published until it was rediscovered in 1830 with the title *Y-King antiquissimus Sinarum liber quem ex Latina interpretation P. Regis aliorumque ex Soc Jesu P.P. edidit Julius Mohl* (Smith 2012, 181).

> There is nothing to indicate [that the primitive phallic symbolism, with all the accompanying connotations, is] in the original meaning of the words *yin* and *yang*. In its primary meaning, *yin* is "the cloudy," "the overcast" and *yang* means actually "banners waving in the sun," that is, something "shone upon," or bright (Wilhelm and Baynes 1967, lvi).

Since Baynes' *Changes*, *yin-yang* entered a new era of Western interpretations. The popularity of her *Changes* alongside her renewal of *yin-yang* allowed future scholars and translators to reinvent the gendered interpretation of the *yin-yang* dichotomy from being a leading and positive *yang* with a subordinate and negative *yin*, to become something basic and equal.

As the topics of gender equality became popular in social and political spheres, so too has the *Changes* become subjected to gendered interpretations. Since *yin* has been considered the subordinate version of the two, terms like *yin*, female, and feminine have become the main focal points for several scholars to argue for them as being equal, if not more important, than their *yang*, male, and masculine counterparts. Christopher Markert (1986) is one of the first anglophone authors to create a feminist transcreation of the *Changes* with some global reach. He does this by emphasizing the importance of the feminine and the harmonious interaction between *yin-yang* where he argues that Western cultures are patriarchal due to their focus on *yang* values (Markert 1986). *Yang* values, then, are understood by Markert to mean that Western cultures praise Heaven, a male god, a male son, and male prophets, while completely disregarding the female and feminine side of creation and humanity. While the influence of Markert's *Changes* is hard to fully determine, it surely had some impact, especially in Scandinavia, where the first *Changes* in both Norwegian and Finnish[2] are renditions of his version.

Since the late 1980s, ideas of the *Changes* like *yin-yang* and important terms found in the *Changes* like *junzi* 君子 and *daren* 大人 have received increased attention by scholars such as Clark and Wang (2004), and Ames (2011) who argue that the terms should be considered gender neutral. In response to the overall development of ideas related to the *Changes* to be gender neutral in the West, Pearson started her research into the original Chinese text to create a new anglophone translation that is updated with contemporary scholarship since Baynes' publication, and which deliberately presents an interpretation liberated from the patriarchal mode of thinking.

In comparison to Markert's *Changes*, which glorifies the feminine and criticizes Western patriarchy, Pearson's *Changes* does not criticize the West directly to the same degree but simply translates the original text while excluding patriarchy from it. Her translation has been appreciated because it provides a platform for females and the feminine. Considering that many previous anglophone *Changes* are patriarchal, and Markert's transcreation is so critical of Western patriarchy, Pearson's *Changes* is a refreshing translation as women can enjoy reading a version of the classic which is respectful of women's gendered perspective. In fact, the main reason

[2] The first rendition of the *Changes* into Finnish is also a rendering of Christopher Markert's English version by a female author (Markert and Jing 1987) that was published a year before Skodvin's Norwegian version. Noticeably, two other Finnish ladies have also published their renditions of the *Changes* (Holitzka and Ljungberg 1998; Heikkilä 2009). However, Finnish renditions will not be discussed in this chapter due to language limitations.

behind Pearson's *Changes* was to make *yin-yang* gender neutral and allow women to have a version of the classic which neither criticizes them nor subjects them to men. She writes, "I believe that all women who read the *Changes* deserve at least one translation by a woman scholar with knowledge of Chinese language and history" (Pearson 2011, 12). Since Pearson published her *Changes*, the 44th hexagram known as *Gou* 姤, which in the *Changes* of Legge and Baynes criticize women for being able and strong, has become an embodiment of great *yin* values and thus a hexagram which empowers women (Wilhelm and Baynes 1967, 170; Pearson 2011, 176). In comparison with previous anglophone translations, Pearson argues that this hexagram discusses women who have optimized their femininity in a positive manner where women are great spouses or are too good for marrying their partner due to their ability and strength.

12.4 The Feminine in Windeleff's and Skodvin's *Changes*

Like Pearson, Windeleff and Skodvin have rendered the *Changes* by focusing on the importance of feminine qualities. In the first Scandinavian *Changes*, Windeleff argues that terms for female or those commonly associated with the feminine in the German *Changes* by Richard Wilhelm should be considered universal features for people. Windeleff argues, in other words, that the Chinese classic is not patriarchal as the feminine aspects of the classic should not be subjected to a patriarchal reading; rather, feminine terms are used due to lingual limitations or for cultural reasons, not classical. Windeleff writes:

> The female in the Book of Changes (in particular, hexagrams 20 and 37), which in our language means different types of "the feminine," should be applied irrespective of gender, as it is a common saying that does not subject its meaning to some traditional gender stereotype.[3]

Windeleff's statement in his introduction suggests that gender inequality related to the *Changes* is due to ancient cultural ideas. These ideas were never intended to separate men and women in a patriarchal hierarchy. To substantiate his argument, Windeleff highlights hexagrams 20 and 37 since he interprets these two hexagrams to present women in a traditionally gendered stereotypical role. For my discussion, I will focus on hexagram 20 *Guan* 觀, which is translated in the most famous English translation of the *Changes* (Wilhelm and Baynes 1967, 82) as *Contemplation (View)*. The most relevant passage of hexagram 20 concerning gender is Baynes' explanation of line two. In her explanation, she unquestionably positions women in a traditional role which is clearly inferior to men:

> [Line two:] Contemplation through the crack of the door. Furthering through the perseverance of a woman.

[3] My translation of: "Da kvinden i Forvandlingernes Bog (det gælder især hexagrammene nr. 20 og 37) i vort sprog ofte betyder 'det kvindelige' i forskellige afskygninger, som man må kunne vedkende sig uanset køn, er der ofte anvendt udtryk der ikke fastlåser meningen til et traditionelt kønsrollemønster" (Wilhelm and Windeleff 1973, 14).

> [Explanation:] Through the crack of the door one has a limited outlook; one looks outward from within. Contemplation is subjectively limited. One tends to relate everything to oneself and cannot put oneself in another's place and understand his motives. This is appropriate for a good housewife. It is necessary for her to be conversant with the affairs of the world. But for a man who must take active part in public life, such a narrow, egotistic way of contemplating things is of course harmful (Ibid., 84).

Windeleff, who also translated his *Changes* based on Wilhelm's *I Ging*, strongly disagrees with the explanation of women in relation to men in hexagram 20. In response, Windeleff rewrites how line two of the hexagram should be perceived by removing the apparent patriarchal hierarchy, while also provoking his readers through the gender equality issues of the text.

Windeleff writes:

> Through the door's crack, one has a limited outlook. One looks from the inside and outward. The method of contemplation is subjectively limited. One attributes everything to oneself and cannot put oneself in another's place and understand his doings. This is appropriate for a good housemother [housewife]; she does not need to be familiar with the problems of the world. But for a human that must take an active part in public life, such a limited, selfish angle is naturally something of evil.[4]

On the surface, these two paragraphs do not appear very different in their overall meaning. However, there are three important combining factors that Windeleff applies to highlight the importance of the feminine as well as revealing himself as a potential feminist translator. The first is by highlighting the hexagram in his introduction as addressing a gender equality issue, thereby making his readers perspicacious to the topic of gender inequality when reading hexagram 20. The second is Windeleff's deliberate replacement of Wilhelm's perfectly translatable German term for "man" (*ein Mann*) in the last sentence with the Danish word for a human (*et menneske*). By making this subtle alteration to the text, Windeleff's explanation of line two in hexagram 20 can no longer be understood as providing a deliberate hierarchy where the housewife's role is second to whatever applies to a man as in Wilhelm's and Baynes' last sentence. Another effect of replacing "man" with "human" is that the role of the housewife is best understood as an individual choice, and for those who choose that lifestyle, it is fine to ignore the "problems of the world." Additionally, since Windeleff uses the term "human" in the last sentence, women can be housewives, but they can also enjoy living an active part in public life since the last part of the sentence specifies "human" as opposed to "man."

The difference between man and human in relation to the housewife between Baynes' and Windeleff's *Changes* is further explicated by the attributes with which these nouns are provided by each author. Whereas Baynes subjects the housewife to the man and demands her to be conversant with the affairs of the world, Windeleff

---

[4] My translation of: "Gennem dørsprækken har man et begrænset udsyn. Man ser indefra og ud. Betragtningsmåden er subjektivt begrænset. Man henfører alt til sig selv, og kan ikke sætte sig selv i en andens sted og forstå hans bevæggrunde. Dette er passende for en god husmoder; hun behøver ikke at være fortrolig med verdens problemer. Men for et menneske der må tage aktiv del i det offentlige liv, er en sådan indskrænket, egoistisk synsvinkel naturligvis af det onde" (Wilhelm and Windeleff 1973, 97).

insinuates that housewives can be ignorant of public life because it is a self-chosen lifestyle. To Windeleff, that housewives exists is not a problem, but any social practice of confining a human within a home (so that it is not an agreed-upon lifestyle) is evil. The word "human" is important in the last sentence because, as Windeleff instructs his readers in his introduction, terms associated with femininity, especially in hexagram 20, should be considered universal values. In other words, Windeleff's "housewife" also includes men who are performing the role in a relationship traditionally assigned to a housewife. Thus, Windeleff deliberately uses the term "housewife" to provoke his readers' attention about the issue of gender equality because he could have used "human" to replace that traditional house-role word as he does in the last sentence.

Windeleff's method of highlighting the issue of gender inequality by criticizing people for a lack of action and his argument of the universal value of femininity is also adopted by Skodvin in her Norwegian translation. In Skodvin's *Changes*, she accuses the West of being *yang*-centric by ignoring the fact that *yin-yang* are perfectly equal pairs of energies, and as a result, the values of *yin*, which is also associated with women and femininity, have become subjected to men and the masculine. Skodvin writes, "Most Western philosophers and holy writings tend to glorify one polarity and ignore the other." In her argument, Skodvin differentiates between the "Heavenly Father" and the "Earthly Mother" whereas the mother has been ignored or subjected to their male counterpart in Western classics and therefore women have become a suppressed gender. She continues, "The most important reason why so many women in the West abandon the female role [is because] they feel feminine qualities are viewed as inferior in [the Western] *yang*-oriented culture."[5] Skodvin argues that the Western focus on *yang* values while neglecting *yin* values is clear evidence that Western cultures are inferior to the Eastern cultures which embrace the complementary equilibrium of *yin-yang*. Skodvin argues for Eastern superiority through the fact that Western languages have not been able to translate *yin-yang* because there simply is no equivalent concept in Western ideologies. Since the Western philosophical and cosmological vocabulary does not have a fundamental notion of equality, Skodvin decides to glorify Chinese philosophy and culture as exemplary, and she wants her readers to reevaluate their own cultural-historical background to reinvent themselves to become more mindful of the Western lack of *yin* values in their ideologies.

To further her argument of the importance of equalizing the *yin* values to the *yang* values, Skodvin emphasizes the feminine aspects of the *Changes*. The most striking example is Skodvin's argument that the commonly placed second hexagram in the Western reception of the *Changes*, *Kun* 坤, should be positioned as the first in the book and followed by the 63 other hexagrams (Markert and Skodvin 2001, 32). To place the second hexagram first might not be as radical as it may seem at first since the excavated *Gui Cang* 歸藏 version of the *Changes*, discovered in the Wangjiatai 王家台 tombs in Hubei, also places *Kun* first in the line of hexagrams (Shaughnessy 2014,

[5] My translation of: "De fleste vestlige filosofier og hellige skrifter har en tendens til å forherlige den ene polen og overse den andre," "Himmelske Far," "Moder Jord," and "Den viktigste grunnen til at så mange kvinner i Vesten forkaster kvinnerollen [er fordi] de føler at kvinnelige egenskaper blir ansett for mindreverdige i [Vestens] *yang*-orienterte kultur" (Markert and Skodvin 2001, 30–31).

161–174). What makes Skodvin's situation unique, however, is that her rendition is the first *Changes* in Norwegian, so not only is the original Norwegian reading with a special focus on the *Kun* hexagram, but it especially highlights the feminine aspects of the classic since Skodvin renders the title of the *Kun* hexagram as "*The Female Principle* (*Det kvinnelige prinsipp*)" (Markert and Skodvin 2001, 79). In comparison, Baynes positions *Kun* as the second hexagram with the title *The Receptive*, and explains it as the perfect complement to the masculine hexagram *Qian* (Wilhelm and Baynes 1967, 10–15). Interestingly, Pearson (2011, 67–69) not only maintains *The Receptive* title but also positions *Kun* as the second hexagram of the 64, which both shows how rooted that order is and how fundamentally different Skodvin is from the established reception in the West.

Skodvin justifies the position of *Kun* as the first hexagram as simply being the most logical arrangement. She writes, "I am convinced that this version is not only more authentic but also more logical because in Chinese cosmology *yin* is traditionally mentioned before *yang*."[6] Deciding this arrangement also strengthens her focus on prioritizing the feminine of the *Changes*. In the explanation of *Kun*'s lines, she offers an argument similar to Windeleff's in how the feminine aspects of the *Changes* should be understood: Namely, that terms often associated with females and values considered feminine should apply equally to men as women. Arguably, she takes the importance of the feminine even further than Windeleff by stating that it is the fundamental value which can bring things to completion. She writes, "Everything achieves its full completion through [the female principle]."[7] Together, Windeleff and Skodvin have established the *Changes* in Denmark and Norway as a classic of feminine values and with a stern message for the importance of gender equality. Whereas Skodvin can be deemed more extreme than Windeleff by restructuring the common hexagram order and textually attack Western culture as *yang*-centric to its very core, Windeleff's priority of gender equality in the *Changes* is further revealed by the way he renders the perfectly translatable German masculine terms in Wilhelm's *I Ging* for *junzi* (*der Edle*) and *daren* (*der große Mann*) to become gender neutral in Danish.

12.5 Windeleff's and Kossman's Translation of *Junzi* and *Daren*

As part of Windeleff's quest to improve gender equality, he decided to essentially reinvent the Western reception of *junzi* and *daren* in his *Changes* by rendering them as the noble human (*det ædle menneske*) and the big human (*det store menneske*). A

[6] My translation of: "Jeg er overbevist om at denne versjonen ikke bare er mer autentisk, men også mer logisk, for i kinesisk kosmologi blir *Yin* tradisjonelt nevnt før *Yang*" (Markert and Skodvin 2001, 32).

[7] My translation of: "Alle ting oppnår sin fylle utfoldelse gjennom [det kvinnlige prinsipp]" (Ibid., 79).

creative rendering of *junzi* is also provided in the first Swedish *Changes* by Kossman who renders the term as "the heightened (*den upphöjde*)." Before Windeleff, Baynes' translation of Wilhelm's *I Ging*, which has dominated the Western reception of the *Changes*, renders *junzi* as "the superior man" and *daren* as "the great man" in English. Basically, the most influential rendering of the *Changes* in the West has prevented women from accomplishing excellence to the prestigious degree granted to men, and arguably, this is not a literal but a contextual interpretation. As expressed by Ivanhoe (2008, 39) about ancient Chinese philosophical culture in relation to *junzi*: "Deplorably, given the patriarchal nature of Kongzi's society, women were not thought capable of achieving the status of *junzi*." This is ironic, because anyone familiar with Chinese characters recognizes that *junzi* 君子 and *daren* 大人 do not possess strokes or sub-characters that undoubtedly relate to a specific gender.

It is clear from contemporary scholarly work that the *Changes* should be considered more gender equal than it is in the popular rendition of the classic by Baynes. This is for instance argued by Redmond and Hon (2014, 72) who state that "while the [*Changes*] was often read as assuming that women should be subordinate to men [...] this reading is not present in the explicit form in the original Western Zhou meanings." A similar argument can be found with Clark and Wang (2004), who point out that the *Changes* has been interpreted with a strong bias to establish a patriarchal reading. In light of the manifold arguments that the original *Changes* text is not patriarchal as previously received in the West, several scholars have provided new translations of important terms such as *junzi*. For instance, Redmond in his recent translation renders *junzi* as "the upright person." (Redmond 2017, 63) Pearson (2011, 64) argues that *junzi* should be understood as "one worthy of power." Other scholars suggest rendering *junzi* as "exemplary person" or "superior person." (Ames 2011, 69; Clark and Wang 2004, 399) In other words, Windeleff and Kossman could be said to have brought back an original meaning of the *Changes* with their "noble human" and "the heightened" in the Danish and Swedish renditions of Wilhelm's *I Ging*.

A question remains why Windeleff and Kossman chose not to translate perfectly translatable terms from German into Danish and Swedish? Neither of their understanding of *junzi* is justified by them in their renditions. Kossman does not provide her own introduction and Windeleff only justifies his alteration of *daren* in his introduction to the *Changes*. Windeleff writes: "The [German] expression '*der große Mann*' is translated as 'the big human' because [a direct translation into] 'the big man' is presumed to connote unfortunate biased associations."[8] With Windeleff's emphasis on the importance of the feminine and this citation, we can analogously assume that Windeleff was deliberate in rendering *junzi* as gender neutral and that the same applies to his "the noble human (*det ædle menneske*)." Kossman, on the other hand, maintains the patriarchy of *daren* by rendering it as "the important man (*den betydande mannen*)," but as will be clear shortly, she goes further than Windeleff with her rendering of *junzi* by phrasing it as "the heightened (*den upphöjde*)."

[8] My translation of: "Udtrykket 'Der grosse mann' er oversat med 'det store menneske,' da 'den store mand' formodes at give uheldige biassociationer" (Wilhelm and Windeleff 1973, 14).

Whereas Windeleff's "the noble human (*the ædle menneske*)" is a direct gender-neutral rendering of Wilhelm's "*der Edle* (masculine article of 'the' in "the noble," which is rendered as "the superior man" in Baynes' rendition)," Kossman completely reinvents the meaning of *junzi* in the Swedish *Changes*. This reinvention is not limited to the phrasing of *junzi* as "the heightened," but also reflected in a natural way to a foreword in Kossman's *Changes* written by Liselotte Weiss. Kossman's *Changes* includes four forewords: one by Per Sörbom, a translation of Carl G. Jung's foreword found in Baynes' *I Ching*, one by Liselotte Weiss, and lastly, a translation of Richard Wilhelm's foreword from the *I Ging*. The foreword by Weiss is important for Kossman's *junzi* as she argues that the *Changes* functions as a practical key for people to realize their true abilities by understanding that our earthly and materialistic reality is inferior to the superior spiritual reality of the *Changes* (Weiss 1991, 5). By connecting Kossman's "the heightened" with what can be rendered as Weiss' heightened reality, the Swedish *junzi* becomes an important goal for either gender to pursue in order to unlock some sort of true knowledge about life and the universe. As a result, Kossman's *Changes* becomes an important source for either gender in their pursuit of achieving *junzi-ness*, whereas her decision to not reinvent *daren* from its patriarchal associations becomes somewhat overshadowed by the much more important role of *junzi* in her rendition.

To compare the different outcomes of the choices made by Baynes, Windeleff, and Kossman in rendering *daren* and *junzi*, I will show their versions of lines two and three in hexagram *Qian* 乾. The *Qian* hexagram is chosen to compare the three renditions because it possesses both *daren* and *junzi* in a clear connection to something else and because it is arguably the most familiar hexagram to most readers of the *Changes* since it is frequently used as an example of how to interpret the classic. Let us start with the familiar rendition of Baynes, who renders line two of the hexagram as "it furthers one to see 'the great man [*daren*]'," and in her rendering of the third line, she writes, "all day long the 'superior man [*junzi*]' is creatively active." (Wilhelm and Baynes 1967, 8)[9] From a feminist perspective, the problem with Baynes' formulation of these two terms is that her *Changes* becomes a classic for males only, especially if we keep in mind how immensely important and influential *daren* and *junzi* are to the *Changes* and Chinese culture in general. By only allowing males the potential to achieve the aristocratic social and political position corresponding to these two terms, women automatically become subjected to a patriarchal hierarchy when reading Baynes' *Changes*. Therefore, the different rendering approaches to *junzi* and *daren* by Kossman and Windeleff will significantly alter how readers of Danish and Swedish understand these essential ideas of the *Changes*.

Kossman decides to render line two of *Qian* as, "it is furthering to see 'the important man [*daren*]'," and line three as, "the heightened [*junzi*] is active and creates all day."[10] Here women enjoy the status of *junzi* but there are still some patriarchal restrictions as only the male gender is emphasized in relation to *daren*. The result of

---

[9] In Chinese: 九二:見龍在田,利見大人。And 九三:君子終日乾乾,夕惕若,厲,无咎。

[10] My translation of: "Det är befrämjande att se den betydande mannen," and "Den upphöjde är verksam och skapar hela dagen" (Wilhelm and Kossman 1991, 31).

Kossman's rendering is, for instance, that a female reader might feel inspired by her possibility to become a *junzi* according to the message in the *Changes*, but that pursuit is arguably more achievable if she is guided by the important man. For example, from reading these passages, a girl might choose to ask for her father's advice instead of her mother's, since male is "the important gender" which is "furthering to see." From a gendered perspective, Kossman brings an improvement to gender equality in the *Changes* when compared with Baynes, but Windeleff is arguably more gender equal with his Danish rendering. His version of line two says "it is beneficial to see 'the big human [*daren*]'," and his line three, "the noble human [*junzi*] is active throughout the day."[11] In the last two versions of *Qian's* line two and three, male and female can achieve the social status of *junzi*, but also in the parental example above, both boy and girl would find either mother and father as a "big human" who it is furthering or beneficial to see (for guidance).

12.6 Conclusion

Windeleff might be the most gender-equal renderer of *junzi* and *daren* of the three Scandinavian versions compared in this chapter, while from a feminist perspective, Windeleff's use of *(menn)-eske*, as in hu-(man), in both *junzi* and *daren* can give rise to criticism. Just as (his)-story and (man)-kind can be argued to support a patriarchal development in the anglophone world from its very fundamental language (Godard 2022, 16), so too can *(menn)-eske* be accused of the same in Danish. However, given Windeleff's focus on the feminine, and how he deliberately accuses Wilhelm's *I Ging* for providing unfortunate patriarchal gender associations with his rendering of *junzi* and *daren*, we can consider Windeleff as a feminist translator when he deliberately removes patriarchal connotations from otherwise perfectly translatable terms. Whether his use of "*menneske* (human)" deserves criticism must be the topic of another research paper on the potentially unfortunate gendering of the Danish language, not of this chapter.

In assessing how feminist Skodvin's *Changes* is, she falls into a similar category as Windeleff. On one hand, her rendition is obviously against patriarchy, since she highlights the importance of the feminine to the degree that it is the most fundamental value. Her formulations, on the other hand, are written within a "he" framework, which results in her version of the classic to primarily relate to men. One can argue that this is deliberate so that men will reevaluate their understanding of their dominant idea of women and femininity, or it can be criticized for at least not alternating between he and she. Additionally, Skodvin did not make many substantial feminist interpretations of the ideas in the *Changes* herself as she decided to render a feminist transcreation of the text. Thus, the primary feminist feature of Skodvin does not consist in rendering, reinventing, arguing, or manipulating the text for the purpose of

[11] My translation of: "Det gavner at se det store menneske,"and "Det ædle menneske er dagen igennem skabende virksom" (Wilhelm and Windeleff 1973, 34).

feminism, rather, she is a feminist translator because she chose to translate a feminist transcreation of the *Changes* instead of other available English versions like James Legge's translation or Baynes' rendering of the classic.

Among the three Scandinavian renditions of the *Changes* discussed in this article, Kossman's version is the only one without any obvious feminist agenda. Whereas she does render the *junzi* of the classic into "the heightened," she ignores the patriarchy of *daren* and does not explicitly seek to revise the *Changes* to become more feminine-friendly as in the cases of the Danish and Norwegian versions. Nevertheless, compared with Windeleff, Kossman arguably provides an even purer rendering of *junzi* because "the heightened" cannot be criticized for possessing fundamental linguistic inequality in the Swedish language. Also, the foreword by Weiss in Kossman's *Changes* is written in a deliberate "she" framework that strongly contrasts with, for instance, Skodvin's usage of "he." However, I understand Kossman's "the heightened" to be related to a general spiritual self-discovery which makes it less likely that the rendering was chosen as a response to gender inequality from reading Wilhelm's *I Ging*. Similarly, using "he" or "she" as a pronoun in sentences might arguably be the result of a person's habitual way of writing than a deliberate statement about gender roles, especially when less is done in the rendering of her *Changes* to further establish a feminist standpoint.

Kossman's style of completely reinventing her *junzi* term makes her approach more similar to Pearson's than is the case with her fellow Scandinavians. For example, Pearson (2011, 64) translates *junzi* as "one worthy of power" and *daren* as "someone wiser than you are." Both Pearson and Kossman use a technique that completely liberates an important term in the *Changes* from naturally belonging to either gender. Despite the similar approaches to *junzi* and due to Kossman's decision to maintain the patriarchy of the *daren* term, rather than for instance, reinventing it as something like "the learned (*den lärde*)," it suggests that she is focused on the *junzi* term for other reasons than purely feminist purposes. Because of her nuanced focus, Kossman's gender-neutral rendering cannot be deemed as deliberately feminist like that of Windeleff, Skodvin, and Pearson. However, despite their different approaches, the Danish, Norwegian, and Swedish reception of the *Changes*, whether deliberate or not, have an apparent focus on how gender is represented in the classic.

References

Adler, Joseph A. 2022. *The Yijing. A guide*. Oxford: Oxford University Press.

Ames, Roger T. 2011. *Confucian role ethics: A vocabulary*. Hong Kong: The Chinese University of Hong Kong Press.

Bonvillain, Nancy. 2007. *Women and men: Cultural constructs of gender*, 4th ed. Upper Saddle River, NJ: Pearson Education Inc.

Camman, Schuyler. 1991. Chinese hexagrams, trigrams, and the binary system. *Proceedings of the American Philosophical Society* 135 (4): 576–589.

Clark, Kelly James, and Robin R. Wang. 2004. A confucian defense of gender equity. *Journal of American Academy of Religion* 72 (2): 395–422.

van Ess, Hans. 2010. Cheng Yi and his ideas about women as revealed in his commentary to the "Yijing." *Oriens Extremus* 49 (1): 63–77.

Fung, Yu-Lan. 1976. *A short history of Chinese philosophy*. Ed. Derk Bodde. New York: The Free Press.

Gatlin, Rochelle. 1987. *American women since 1945*. London: Macmillan.

Godard, Barbara. 2022. Language and sexual difference: The case of translation. In *Translation, semiotics, and feminism: Selected writings of Barbara Godard*, ed. C. Eva, 10–16. Karpinski and Elena Basile. New York: Routledge.

Graham, Angus Charles. 1986. *Yin-Yang and the nature of correlative thinking*. Singapore: Institute of East Asian Philosophies.

Heikkilä, Margit. 2009. *I Ching: Muutosten kirja*. Helsinki: Books on Demand.

Hinsch, Bret. 2006. The criticism of powerful women by western Han dynasty portent experts. *Journal of the Economic and Social History of the Orient* 49 (1): 96–121.

Holitzka, Marlies and Tuikku Ljungberg (Trans.). 1998. *I Ching: Avain muutokseen*. Helsinki: Karisto.

Hon, Tze-Ki. 2019. Chinese philosophy of change (*Yijing*). In *Stanford encyclopedia of philosophy*. Ed. Edward N. Zalta.

Ivanhoe, Philip J. 2008. The shade of confucius: Social roles, ethical theory, and the self. In *Polishing the Chinese mirror: Essays in honor of Henry Rosemont Jr*, ed. Ronnie L. Littlejohn, and Marthe Chandler, 34–49. New York: Global Scholarly Publications.

Legge, James. 1899. *The Yi King*. Oxford: Clarendon Press.

Markert, Christopher. 1986. *I Ching the no. 1 success formula*. New York: Aquarian Press.

Markert, Christopher, and Eva Skodvin (Trans.). 2001. *I Ching forvandlingenes Bok*. Oslo: Hilt & Hansteen.

Markert, Christopher, and Jatta-Lisa Jing (Trans.). 1987. *I Ching: Muutosten kirja*. Helsinki: Tammi.

McClatchie, Rev. Canon Thomas. 1876. *A translation of the Confucian YIJING or the "classic of change" with notes and appendix*. Shanghai: American Presbyterian Mission Press.

Nielsen, Mathias Wullum. 2014. Justification of gender equality in academia: Comparing gender equality in six Scandinavian Universities. *NORA—Nordic Journal of Feminist and Gender Research* 22(3): 187–203.

Redmond, Geoffrey. 2017. *The I Ching (Book of Changes). A critical translation of the ancient text*. New York: Bloomsbury.

Redmond, Geoffrey. 2021. The *Yijing* in early postwar counterculture in the west. In *The making of the global Yijing in the modern world*, ed. Benjamin Wai-ming, 197–221. Ng. Singapore: Springer.

Redmond, Geoffrey, and Tze-Ki. Hon. 2014. *Teaching the I Ching (Book of Changes)*. Oxford: Oxford University Press.

Robinson, Christa. 2018. The I Ching and analytical philosophy: How the east met west through C. G. Jung. *Zhouyi Studies* 9 (1): 139–154.

Rongen, Ole Bjørn. 2006. *Yijing Forandringenes Bok*. Oslo: Bokklubben.

Ryan, James A. 1996. Leibniz' binary system and shao yong's "*Yijing*". *Philosophy East and West* 46 (1): 59–90.

Pearson, Margaret J. 2011. *The original I Ching: An authentic translation of the book of changes based on recent discoveries.* North Clarendon, VT: Tuttle Publishing.

Shaughnessy, Edward L. 2014. *Unearthing the changes: recently discovered manuscripts of the Yi Jing (I Ching) and related texts.* New York: Columbia University Press.

Smith, Richard J. 2012. *The I Ching: A biography.* Princeton, NJ: Princeton University Press.

Wang, Robin R. 2005. Dong Zhongshu's transformation of "Yin-Yang" theory and contesting of gender identity. *Philosophy East and West* 55 (2): 209–231.

Weiss, Liselotte. 1991. "Foreword." In *I Ching Förvandlingarnas eller Växlingarans bok.* Trans. Richard Wilhelm, and Christine Tranmark Kossman, 5–9. Stockholm: Berghs Förlag AB.

Wilhelm, Richard. 1924. *I Ging: Das Buch der wandlungen.* Schule des Rades: https://schuledesrades.org/public/iging/buch/.

Wilhelm, Richard, and Cary F. Baynes (Trans.). 1967. *The I Ching or the book of changes.* Princeton, NJ: Princeton University Press.

Wilhelm, Richard, and Christine Tranmark Kossman (Trans.). 1991. *I Ching Förvandlingarnas eller Växlingarans bok.* Stockholm: Berghs Förlag AB.

Wilhelm, Richard, and Jens Windeleff (Trans.). 1973. *I Ching Forvandlingernes Bog I–II.* Copenhagen: Thaning & Apple.

Wu, Li-Jing. 2021. Historicizing the *Yijing* in the Anglophone world. In *The making of the global Yijing in the modern world.* Ed. Benjamin Wai-ming Ng, 41–61. Singapore: Springer.

Zhang, Dainian. 2019. "Preface." In *An introduction to the Zhouyi (book of changes).* Trans. Liu Dajun, and Zhang Wenzhi, 7–10. Asheville, NC: Chiron Publications.

